Advances in Molecular and Cellular Microbiology 21

Tuberculosis: Laboratory Diagnosis and Treatment Strategies

Edited by

Timothy D. McHugh

University College London, UK

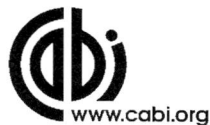

www.cabi.org

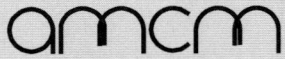

omcm Advances in Molecular and Cellular Microbiology

Through the application of molecular and cellular microbiology, we now recognize the diversity and dominance of microbial life forms on our planet, which exist in all environments. These microbes have many important planetary roles, but for us humans a major problem is their ability to colonize our tissues and cause disease. The same techniques of molecular and cellular microbiology have been applied to the problems of human and animal infection during the past two decades and have proved to be immensely powerful tools in elucidating how microorganisms cause human pathology. This series has the aim of providing information on the advances that have been made in the application of molecular and cellular microbiology to specific organisms and the diseases that they cause. The series is edited by researchers active in the application of molecular and cellular microbiology to human disease states. Each volume focuses on a particular aspect of infectious disease and will enable graduate students and researchers to keep up with the rapidly diversifying literature in current microbiological research.

Series Editor

Professor Michael Wilson
University College London

Titles Available from CABI

17. *Helicobacter pylori* in the 21st Century
Edited by Philip Sutton and Hazel M. Mitchell

18. Antimicrobial Peptides: Discovery, Design and Novel Therapeutic Strategies
Edited by Guangshun Wang

19. Stress Response in Pathogenic Bacteria
Edited by Stephen P. Kidd

20. Lyme Disease: an Evidence-based Approach
Edited by John J. Halperin

21. Tuberculosis: Laboratory Diagnosis and Treatment Strategies
Edited by Timothy McHugh

22. Antimicrobial Drug Discovery: Emerging Strategies
Edited by George Tegos and Eleftherios Mylonakis

24. Bacteriophages in Health and Disease
Edited by Paul Hyman and Stephen T. Abedon

Titles Forthcoming from CABI

Microbial Metabolomics
Edited by Silas Villas-Bôas and Katya Ruggiero

The Human Microbiota and Microbiome
Edited by Julian Marchesi

Meningitis: Cellular and Molecular Basis
Edited by Myron Christodoulides

Earlier titles in the series are available from Cambridge University Press (www.cup.cam.ac.uk).

CABI is a trading name of CAB International

CABI
Nosworthy Way
Wallingford
Oxfordshire, OX10 8DE
UK

CABI
Chauncey Street
Suite 1002
Boston, MA 02111
USA

Tel: +44 (0)1491 832111
Fax: +44 (0)1491 833508
E-mail: info@cabi.org
Website: www.cabi.org

T: +1 800 552 3083 (toll free)
T: +1 (0)617 395 4051
E-mail: cabi-nao@cabi.org

A catalogue record for this book is available from the British Library, London, UK.

Library of Congress Cataloging-in-Publication Data

Tuberculosis : laboratory diagnosis and treatment strategies / edited by
Timothy D. McHugh.
    p. ; cm. -- (Advances in molecular and cellular microbiology ; 21)
  Includes bibliographical references and index.
  ISBN 978-1-84593-807-9 (alk. paper)
  I. McHugh, Timothy D. (Timothy Daniel) II. Series: Advances in molecular
and cellular microbiology ; 21.
  [DNLM: 1. Tuberculosis--diagnosis. 2. Antitubercular Agents. 3. Drug Discovery.
  4. Molecular Diagnostic Techniques. WF 220]

  616.99'5075--dc23
                        2012030958

ISBN-13: 978 1 84593 807 9

Commissioning editor: Rachel Cutts
Editorial assistant: Alexandra Lainsbury
Production editor: Simon Hill

Typeset by Columns Design XML Ltd, Reading, UK.
Printed and bound by CPI Group (UK) Ltd, Croydon, CR0 4YY.

Contents

Contributors

Leonard Amaral, Unit of Mycobacteriology, Instituto de Higiene e Medicina Tropical, Universidade Nova de Lisboa, Rua da Junqueira, 100, 1349-008 Lisbon, Portugal. E-mail: lamaral@ihmt.unl.pt

M.R. Barer, Department of Infection, Immunity and Inflammation, University of Leicester College of Medicine, Biological Sciences and Psychology, Maurice Shock Building, Leicester, UK. E-mail: mrb19@le.ac.uk

Anna L. Bateson, Centre for Clinical Microbiology, Department of Infection, Royal Free Campus, University College London, Rowland Hill Street, London NW3 2PF, UK. E-mail: a.bateson@ucl.ac.uk

Pablo Bifani, The Novartis Institute for Tropical Diseases, Singapore. E-mail: pablo.bifani@novartis.com

Martin J. Boeree, Associate Professor, Radboud University Nijmegen Medical Centre, Nijmegen, The Netherlands. E-mail: M.Boeree@uccz.umcn.nl

Ronan Breen, Department of Respiratory Medicine, Guys' & St Thomas' NHS Trust, Westminster Bridge Road, London SE1 7EH, UK. E-mail: Ronan.breen@gsst.nhs.uk

Philip D. Butcher, Centre for Infection and Immunity, Division of Clinical Sciences, St George's University of London, London SW17 0RE, UK. E-mail: butcherp@sgul.ac.uk

Simeon Cadmus, Tuberculosis Research Laboratory, Department of Veterinary Public Health and Preventive Medicine, University of Ibadan, Nigeria.

Isabel Couto, Unit of Mycobacteriology, Instituto de Higiene e Medicina Tropical, Universidade Nova de Lisboa, Rua da Junqueira, 100, 1349-008 Lisbon, Portugal.

Geoff Coxon, Strathclyde Institute of Pharmacy and Biomedical Sciences, John Arbuthnott Building, University of Strathclyde, 27 Taylor Street, Glasgow G4 0NR, UK. E-mail: geoff.coxon@strath.ac.uk

G.R. Davies, Senior Lecturer in Infectious Diseases, Institute of Translational Medicine, University of Liverpool, Liverpool, UK. E-mail: gerrydavies@doctors.org.uk

N.J. Garton, Department of Infection, Immunity and Inflammation, University of Leicester College of Medicine, Biological Sciences and Psychology, Maurice Shock Building, Leicester, UK. E-mail: njg17@le.ac.uk

Stephen H. Gillespie, The Bute Medical School, St Andrews University, North Haugh, St Andrews KY16 9TF, UK. E-mail: shg3@st-andrews.ac.uk

Leonid Heifets, Mycobacteriology Reference Laboratory, National Jewish Health, Denver, Colorado, USA. E-mail: heifetsl@njhealth.org

Isobella Honeyborne, Centre for Clinical Microbiology, Department of Infection, Royal Free Campus, University College London, Rowland Hill Street, London NW3 2PF, UK. E-mail: i.honeyborne@ucl.ac.uk

Ajit Lalvani, Tuberculosis Research Unit, Department of Respiratory Medicine, National Heart and Lung Institute, Imperial College London, London, UK. E-mail: a.lalvani@imperial.ac.uk

Marc Lipman, Centre for Respiratory Medicine, Royal Free Campus, University College London, Rowland Hill Street, London NW3 2PF, UK. E-mail: marclipman@nhs.net

Diana Machado, Unit of Mycobacteriology, Instituto de Higiene e Medicina Tropical, Universidade Nova de Lisboa, Rua da Junqueira, 100, 1349-008 Lisbon, Portugal.

Ruth McNerney, Department of Pathogen Molecular Biology, London School of Hygiene and Tropical Medicine, London, UK. E-mail: Ruth.Mcnerney@lshtm.ac.uk

Helen McShane, Professor of Vaccinology and Wellcome Senior Fellow, The Jenner Institute, University of Oxford, Old Road Campus Research Building, Roosevelt Drive, Oxford OX3 7DQ, UK. E-mail: helen.mcshane@ndm.ox.ac.uk

Marta Martins, Unit of Mycobacteriology and UPMM, Instituto de Higiene e Medicina Tropical, Universidade Nova de Lisboa, Rua da Junqueira, 100, 1349-008 Lisbon, Portugal.

Barun Mathema, Tuberculosis Center, Public Health Research Institute, University of Medicine and Dentistry, Newark, New Jersey, USA.

Vanessa Mathys, Tuberculosis and Mycobacteria, Communicable and Infectious Diseases, Scientific Institute of Public Health, Belgium.

G.V. Mukamolova, Department of Infection, Immunity and Inflammation, University of Leicester College of Medicine, Biological Sciences and Psychology, Maurice Shock Building, Leicester, UK. E-mail: gvm4@le.ac.uk

Justin O'Grady, Norwich Medical School, NRP Innovation Centre, Norwich Research Park, Colney Lane, Norwich, NR4 7GJ, UK. E-mail: justin.ogrady@ued.ac.uk

Denise M. O'Sullivan, Molecular and Cell Biology Team, LGC, Queens Road, Teddington, Middlesex TW11 0LY, UK. E-mail: denise.osullivan@lgcgroup.com

Madhukar Pai, Department of Epidemiology, Biostatistics and Occupational Health, McGill University, Montreal, Canada. E-mail: Madhukar.pai@mcgill.ca

Manish Pareek, Department of Infection, Immunity and Inflammation, University of Leicester, Leicester, UK. E-mail: mp426@le.ac.uk

Andrew Ramsay, UNICEF/UNDP/World Bank/WHO Special Programme for Research and Training in Tropical Diseases (TDR), World Health Organization, Geneva, Switzerland. E-mail: ramsaya@who.int

Kate Reddington, Molecular Diagnostics Research Group, Microbiology, School of Natural Sciences, National University of Ireland Galway, Galway, Ireland. E-mail: k.reddington1@nuigalway.ie

Karen R. Steingart, University of Washington School of Public Health, Seattle, USA.

Claire Turner, Department of Life, Health and Chemical Sciences, The Open University, Milton Keynes, UK.

Dick van Soolingen, Mycobacteria Reference Laboratory, National Institute of Public Health and the Environment (RIVM), The Netherlands. E-mail: dick.van.soolingen@rivm.nl

Miguel Viveiros, Unit of Mycobacteriology, Instituto de Higiene e Medicina Tropical, Universidade Nova de Lisboa, Rua da Junqueira, 100, 1349-008 Lisbon, Portugal.

Simon J. Waddell, Brighton and Sussex Medical School, University of Sussex, Brighton BN1 9PX, UK. E-mail: s.waddell@bsms.ac.uk

Abbreviations

AFB	Acid-fast bacilli
Anti-TNF	Anti-tumour necrosis factor
BAL	Bronchoalveolar lavage
BCG	Bacillus Calmette–Guérin
CFP-10	Culture filtrate protein-10
CFU	Colony-forming units
DOTS	Direct observed therapy short course
DST	Drug susceptibility testing
EBA	Early bactericidal activity
ELISA	Enzyme-linked immunosorbent assay
ELISpot	Enzyme-linked immunosorbent spot
ESAT-6	Early secretory antigen target-6
GC-MS	Gas chromatography–mass spectrometry
GTC	Guanidine thiocyanate
GUs	Growth units
IFN-γ	Interferon-gamma
IGRAs	Interferon-gamma release assays
IL-12	Interleukin-12
IMIDs	Immune-mediated inflammatory diseases
LAMP	Loop-mediated isothermal amplification
LBs	Lipid bodies
LEDs	Light-emitting diodes
LJ	Löwenstein–Jensen
LMIC	Low- and middle-income country
LPAs	Line probe assays
LTBI	Latent tuberculosis infection
MDR-TB	Multidrug-resistant tuberculosis
MGIT	Mycobacterial growth indicator tube
MIC	Minimum inhibitory concentration
MPN	Most probable number
MTC	*Mycobacterium tuberculosis* complex
NAAT	Nucleic acid amplification assay
NASBA	Nucleic acid sequence-based amplification
NO	Nitric oxide
NTM	Non-tuberculous mycobacteria

PBMCs	Peripheral blood mononuclear cells
PD	Pharmacodynamic
PK	Pharmacokinetic
POC	Point of care
PPD	Purified protein derivative
qPCR	Quantitative PCR
RD	Region of difference
Rpf	Resuscitation-promoting factor
RR	Resistance ratio method
RRDR	Rifampicin resistance-determining region
RT-PCR	Reverse transcription polymerase chain reaction
SARs	Structure–activity relationships
SDA	Strand displacement amplification
SSCC	Sputum serial colony counting
TAG	Triacylglycerol
TDR-TB	Totally drug-resistant tuberculosis
Th1	T-helper cell type 1
TLRs	Toll-like receptors
TMA	Transcription-mediated amplification
TNF-α	Tumour necrosis factor alpha
TST	Tuberculin skin test
TTP	Time to positivity
VOC	Volatile organic compounds
WE	Wax ester
XDR-TB	Extremely drug-resistant tuberculosis
ZN	Ziehl–Neelsen stain

DRUGS

Amikacin	AK
Aminoglycocide	AG
Aminothiazole carboxylate	ATC
Benzothiazinone	BTZ
Capreomycin	CM or CAP
Chlorpromazine	CPZ
Ciprofloxacin	CIP
Clofazimine	CF
Cycloserine	CS
Dithiothreitol	DTT
Ethambutol	EMB or E
Ethionamide	ETA
Fluoroquinolone	FQ
Gatifloxacin	GAT
Isoniazid	INH or H
Kanamycin	KM
Levofloxacin	LEVO
Moxifloxacin	MOX or M
Ofloxacin	OFLOX
Para-amino-salicylic acid	PAS
Pyrazinamide	PZA or Z
Rifabutin	RBT
Rifampicin (rifampin)	RIF, RMP or R
Rifapentine	RPT
Sparfloxacin	SPA
Streptomycin	SM or S
Thioridazine	TZ

Introduction

Tuberculosis is a disease of poverty affecting adults in their most productive years. In 2010, there were 8.8 million incident cases with 1.1 million tuberculosis deaths in patients not infected with HIV. A further 0.35 million deaths were associated with HIV-positive patients (WHO, 2011). These oft-quoted figures demonstrate the challenge that tuberculosis control presents and this book highlights the state of the art in the mainstays of tuberculosis control: laboratory diagnosis and treatment.

Tuberculosis control is a multifaceted problem, but positive identification of the tubercle bacillus and assessment of its drug susceptibility are essential components in the strategy. It is telling that in 2010, 8 out of 22 high-burden countries did not meet the benchmark of 1 microscopy unit per 100,000 population. Furthermore, in a combined list of 36 countries that were high-burden countries and/or high MDR-TB burden countries, 20 had less than the benchmark of one laboratory capable of culture and drug sensitivity testing per 5 million population (WHO, 2011). It is hoped that the rational approach to conventional testing and roll-out of novel technologies described here will serve to provide cost-effective and robust technologies that will improve delivery of diagnostic services in resource-poor settings.

For many years, there was stasis in the development of drugs for the treatment of tuberculosis. The HIV pandemic and, more recently, the development of MDR- and XDR-TB (and indeed now TDR-TB) have changed our perspective. New drugs are being developed and our approaches to evaluating them require review. The spectrum of this activity is outlined in chapters covering the fundamental biology of drug action (Chapters 12 and 13), as well those focused on clinical trial methodology (Chapters 10, 11 and 15).

I have included three examples of approaches to new drug development; the ATC compounds (Chapter 16) represent a design-based approach in which the ATC scaffold is designed to inhibit the fatty acid synthase pathway. By comparison, Chapters 17 and 18 discuss repurposing established drugs: in Chapter 17 the rifamycins are revisited and Chapter 18 discusses how the imperative of MDR-TB has driven the reconsideration of thioridazine. Of course, matching these developments are exciting developments in vaccine design and these are captured in Chapter 19.

In the past 10 years, the pace of research into new diagnostic tools and treatments has increased, there is a new enthusiasm for tuberculosis research and while this book captures the zeitgeist, it also aims to provide underlying information for future developments.

Tim McHugh
UCL

Reference

WHO (2011) Global Tuberculosis Report 2011.

Part I

Diagnosis

1 Improving on Sputum Smear Microscopy for Diagnosis of Tuberculosis in Resource-poor Settings

Andrew Ramsay,[1] Karen R. Steingart[2] and Madhukar Pai[3]

[1]*UNICEF/UNDP/World Bank/WHO Special Programme for Research and Training in Tropical Diseases (TDR), World Health Organization, Geneva, Switzerland;* [2]*University of Washington School of Public Health, Seattle, USA;* [3]*Department of Epidemiology, Biostatistics and Occupational Health, McGill University, Montreal, Canada*

1.1 Introduction

In 2011, despite the long-established tradition of solid culture for *Mycobacterium tuberculosis* and the numerous more recent advances in tuberculosis diagnosis, direct sputum smear microscopy remains the cornerstone of global tuberculosis control. However, direct sputum smear microscopy has major limitations. It is associated with low and variable sensitivity, particularly in HIV-associated tuberculosis. It gives no information regarding the drug resistance of the infecting tuberculosis bacilli. It is, however, to date, the only diagnostic method for tuberculosis that has been shown to be implementable and sustainable in resource-poor health-care facilities in low- and middle-income countries (LMICs). The dire situation is well recognized by national tuberculosis programmes, technical agencies and donors. The World Health Organization (WHO), in an effort to improve diagnosis, has made more than 15 global recommendations related to tuberculosis diagnosis in the past 4 years, and yet little has changed on the ground (WHO, 2011a). This chapter will discuss the limitations of direct sputum smear microscopy as practised currently, review the recent WHO recommendations and discuss how the performance of sputum smear microscopy may be improved, explore how sputum smear microscopy services may be complemented by add-on tests and identify which tests (now and in the future) may replace smear microscopy in certain defined situations.

1.2 Direct Sputum Smear Microscopy

Direct sputum smear microscopy is inherently insensitive since the typical acid-fast bacilli (AFB) can only be detected when large numbers of them are present in the sputum ($>10^5$ organisms/ml). This impacts particularly on the diagnosis of HIV-associated tuberculosis, which is often paucibacillary, as well as the diagnosis of tuberculosis in children, who are often unable to produce a sputum specimen. Moreover, well-trained and dedicated microscopists are needed to ensure a good quality service. Ziehl–Neelsen (ZN) stained smears require examination under the microscope for 5–10 min before being declared negative (IUATLD, 2000). To counter the inherent lack of sensitivity of the method, the WHO recommended that three sputum specimens (including an early morning specimen) be collected for examination from each suspected tuberculosis patient over 2 days. This clearly has implications for the laboratory workload. A microscopist can only examine some 20–25 smears/day (IUATLD, 2000). Smear microscopy workloads heavier than that impact adversely on service quality. The requirement for three sputum specimens also places a burden on the suspected tuberculosis patient, since they have to make repeated visits to the health-care facility to submit specimens, receive results and start any treatment indicated. This is particularly burdensome if the patient is poor, weak or has travelled a long distance to the health-care facility. Patient dropout during the diagnostic process is common (Kemp, 2007; Botha, 2008).

The three-specimen, multi-day standard approach above, which has been devised to improve the sensitivity of sputum smear microscopy, also includes, paradoxically, a requirement that reduces the sensitivity of the technique further. A patient must have two positive smears to be defined as a smear-positive tuberculosis case, and one of these smears must contain at least 10 bacilli/100 high-power microscopic fields (HPF). These last requirements were introduced to maximize the specificity of direct sputum smear microscopy. The requirement dates back to the times when treatment regimens were longer and rifampicin was very expensive and was likely a measure to reduce costs and inconvenience to patients resulting from unnecessary treatment. Today, first-line treatment for tuberculosis is shorter, but 6-month regimens are still a considerable undertaking for patients. The cost of all the drugs for the standard 6-month first-line regimen is now approximately US$10–30 (Management Sciences for Health, 2005).

Sputum smear microscopy gives no information on the drug susceptibility of tuberculosis bacilli detected in the sputum smear of new tuberculosis patients and therefore cannot diagnose multidrug-resistant tuberculosis (MDR-TB) or extremely drug-resistant tuberculosis (XDR-TB).

In addition to the diagnosis of new cases, direct sputum smear microscopy repeated at different time points following initiation of anti-tuberculosis treatment is used to monitor patients' response (Gilpin *et al.*, 2007). Continued presence of AFB in sputum may indicate treatment failure, but this may be due to causes other than drug resistance, such as failure to take medication as indicated.

The recommended system for external quality assessment (EQA) of smear microscopy services requires the blinded rechecking of a sample of the slides examined by each laboratory. Usually, the national tuberculosis reference laboratory is expected to take on this monumental task. It is recommended that blinded rechecking is complemented by regular visits to microscopy laboratories to ensure a proper staining technique is used and to check the condition of microscopes (Association of Public Health Laboratories, 2002). Microscopes can be damaged or impaired by rough handling. In hot, humid climates, the lenses of microscopes are prone to colonization by algae or mould, which can render them worse than useless. A fully functional national EQA scheme based on this system is rarely achieved or sustained.

Nevertheless, most district hospitals and large health centres in countries with a high prevalence of tuberculosis can offer a sputum smear microscopy service of some kind. It is estimated that more than 50 million smear microscopy examinations are conducted globally each year (TDR/FIND, 2006). The only equipment required is a microscope (relatively inexpensive as laboratory equipment goes) and a gas, or spirit, burner. Microscopes generally need an electricity supply, but they can accommodate some fluctuation in power without damage. Microscopes may also be powered off car batteries or solar cells or, with a mirror and some experience, can be operated using directed daylight. The only consumables and reagents required are low cost and include specimen pots, applicator sticks for making smears, glass slides, a simple set of heat-stable stains with very long shelf lives and small amounts of microscope immersion oil to use with the ×100 oil objective lens. Training of staff is straightforward and relatively short and, importantly, is a well-established module in laboratory assistant and laboratory technician training courses and given importance in all countries where tuberculosis is a public health problem.

1.3 Optimized Sputum Smear Microscopy

In the absence of simple, low-cost alternatives to sputum smear microscopy much effort has been expended in recent years in developing optimized smear microscopy procedures. Much of this effort was catalysed by a series of systematic reviews of smear microscopy conducted in 2005–2006 and which led to the development of a prioritized international research agenda and to five global policy changes by the WHO in 2007–2009 (Steingart, 2006a,b, 2007a; Mase, 2007; WHO, 2007b,c, 2010b,c).

These systematic reviews focused on methods of improving sputum microscopy services in LMICs through more efficient and patient-friendly specimen collection, the use of fluorescence microscopy and the chemical digestion of sputum followed by a physical sputum concentration method.

The main findings of the systematic reviews were as follows.

1.3.1 Serial sputum smear examination (Mase, 2007; Steingart, 2007a)

The average increase in sensitivity/incremental yield of tuberculosis cases through examination of the third specimen was only 2–5%. Thus, evaluating 1000 persons suspected of having tuberculosis in a setting with 10% prevalence of the disease would require examination of 900 third specimens to yield an additional two–five cases. However, the analysis defined a smear-positive case as one with only one or more positive smears (≥3 AFB/100 HPF). The examination of only

two specimens decreased the number of sputum smear-positive cases defined as having two positive smears (≥10 AFB/100 HPF). A service that examined only two specimens might be more efficient and less onerous for laboratory staff. However, such a policy decision would require reassessment of the standard definition of a smear-positive case. If both specimens could be collected (and preferably examined) on the same day, this could reduce the number of patient visits required, reduce patient expenditure and possibly reduce default during the diagnostic process.

1.3.2 Fluorescence microscopy (Steingart, 2006a, 2007a)

Fluorescence microscopy (FM) was, on average, 10% more sensitive than ZN microscopy, with similar (98%) specificity. FM was also much quicker than ZN microscopy, with FM examination for 1 min being associated with a higher sensitivity and similar specificity to ZN examination for 4 min. The systematic review was conducted prior to the recent work on FM based on light-emitting diodes (LEDs). Conventional FM was dependent on very expensive, sophisticated equipment considered inappropriate for use outside of high throughput reference laboratories in LMICs. However, the authors noted that simple, low-cost LED-FM systems were being developed and should be evaluated in resource-poor settings (Gilpin, 2007).

1.3.3 Specimen processing (Steingart, 2006b, 2007a)

The systematic review indicated that, in comparison with direct smears, centrifugation preceded by digestion with any one of several different chemicals (including household bleach) was more sensitive. The review also revealed that overnight sedimentation preceded by chemical processing (including with household bleach) was more sensitive and specificity was similar. The latter method, since it did not require an expensive centrifuge, was considered to be more appropriate to basic laboratories in resource-poor settings.

A 5-year long, multi-partner, internationally coordinated programme of research followed, which provided evidence that (Ramsay, 2011):

1. 'Scanty' smears (i.e. with less than 10 AFB/100 HPF) were 'true positive' smears and considering these as positives increased the sensitivity of sputum smear microscopy without reducing specificity.
2. A single positive smear (including scanty smears) was sufficient to confirm a patient as a smear-positive tuberculosis case and increased the sensitivity of sputum smear microscopy without reducing specificity.
3. Reducing the number of specimens examined from three to two resulted in more efficient detection of cases, with only marginal reductions in sensitivity (2–5%).
4. Examining two specimens collected 1 h apart on the same day was equivalent to examination of two or three specimens collected over 2 days (Ramsay, 2009; Cuevas, 2012a).
5. Sensitivity and specificity of LED-FM was comparable to that of conventional FM.[21,22] The use of LED-FM was more sensitive than ZN microscopy, and if sufficient attention was paid to proper training of microscopists, it had similar specificity (including when used with a same-day specimen collection approach) (Cuevas, 2012b).
6. Bleach digestion followed by overnight sedimentation led to only small increases in sensitivity (9%), with associated small decreases in specificity (–3%).
7. LED-FM combined with bleach digestion and overnight sedimentation had the same sensitivity and slightly lower specificity than direct LED-FM alone (Bonnet, 2011).

Between 2007 and 2010, the WHO endorsed a new definition of a positive smear, a new definition of a smear-positive case, a reduction in the number of sputum specimens to be examined in the investigation of pulmonary tuberculosis, same-day microscopy and direct LED-FM (Ramsay, 2011).

A pragmatic randomized trial in Pakistan showed that simple standardized instructions on how to produce good quality sputum specimens increased significantly the number of smear-positive cases detected among women (Khan, 2007).

Thus, an optimized sputum smear microscopy service would incorporate simple standardized instruction on sputum specimen production, collection (and examination) of two specimens on the same day, use of LED-FM and new definitions of a positive smear and a smear-positive case. Wherever possible, smear results should be reported on the same day and treatment initiated to reduce initial default.

1.4 Serological Tests as Add-on or Replacement Tests

A series of systematic reviews have evaluated the performance of various serological (antibody detection) tests for the diagnosis of tuberculosis (Steingart, 2007b,c,d, 2009, 2011a; WHO, 2008). These tests used formats that required laboratory infrastructure such as enzyme-linked immunosorbent assays (ELISAs), as well as rapid immunochromatographic test platforms. The latter tests, if they could perform as well as smear microscopy, potentially could replace it, making diagnosis simpler and quicker. Moreover, the tests, being simple and robust, could be performed by non-specialized staff in health centres without laboratories and closer to the community. If performance did not compare with smear microscopy, there was the possibility that their use might complement smear microscopy and serological testing of smear-negative patients might result in an incremental gain in tuberculosis cases detected. A laboratory-based head-to-head evaluation of 19 commercially available rapid antibody detection tests for tuberculosis was included in the systematic review (WHO, 2008a).

The systematic reviews and meta-analyses concluded that diagnostic accuracy data indicated that none of the tests could replace sputum smear microscopy, nor could they be used as an add-on test to complement sputum smear microscopy (Steingart, 2011).

The wide availability of these tests in India, particularly in the private health sector, has recently been reported (Grenier, 2012; Steingart, 2012). Modelling of data from these studies has indicated enormous economic, social and public health costs associated with the use of these inadequate tests. Most of these tests are produced by companies based in Western countries (such as France, the UK, Germany and the USA), where these tests are not approved for use but the companies market and sell them in LMICs with high tuberculosis prevalence rates and poor regulatory oversight of imported diagnostics (Steingart, 2012). A very recent study has confirmed that these tests are widely used in the private sector of most of the 22 countries with the highest burdens of tuberculosis (high-burden countries). In about one-third of high-burden countries, the tests were also widely used in the public sector (Grenier, 2012).

Based on expert consideration of the evidence presented in the systematic reviews, the WHO released a policy statement in 2011 actively discouraging the use of all commercially available serological tests for tuberculosis, whether as a smear microscopy replacement test or as an add-on test (WHO, 2011b).

1.5 WHO-endorsed Replacement or Add-on Tests (Culture Based)

The WHO has endorsed only one culture-based test, liquid culture, for tuberculosis diagnosis. The term 'liquid culture' can be confusing since a number of culture-based tests that have not been endorsed by WHO could reasonably be described as 'liquid culture'. The WHO endorsement, however, refers specifically to commercially available broth-based culture systems, and most of the evidence which the WHO reviewed prior to the endorsement was specific to the Mycobacterial Growth Indicator Tube (MGIT) system produced by Becton Dickinson (USA) (WHO, 2007a). These commercially available broth-based culture systems can be manual or automated. They are expensive and require sophisticated biosafety laboratories. They are 20–25% more sensitive than solid culture and the time to positivity is reduced by an average of about 1 week (Chihota, 2010). Their application in tuberculosis reference laboratories in LMICs has frequently been problematic, and extensive international technical expertise has been required for implementation (Muyoyeta, 2009). Unacceptably high culture contamination rates have proved a common and difficult problem (Peres, 2011).

Even when implemented satisfactorily in the laboratory, the impact of tuberculosis culture on patient management is frequently uncertain (Stall, 2011). Mathematical modelling has indicated the key importance of patient access to diagnostics in determining their public health impact (Keeler, 2006). Diagnostic testing in central or national reference laboratories far from the health facilities where patients present is unlikely to be associated with any major public health impact unless equitable services can be developed with well-organized specimen transport, rapid turnaround times in the laboratory and prompt, efficient communication of results. Such systems are difficult to build and sustain in LMICs, even when funding is available. Experience to date has largely confirmed these predictions (Harries, 2004).

Several other culture-based tests have been endorsed by the WHO in recent years; these include the microscopic observation drug susceptibility (MODS) assay, redox indicator colorimetric drug susceptibility tests and the nitrate reductase (Greiss) test (WHO, 2011c). However, these alternative tests have only been endorsed, as interim measures, for the direct and/or indirect screening for drug resistance and until capacity for commercially available broth-based culture has been built. The alternative tests, like the commercially available broth-based culture, also require sophisticated biosafe laboratories and are subject to the same concerns about a lack of major public health impact.

The recent development of mobile shipping container based culture laboratories may help to improve patient access to these tests (WHO, 2009).

1.6 WHO-endorsed Replacement or Add-on Tests (Nucleic Acid Amplification Tests)

To date, the WHO has endorsed two nucleic acid amplification tests for tuberculosis. The first, endorsed in 2008, was the line probe assay (Hains test, or Inno-LiPa) (WHO, 2008b). This was endorsed for rapid screening of patients at risk of MDR-TB. These line probe assays, which detect rifampicin resistance (Inno-LiPa) or rifampicin and isoniazid resistance, are endorsed for use indirectly on isolates obtained from tuberculosis cultures or directly on smear-positive patients only. Clearly, then, sputum smear microscopy (particularly the more sensitive optimized sputum smear microscopy) could be combined with line probe assays for MDR screening in line with WHO recommendations.

If line probe assays are to be performed on culture isolates, the procedures need to be conducted in the same standard of biosafe laboratory required for the handling of tuberculosis culture systems. If, however, the sputum from smear-positive patients will not be cultured but processed directly for line probe assay, the biosafety requirements may be less stringent (WHO, 2010d). It may be possible, therefore, to conduct the line probe assay testing at intermediate laboratories closer to the sputum smear microscopy centre. The closer proximity of the advanced secondary testing site (for drug resistance) to the site of the primary smear-based diagnosis may facilitate better interaction and promote a more rapid patient-centred service. Unfortunately, in most cases, the implementation of line probe assays has not followed this model and secondary testing is usually confined to reference laboratories, sometimes considerable distances from the site of primary screening. The issues around access that applied to the culture-based systems would also apply here.

In 2010, the WHO endorsed the GeneXpert MTB/RIF, a cartridge-based real-time PCR for the simultaneous diagnosis of tuberculosis and detection of rifampicin resistance (WHO, 2011d). This closed system does not require biosafety laboratories, as the culture-based tests and line probe assays do. It is simple and results can be available within 2 h. Recent studies confirm earlier reports of good specificity and a sensitivity (using one cartridge) greater than smear microscopy but less than liquid culture (Banada, 2009; Blakemore, 2010; Boehme 2010, 2011). Sensitivity increases and approaches that of liquid culture if three specimens (and three cartridges) are used. One of the major drawbacks of this technology is its cost. Even at prices specially negotiated with the company for the public sector in high tuberculosis burden countries, each cartridge costs at least US$15. Each four-berth instrument, which can process only 20 cartridges in an average working day, currently costs US$15–17,000 at the specially negotiated price. The instruments are very sensitive to fluctuations in power supply and must be protected electrically with an uninterruptible power supply (UPS). At present, each instrument needs to be sent to Europe once a year for recalibration. The simplicity of this technology undoubtedly could bring more sensitive tuberculosis diagnosis and MDR-tuberculosis screening closer to where patients are seeking medical care and reduce time to diagnosis and to appropriate treatment. It is likely that this test could be used in health centres in some middle-income countries and perhaps at district hospital level in parts of sub-Saharan Africa. The WHO currently recommends that the MTB/RIF is used as the initial diagnostic test (i.e. smear microscopy replacement) in areas with high rates of MDR-TB or high rates of HIV-associated tuberculosis. The WHO further suggests that in areas where MDR-TB or HIV-associated tuberculosis is of less importance, the MTB/RIF is used as an add-on test (following smear microscopy) to detect smear-negative tuberculosis (WHO, 2011d). Cost-effectiveness models have been developed around these two applications (replacement and add-on) (WHO, 2011e). The problem with the use of the MTB/RIF on smear negatives only is that smear-positive patients will be systematically denied a rapid rifampicin resistance test. Concerns have also been raised about false positive rifampicin-resistant results with the test and the associated low positive predictive value, even in areas with relatively high MDR-TB prevalence (Lawn, 2011). The most pressing issue, of course, is the cost of the technology. Over 50 million smear microscopy investigations are conducted annually around the world. Even if the MTB/RIF is to be an add-on test for smear negatives, the volume of testing will be immense, and very costly.

1.7 The Current Tuberculosis Diagnostics Pipeline

There is little new expected from tuberculosis diagnostics in the coming 5 years. The LAMP assay has been proposed as a nucleic acid amplification test suitable for the peripheral laboratory. Demonstration studies have been ongoing for several years.

Progress is being made in our understanding of humoral immune responses to *M. tuberculosis* in different stages of the disease and the importance of multiple antigen testing and immunoresponse signatures in interpreting test results (Steingart, 2009; Kumnath-Velayudhan, 2010).[4] These may result in serological tests that would fit a point-of-care (POC) test format. Technological platforms suitable for POC application are currently being revolutionized through the use of microfluidics and nanoparticles (Chin, 2011). A number of groups are working on breath analysers that detect volatile organics associated with tuberculosis disease in sampled breath (Syhre, 2009; McNerney, 2010; Phillips, 2010).

1.8 The Future

It is unlikely that tuberculosis control activities in resource-poor settings will come to rely on a single new test in the near future. It is more probable that diagnostic services will be dependent on multiple diagnostic technologies with different roles at different levels of the tiered health service structure (Ramsay, 2009). Test evaluations to date have been largely diagnostic accuracy studies (Pai,

2010). Very few have looked at patient-important outcomes. Nearly all studies, to date, have evaluated a single diagnostic test rather than a real-world diagnostic service based on multiple tests at different health service levels (Squire, 2011). It is recognized that the current evidence on which the WHO is endorsing new diagnostic tools is sufficient only for a 'technical endorsement' – that this tool performs with this diagnostic accuracy when used in ideal conditions and may be useful in tuberculosis control programme activities (Ramsay, 2010). More research and more evidence is required on the performance of these tests when used in routine programmatic settings in combination with other diagnostic tests. This would allow the development of a process for the 'programmatic endorsement' of a new tool, which would be accompanied by evidence-based guidance on how to implement the test and scale-up use (Wilson, 2011).

1.9 Conclusion

Despite exciting advances in diagnostic technologies for tuberculosis and the creation of a tuberculosis diagnostic toolbox of several WHO-endorsed diagnostic technologies and approaches, global tuberculosis control for the time being is reliant on sputum smear microscopy. It is important that these sputum smear microscopy services are optimized as described above to:

- provide improved diagnostic services to patients in LMICs while the MTB/RIF and other diagnostic tools are rolled out. This roll-out may take several years before adequate service coverage is achieved;
- provide enhanced performance of the diagnostic service in areas where new diagnostics such as MTB/RIF are being considered as an add-on test to sputum smear microscopy;
- provide the best possible baseline data on which to judge the performance and added value of new technologies as they are introduced.

References

Association of Public Health Laboratories (2002) *External Quality Assessment for AFB Smear Microscopy.* Washington, USA.

Banada, P.P., Sivasubramani, S.K., Blakemore, R., Boehme, C., Perkins, M.D., Fennelly, K., *et al.* (2009) Containment of bioaerosol infection risk by the Xpert MTB/RIF assay and its applicability to point-of-care settings. *Journal of Clinical Microbiology* 48(10), 3551–3557.

Blakemore, R., Story, E., Helb, D., Kop, J., Banada, P., Owens, M.R., *et al.* (2010) Evaluation of the analytical performance of the Xpert MTB/RIF assay. *Journal of Clinical Microbiology* 48(7), 2495–2501.

Boehme, C.C., Nabeta, P., Hillemann, D., Nicol, M.P., Shenai, S., Krapp, F., *et al.* (2010) Rapid molecular detection of tuberculosis and rifampicin resistance. *The New England Journal of Medicine* 363(11), 1005–1115.

Boehme, C.C., Nicol, M.P., Nabeta, P., Michael, J.S., Gotuzzo, E., Tahirli, R., *et al.* (2011) Feasibility, diagnostic accuracy, and effectiveness of decentralized use of the Xpert MTB/RIF test for diagnosis of tuberculosis and multidrug resistance: a multicentre implementation study. *The Lancet* 377(9776), 1495–1505.

Bonnet, M., Gagnidze, L., Githui, W., Guerin, P.J., Bonte, L., Varaine, F., *et al.* (2011) Evaluation of LED-based fluorescence microscopy for diagnosis of tuberculosis in a peripheral laboratory of a high HIV prevalence country. *PLoS ONE* 6(2), e17214.

Bonnet, M., Gagnidze, L., Guerin, P.J., Bonte, L., Ramsay, A., Githui, W., *et al.* (2011) Evaluation of combined LED-fluorescence microscopy and bleach sedimentation for diagnosis of tuberculosis at peripheral health service level. *PLoS ONE* 6, e20175.

Botha, E., den Boon, S., Lawrence, K.A., Reuter, H., Verver, S., Lombard, C.J., *et al.* (2008) From suspect to patient: tuberculosis diagnosis and treatment initiation in health facilities in South Africa. *International Journal of Tuberculosis and Lung Diseases* 12(8), 936–941.

Chihota, V.N., Grant, A.D., Fielding, K., Ndibongo, B., van Zyl, A., Muirhead, D., *et al.* (2010) Liquid vs solid culture for tuberculosis: performance and cost in a resource-constrained setting. *International Journal of Tuberculosis and Lung Diseases* 14(8), 1024–1031.

Chin, C.D., Laksanasopin, T., Cheung, Y.K., Steinmiller, D., Linder, V., Parsa, H., *et al.* (2011) Microfluidics-based diagnostics of infectious diseases in the developing world. *Nature Medicine* 17, 1015–1019.

Cuevas, L.E., Al-Sonboli, N., Lawson, L., Yassin, M.A., Arbide, I., Al-Aghbari, N., *et al.* (2011) A multi-country evaluation of LED-fluorescence microscopy for the diagnosis of pulmonary tuberculosis. *PLoS Medicine* 8, e1001057.

Cuevas, L.E., Yassin, M.A., Al-Sonboli, N., Lawson, L., Arbide, I., Al-Aghbari, N., *et al.* (2011) A multi-country non-inferiority cluster randomized trial of frontloaded smear microscopy for the diagnosis of pulmonary tuberculosis. *PLoS Medicine* 8, e1000443.

Gilpin, C., Kim, S.J., Lumb, R., Reider, H.L. and Van Deun, A. (2007) Working Group on Smear Microscopy. Critical appraisal of current recommendations and practice for tuberculosis sputum smear microscopy. *International Journal of Tuberculosis and Lung Diseases* 11(9), 946–952.

Grenier, J., Pinto, L., Nair, D., Steingart, K., Dowdy, D., Ramsay, A., *et al.* (2012) Widespread use of serological tests for tuberculosis: data from 22 high-burden countries. *European Respiratory Journal* 39, 502–505.

Harries, A.D., Michongwe, J., Nyirenda, T.E., Kemp, J.R., Squire, S.B., Ramsay, A.R., *et al.* (2004) Using a bus service for transporting sputum specimens to the central reference laboratory: effect on the routine TB culture service in Malawi. *International Journal of Tuberculosis and Lung Diseases* 8(2), 204–210.

IUATLD [International Union Against Tuberculosis and Lung Diseases] (2000) *Technical Guide. Sputum Examination for Tuberculosis by Direct Microscopy in Low-income Countries.* 5th edn. IUATLD, Paris.

Keeler, E., Perkins, M.D., Small, P., Hanson, C., Reed, S., Cunningham, J., *et al.* (2006) Reducing the global burden of tuberculosis: the contribution of improved diagnostics. *Nature* 444, Suppl 1, 49–57.

Kemp, J.R., Mann, G., Simwaka, B.N., Salaniponi, F.M. and Squire, S.B. (2007) Can Malawi's poor access free tuberculosis services? Patient and household costs associated with a tuberculosis diagnosis in Lilongwe. *Bulletin World Health Organization* 85(8), 580–585.

Khan, M.S., Dar, O., Sismanidis, C., Shah, K. and Godfrey-Faussett, P. (2007) Improvement of tuberculosis case-detection and reduction of discrepancies between men and women by simple sputum submission instructions: a pragmatic randomised controlled trial. *The Lancet* 369(9577), 1955–1960.

Kunnath-Velayudhan, S., Salamon, H., Wang, H.Y., Davidow, A.L., Molina, D.M., Huynh, V.T., *et al.* (2010) Dynamic antibody responses to the *Mycobacterium tuberculosis* genome. *Proceed-*

ings of the National Academy of Sciences 107(33), 14703–14708.

Lawn, S.D., Brooks, S.V., Kranzer, K., Nicol, M.P., Whitelaw, A., Vogt, M., et al. (2011) Screening for HIV-associated tuberculosis and rifampicin resistance before antiretroviral therapy using the Xpert MTB/RIF assay: a prospective study. PLoS Medicine 8(7).

McNerney, R., Wondafrash, B.A., Amena, K., Tesfaye, A., McCash, E.M. and Murray, N.J. (2010) Field test of a novel detection device for Mycobacterium tuberculosis antigen in cough. BMC Infectious Diseases 8(10), 161.

Managing Pharmaceuticals and Commodities for Tuberculosis: A Guide for National Tuberculosis Programmes (2005) Virginia, USA.

Mase, S.R., Ramsay, A., Henry, M., Ng, V., Hopewell, P.C., Cunningham, J., et al. (2007) The incremental yield of serial sputum smears in the diagnosis of tuberculosis: a systematic review. International Journal of Tuberculosis and Lung Diseases 11(5), 485–495.

Muyoyeta, M., Schaap, J.A., De Haas, P., Mwanza, W., Muvwimi, M.W., Godfrey-Faussett, P., et al. (2009) Comparison of four culture systems for Mycobacterium tuberculosis in the Zambian National Reference Laboratory. International Journal of Tuberculosis and Lung Diseases 13(5), 460–465.

Pai, M., Minion, J., Steingart, K.R. and Ramsay, A. (2010) New and improved tuberculosis diagnostics: evidence, policy, practice and impact. Current Opinion in Pulmonary Medicine 16, 271–284.

Peres, R.L., Palaci, M., Loureiro, R.B., Dietze, R., Johnson, J.L. and Maciel, E.L. (2011) Reduction of contamination of mycobacterial growth indicator tubes using increased PANTA concentration. International Journal of Tuberculosis and Lung Diseases 15(2), 281–283.

Phillips, M., Basa-Dalay, V., Bothamley, G., Cataneo, R.N., Lam, P.K., Natividad, M.P., et al. (2010) Breath biomarkers of active pulmonary tuberculosis. Tuberculosis 90(2), 145–151.

Ramsay, A. and Harries, A.D. (2009) The clinical value of new diagnostic tools for tuberculosis. F1000 Medical Reports. Part ii, 36.

Ramsay, A., Yassin, M.A., Cambanis, A., Hirao, S., Almotawa, A., Gammo, M., et al. (2009) Front-loading sputum smear microscopy services: an opportunity to optimize smear-based case detection of tuberculosis in high prevalence countries. Journal of Tropical Medicine 2009, 398767.

Ramsay, A., Steingart, K.R. and Pai, M. (2010) Assessing the impact of new diagnostics on tuberculosis control. International Journal of

Tuberculosis and Lung Diseases 14(12), 1506–1507.

Ramsay, A., Steingart, K.R., Cunningham, J. and Pai, M. (2011) Translating tuberculosis research into global policies. International Journal of Tuberculosis and Lung Diseases 15, 1283–1293.

Squire, S.B., Ramsay, A., van den Hof, S., Millington, K.A., Langley, I., Bello, G., et al. (2011) Making innovations work for the poor through implementation by research. International Journal of Tuberculosis and Lung Diseases 5(7), 862–870.

Stall, N., Rubin, T., Michael, J.S., Mathai, D., Abraham, O.C., Mathews, P., et al. (2011) Does solid culture for tuberculosis influence clinical decision-making in India? International Journal of Tuberculosis and Lung Diseases 15(5), 641–646.

Steingart, K.R., Henry, M., Ng, V., Hopewell, P.C., Ramsay, A., Cunningham, J., et al. (2006a) Fluorescence versus conventional sputum smear microscopy for tuberculosis: a systematic review. Lancet Infectious Diseases 6(9), 570–581.

Steingart, K.R., Ng, V., Henry, M., Hopewell, P.C., Ramsay, A., Cunningham, J., et al. (2006b) Sputum processing methods to improve the sensitivity of smear microscopy for tuberculosis: a systematic review. The Lancet Infectious Diseases 6(10), 664–674.

Steingart, K.R., Ramsay, A. and Pai, M. (2007a) Optimizing sputum smear microscopy for the diagnosis of pulmonary tuberculosis. Expert Reviews in Anti-Infective Therapy 5(3), 327–331.

Steingart, K.R., Henry, M., Hopewell, P.C., Laal, S., Ramsay, A., Menzies, R., et al. (2007b) Commercial serological antibody detection tests for the diagnosis of pulmonary tuberculosis: a systematic review. PLoS Medicine 4(6), e202.

Steingart, K.R., Henry, M., Hopewell, P.C., Laal, S., Ramsay, A., Menzies, R., et al. (2007c) A systematic review of commercial serological antibody detection tests for the diagnosis of extrapulmonary tuberculosis. Thorax 62(10), 911–918.

Steingart, K.R., Ramsay, A. and Pai, M. (2007d) Commercial serological tests for tuberculosis: do they work? Future Microbiology 2(4), 355–359.

Steingart, K.R., Dendukuri, N., Henry, M., Schiller, I., Nahid, P., Hopewell, P.C., et al. (2009) Performance of purified antigens for serodiagnosis of pulmonary tuberculosis: a meta-analysis. Clinical and Vaccine Immunology 16(2), 260–276.

Steingart, K.R., Flores, L.L., Dendukuri, N., Schiller,

I., Laal, S., Ramsay, A., *et al.* (2011) Commercial serological antibody detection tests for the diagnosis of tuberculosis: an updated systematic review and meta-analysis. *PLoS Medicine* 8, e1001062.

Steingart, K.R., Ramsay, A., Dowdy, D.W. and Pai, M. (2012) Serological tests for the diagnosis of active tuberculosis: relevance for India. *Indian Journal of Medical Research* 135, 695–702.

Syhre, M., Manning, L., Phuanukoonnon, S., Harino, P. and Chambers, S.T. (2009) The scent of *Mycobacterium tuberculosis*: Part II breath. *Tuberculosis* 89(4), 263–236.

TDR/FIND (2006) WHO diagnostics for tuberculosis: global demand and market potential (http://apps.who.int/tdr/svc/publications/tdr-research-publications/diagnostics-tuberculosis-global-demand, accessed 11 April 2011).

Wilson, N., Chadha, S., Beyers, N., Claassens, M. and Naidoo, P. (2011) Helping the poor access innovation in tuberculosis control: using evidence from implementation research. *International Journal of Tuberculosis and Lung Diseases* 15(7), 853.

WHO [World Health Organization] (2007a) The use of liquid medium for culture and DST, Geneva (http://www.who.int/tb/laboratory/policy_liquid_medium_for_culture_dst/en/index.html, accessed 11 March 2013).

WHO (2007b) Definition of a new sputum smear positive TB case (http://www.who.int/tb/laboratory/policy_sputum_smearpositive_tb_case/en/index.html, accessed 11 April 2011).

WHO (2007c) Reduction of number of smears for the diagnosis of pulmonary TB, 2007 (http://www.who.int/tb/laboratory/policy_diagnosis_pulmonary_tb/en/index.html, accessed 11 April 2011).

WHO (2008a) Laboratory-based evaluation of 19 commercially-available rapid diagnostic tests for tuberculosis. UNICEF/UNDP/World Bank/WHO Special Programme for Research and Training in Tropical Diseases.

WHO (2008b) Molecular line-probe assays for rapid screening of patients at risk of multi-drug resistant tuberculosis: policy statement, Geneva (http://www.who.int/tb/features_archive/policy_statement.pdf, accessed 11 March 2013).

WHO (2009) Non-commercial culture methods and mycobacteriophage-based assays for rapid screening of patients at risk of drug-resistant tuberculosis. Expert Group Meeting Report (http://www.who.int/tb/laboratory/egmreport_non-commercial_rapid_dst_nov09.pdf, accessed 11 March 2013).

WHO (2010a) *WHO Report 2010. Global Tuberculosis Control.* WHO, Geneva, Switzerland.

WHO (2010b) Same-day diagnosis of tuberculosis by smear microscopy. Policy Statement, 2010 (http://www.who.int/tb/laboratory/whopolicy_same_day_diagnosis_bymicroscopy_mar2011.pdf, accessed 11 April 2011).

WHO (2010c) Fluorescent light-emitting diode (LED) microscopy for diagnosis of tuberculosis. Policy Statement, 2010 (http://www.who.int/tb/laboratory/whopolicy_led_microscopy_mar2011.pdf, accessed 11 April 2011).

WHO (2010d) Policy framework for implementing new tuberculosis diagnostics (http://www.who.int/tb/laboratory/whopolicyframework_rev_june2011.pdf, accessed 11 March 2013).

WHO (2011a) Stop TB department. TB diagnostics and laboratory strengthening (http://www.who.int/tb/laboratory/policy_statements/en/index.html, accessed 3 August 2011).

WHO (2011b) WHO policy statement: commercial serodiagnostic tests for diagnosis of tuberculosis, Geneva (http://whqlibdoc.who.int/publications/2011/9789241502054_eng.pdf, accessed 3 August 2011).

WHO (2011c) Non-commercial culture and drug susceptibility testing methods for screening of patients at risk for multi-drug resistant tuberculosis: policy statement, Geneva (http://whqlibdoc.who.int/publications/2011/9789241501620_eng.pdf, accessed 11 March 2013).

WHO (2011d) Automated real-time nucleic acid amplification technology for rapid and simultaneous detection of tuberculosis and rifampicin resistance: Xpert MTB/RIF system. Policy statement (http://whqlibdoc.who.int/publications/2011/9789241501545_eng.pdf, accessed 11 March 2013).

WHO (2011e) Rapid implementation of the Xpert MTB/RIF diagnostic test: technical and operational 'how-to' considerations (http://whqlibdoc.who.int/publications/2011/9789241501569_eng.pdf, accessed 11 March 2013).

2 Molecular Diagnosis of Active Pulmonary Tuberculosis

Anna L. Bateson,[1] Kate Reddington[2] and Justin O'Grady[3]

[1]*Centre for Clinical Microbiology, Department of Infection, University College London, UK;* [2]*Molecular Diagnostics Research Group, Microbiology, School of Natural Sciences, National University of Ireland Galway, Ireland;* [3]*Norwich Medical School, Norwich, UK*

2.1 Introduction

Accurate and rapid diagnosis of tuberculosis is of paramount importance in establishing appropriate clinical management and infection control measures (Migliori *et al.*, 2010; Wallis *et al.*, 2010; O'Grady *et al.*, 2011). The most common method for diagnosing tuberculosis worldwide is sputum smear microscopy, a technology that is over a century old and the sensitivity of which is notoriously poor, particularly in human immunodeficiency virus (HIV)-positive patients. Culture, the gold standard diagnostic method, is now available in most countries, but typically only centrally in resource-poor settings (WHO, 2011b). Culture is highly sensitive but takes between 2 and 6 weeks to obtain a result. Rapid and sensitive tools for the diagnosis of tuberculosis are required, due to the increased incidence of tuberculosis worldwide, particularly in HIV-endemic regions, and the length of time required for classical diagnostic tests. Increasingly, rapid molecular tests are being used for the detection of pulmonary tuberculosis.

Since the turn of the century, there have been significant advances in diagnostic technologies for tuberculosis. Increase in both public and private investment and the joint efforts of agencies such as the World Health Organization (WHO), Stop TB Partnership's New Diagnostics Working Group (NDWG) and the Foundation for Innovative New Diagnostics (FIND) have facilitated this process (Wallis *et al.*, 2010). Liquid media for culture and drug susceptibility testing (DST), molecular line probe assays (LPAs) for screening people at risk of multidrug-resistant tuberculosis (MDR-TB), light-emitting diode microscopy, non-commercial culture and DST and automated real-time PCR technology for the simultaneous detection of tuberculosis and rifampicin (RIF) resistance (Xpert MTB/RIF assay) have all been endorsed by the WHO since 2007 (Fig. 2.1). Endorsement of technology by the WHO, combined with FIND's negotiations on pricing with industry has made new and improved diagnostic tests more affordable and feasible for developing countries (Wallis *et al.*, 2010; O'Grady *et al.*, 2011).

Molecular diagnostic methods for the detection of pulmonary tuberculosis have been commercially available since the 1990s. The amplified MTD (Gen-Probe, Inc, San Diego, USA) test was the first nucleic acid amplification test (NAAT) to get US Food and Drug Administration (FDA) approval for detection of pulmonary tuberculosis, in 1996,

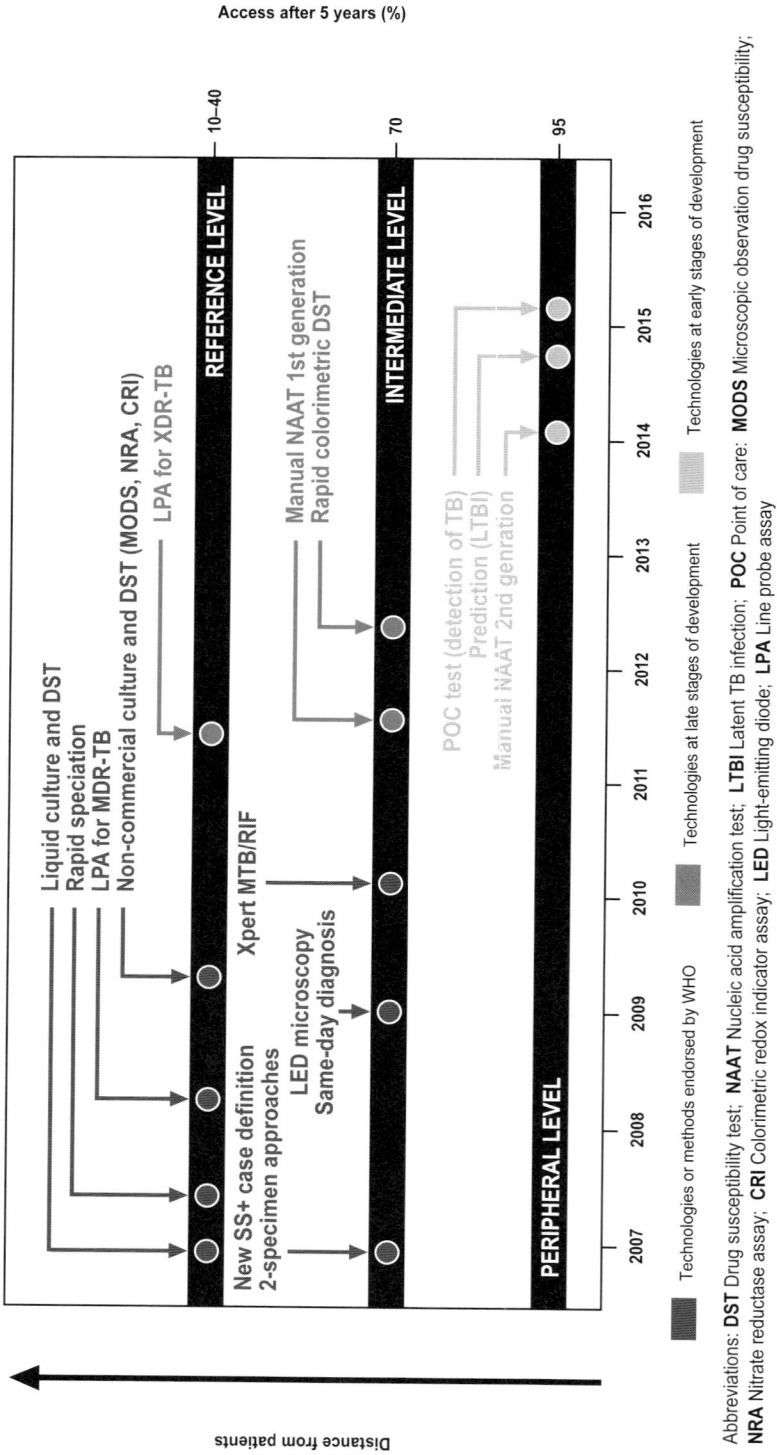

Fig. 2.1. The tuberculosis diagnostics pipeline in 2011 (reproduced with permission from WHO (WHO, 2011b).

Abbreviations: **DST** Drug susceptibility test; **NAAT** Nucleic acid amplification test; **LTBI** Latent TB infection; **POC** Point of care; **MODS** Microscopic observation drug susceptibility; **NRA** Nitrate reductase assay; **CRI** Colorimetric redox indicator assay; **LED** Light-emitting diode; **LPA** Line probe assay shortly followed by the Roche Amplicor MTB test (Nyendak *et al.*, 2009). Early molecular methods were designed to detect the *Mycobacterium tuberculosis* complex (MTC) only. These tests were followed by the introduction of LPAs, which combined nucleic acid amplification with hybridization. LPAs have a higher capacity for multi-parametric detection and have been designed to detect both MTC and first- and second-line anti-*M. tuberculosis* drug resistance. The most recent commercially available WHO endorsed NAAT is the Xpert MTB/RIF assay, which utilizes real-time PCR for the simultaneous detection of MTC and RIF resistance. The major technological advance of this method is the automation of the sample analysis, from nucleic acid extraction to result readout. Molecular diagnosis for tuberculosis is not limited to those tests that are commercially available and endorsed by the WHO. There have been numerous in-house molecular diagnosis assays developed over the past two decades, with varying specificities and sensitivities.

Resistance to anti-*M. tuberculosis* drugs arises as a result of spontaneous mutations in genes encoding either the target of the drug or enzymes involved in drug activation (Parsons *et al.*, 2011). Resistance-associated mutations have been described for all first-line drugs. MDR-TB develops through the sequential acquisition of mutations at multiple loci (Parsons *et al.*, 2011). The most common mutations associated with drug resistance have been described and are publicly available on the tuberculosis drug resistance mutation database (Sandgren *et al.*, 2009). Genotypic DST methods target these well-characterized resistance-associated mutations to identify drug-resistant *M. tuberculosis*. One of the most important drugs in the treatment of tuberculosis is rifampicin (RIF). RIF resistance is particularly suitable for genotypic DST because 95% of RIF resistance-associated mutations are present in an 81-bp region of the *rpoB* gene known as the rifampicin resistance-determining region (RRDR) (Blakemore *et al.*, 2010; O'Grady *et al.*, 2011; Parsons *et al.*, 2011). Molecular methods, such as LPAs and Xpert MTB/RIF assay, targeting this

region have excellent correlation with phenotypic DST results, with specificities and sensitivities >90%, and have been endorsed by the WHO (WHO, 2008, 2011a). Molecular detection of resistance to other anti-*M. tuberculosis* drugs, such as isoniazid (INH) and ethambutol (EMB), is more complex and requires detection of mutations in multiple genes for a good correlation with phenotypic results (O'Grady *et al.*, 2011). INH resistance-associated mutations have been found in the *katG* and *inhA* genes; however, approximately 15–25% of INH-resistant isolates do not contain mutations in these regions, indicating that other sites must also be involved in resistance (Parsons *et al.*, 2011). Accurate genotypic DST for first- and second-line anti-*M. tuberculosis* drugs is, therefore, technically challenging. Increased under-standing of the molecular mechanisms of anti-*M. tuberculosis* drug resistance and improved multi-parametric detection technology will make genotypic DST a more powerful technique in the future.

Tuberculosis in humans can be caused by any of the members of the MTC. The eight closely related species of the MTC have a wide range of natural hosts, including human hosts (*M. tuberculosis, M. africanum, M. canettii*), bovine hosts (*M. bovis*), caprine hosts (*M. caprae*), rodent hosts (*M. microti*) and pinniped hosts (*M. pinnipedii*), along with *M. bovis* Bacillus Calmette–Guérin (BCG), the commonly used vaccine strain. All species of the MTC have been implicated in human infection, regardless of the natural host (Reddington *et al.*, 2011). While *M. tuberculosis* is responsible for the majority of cases of human tuberculosis, accurate identification of other members of the MTC causing infection is not performed routinely (Pinsky and Banaei, 2008). As a result, the global frequency and distribution of each member of the MTC remains largely unknown, with some studies suggesting that tuberculosis caused by members of the MTC other than *M. tuberculosis* are under-represented (Somoskovi *et al.*, 2009; Allix-Béguec *et al.*, 2010). *M. africanum*, for example, has been identified as the causative agent of up to 50% of human tuberculosis infections in West African countries (Kallenius *et al.*, 1999) and *M. canettii* was responsible for 10% of tuberculosis cases in a recent study performed in the Republic of Djibouti (Koeck *et al.*, 2010). Furthermore, *M. bovis* remains an important cause of zoonotic tuberculosis worldwide and should not be overlooked in a clinical setting (Hlavsa *et al.*, 2008; Allix-Béguec *et al.*, 2010). In developing countries, where there is a paucity of data, one study suggests that the prevalence of bovine tuberculosis in humans may be as high as 15% (de la Rua-Domenech, 2006). Some members of the MTC (*M. bovis*, *M. bovis* BCG and *M. canettii*) are intrinsically resistant to pyrazinamide, an important first-line anti-*M. tuberculosis* drug (Somoskovi *et al.*, 2009). Therefore, specific identification of these members of the MTC is clinically important for treatment management decisions. The accurate molecular identification of species of the MTC is therefore required to guide public health and clinical decisions more effectively.

For the purposes of this chapter, molecular diagnostic methods for tuberculosis are divided into three groups: NAATs, LPAs and sequencing assays. The chapter covers both commercial and in-house methods for the detection of the MTC, differentiation of the MTC and molecular DST for anti-*M. tuberculosis* drugs. The advantages, disadvantages and future of molecular diagnosis for tuberculosis, including point-of-care (POC) diagnostic tests, are also discussed.

2.2 Nucleic Acid Amplification Tests

2.2.1 NAATs for the detection of the MTC

A significant number of studies have been published describing both commercial and in-house NAATs for the diagnosis of pulmonary tuberculosis in clinical samples. In-house tests have targeted a wide range of DNA sequences specific for the MTC, including rRNA (16S and 23S); genes encoding the proteins MPB64, MTP40 and protein antigen b; resistance-determining genes such as *gyrB* and *rpoB*; insertion sequences IS*6110* and IS*986* and repetitive elements (De Wit *et al.*, 1990; Soini *et al.*, 1992;

Walker *et al.*, 1992a; Andersen *et al.*, 1993; Verma *et al.*, 1994; Beige *et al.*, 1995; Del Portillo *et al.*, 1996; Iwamoto *et al.*, 2003; Flores *et al.*, 2005; Cui *et al.*, 2012). A published meta-analysis, which focused on PCR-based amplification techniques, showed estimates of the accuracy of in-house NAATs were highly heterogeneous, with sensitivity ranging from 9.4% to 100% and specificity estimates of 5.6–100% (Flores *et al.*, 2005). Several commercial NAATs are available which use different amplification methods. These include the Roche Amplicor *M. tuberculosis* test (Amplicor MTB), the Gen-Probe Amplified *M. tuberculosis* Direct (AMTD) test, the Beckton Dickinson ProbeTec test and, most recently, the Eiken loop mediated isothermal amplification (LAMP) test (Parsons *et al.*, 2011). This chapter is not an exhaustive review of all commercial NAATs and will focus on the tests listed above, as they are the most widely used and have the most published clinical data available. NAATs that also assess drug resistance are covered in a separate section.

The Amplicor MTB test (Roche Diagnostic Systems, New Jersey, USA) is a PCR-based amplification test which targets the 16S rRNA gene, and the amplified product is detected by a colorimetric reaction after hybridization to oligonucleotide probes (Palomino, 2009). An automated version of the test, the COBAS Amplicor MTB test, allows fully automated amplification and detection in the same system using the COBAS Amplicor analyser. Assay results for the COBAS Amplicor MTB test are available in 6–7 h. This method is intended for use on decontaminated, concentrated samples and has FDA approval for testing of smear-positive respiratory specimens. More recently, the COBAS TaqMan MTB test has also been introduced using real-time PCR and hybridization in the COBAS TaqMan 48 analyser that can run 48 samples in 2.5 h (Kim *et al.*, 2011; Yang *et al.*, 2011). Many studies have evaluated the performance of the Amplicor MTB test (Piersimoni and Scarparo, 2003; Greco *et al.*, 2006; Ling *et al.*, 2008a), with overall reported sensitivity ranging from 90% to 100% in smear-positive samples and from 50% to 95.9% in smear-negative samples, and overall specificity ranging from 91.3% to 100% (Palomino, 2009; Parsons *et al.*, 2011).

The AMTD assay (Gen-Probe) is an isothermal transcription-mediated amplification (TMA) method which also targets 16S rRNA. The Gen-Probe TMA method amplifies a specific rRNA target by transcription of DNA intermediates, yielding multiple copies of mycobacterial RNA (Piersimoni and Scarparo, 2003). These RNA amplicons are then detected by binding to a single-stranded, acridinium ester-labelled DNA probe, giving a chemoluminesence signal that is read in a luminometer (Piersimoni and Scarparo, 2003). Amplification and detection are performed in a single tube and test results are available within 2.5 h. This method is approved by the FDA for testing on both smear-positive and smear-negative respiratory samples (Piersimoni and Scarparo, 2003). The reported sensitivities ranged from 91.7% to 100% in smear-positive samples and from 65.5% to 92.9% in smear-negative samples, with a specificity of 92.1–100% (Palomino, 2009; Parsons *et al.*, 2011). A recent prospective study has evaluated the AMTD in a high HIV prevalence population in Uganda and showed that even a moderate sensitivity of 39% in smear-negative patients had a substantial clinical impact in this population (Davis *et al.*, 2011).

The ProbeTec MTB and newer ProbeTec ET Direct TB tests (Beckton Dickinson, Sparks, Maryland, USA) use strand displacement amplification (SDA) to co-amplify the target DNA sequences of IS*6110* and the 16S rRNA gene, and real-time detection of fluorescent labelled detector probes using a ProbeTec instrument. SDA is an isothermal reaction that involves nicking of the DNA by a restriction endonuclease and extension by a DNA polymerase with strand displacement activity (Walker *et al.*, 1992b). The newly replicated and displaced strands are then substrates for repeated rounds of primer annealing, nicking and strand displacement (Walker *et al.*, 1992b; Piersimoni and Scarparo, 2003). The ProbeTec MTB test assay is a closed system and takes approximately 3–4 h to perform. It is recommended for use on digested, decontaminated respiratory specimens, but is not currently approved by the FDA (Piersimoni and Scarparo, 2003). Many studies have evaluated the ProbeTec assay (Piersimoni and Scarparo, 2003; Greco *et al.*, 2006; Ling *et al.*, 2008a), with sensitivities ranging from 98.5% to 100% in smear-positive samples and from 33% to 85.7% in smear-negative samples, and an excellent overall specificity of 98.9–100% (Piersimoni and Scarparo, 2003; Parsons *et al.*, 2011).

The newest NAAT is the LAMP assay (Eiken Chemical Co Ltd, Tokyo, Japan), which is soon to be made commercially available. This is a novel, isothermal molecular method with high amplification efficacy. The target of the Eiken LAMP assay is an *M. tuberculosis* specific region of the *gyrB* gene, encoding DNA gyrase subunit B. The test is a closed system and, importantly, the amplified product can be seen by direct visual inspection of turbidity or fluorescence in the tube (Neonakis *et al.*, 2011).

A full description of the LAMP methodology is available in full elsewhere (Tomita *et al.*, 2008) and a helpful animation can be viewed online (Eiken). The LAMP assay requires four specially designed primers that recognize six distinct sites – one pair of standard primers each recognizing a single domain and one pair of composite primers that each recognize a double domain (two consecutive sequences). The reaction has two phases: the starting structure-producing step and the cycle-amplification step. To generate the starting structure, all four of the primers are required in sequence, initiating rounds of strand displacement DNA synthesis and resulting in a single-stranded dumbbell structure with loops at either end. The amplification stage requires only the two composite primers and results in various-sized stem-loop structures, consisting of alternatively inverted repeats of the target sequence, and cauliflower-like structures with multiple loops formed by annealing of the repeat sequences on the same strand (Notomi *et al.*, 2000; Neonakis *et al.*, 2011). The LAMP reaction can also be used with RNA as the target, with the addition of reverse transcriptase (RT-LAMP). Visualizing of LAMP amplified DNA can be performed in two ways. As the reaction progresses, a white precipitate of magnesium pyrophosphate is formed as a by-product (Tomita *et al.*, 2008). The precipitate can be observed directly by visual inspection or by reading tubes in a turbidometer. Alternatively, calcein, a chelating agent that yields strong fluorescence when combined with metallic ions such as magnesium, can be added to the reaction and the amplified product detected by visual examination under UV light or using a spectrophotometer (Tomita *et al.*, 2008).

The first comprehensive clinical evaluation of the LAMP assay for the detection of pulmonary tuberculosis showed a sensitivity of 97.7% in smear-positive sputum samples and 48.8% in smear-negative samples, and a specificity of 99% (Boehme *et al.*, 2007). Modifications were made to the LAMP kit by Eiken Chemicals to simplify the DNA extraction process, and a recent study in Japan has confirmed this new kit has similar diagnostic performance (Mitarai *et al.*, 2011). A comparison of LAMP to other molecular methods showed performance was similar to other molecular tests for smear-positive samples but was slightly lower for smear negatives, particularly in treated sputum pellets (Mitarai *et al.*, 2011).

Overall, the Eiken LAMP assay is simple (no special reagents or equipment required), rapid (a turnaround time of 60–90 min including DNA extraction) and robust (yields reproducible results across a range of set up temperatures, pH and in the presence of known PCR inhibitors) (Boehme *et al.*, 2007; Francois *et al.*, 2011). Feasibility studies in microscopy centres also showed minimal technical training was required (Boehme *et al.*, 2007). Together, these practical considerations suggest the platform is applicable for use in a resource-poor, peripheral laboratory setting. However, the inferior performance in smear-negative patients (see Table 2.1; Boehme *et al.*, 2010) may suggest limited utility in tuberculosis populations with high rates of smear-negative tuberculosis, such as HIV-positive individuals and children, without further modifications. More clinical data are required to assess the commercial LAMP assay in these groups. For a test to have maximal diagnostic impact in remote, resource-poor settings, it may be a trade-off between practical operational characteristics and performance until the next generation of tests that satisfy both are available.

2.2.2 NAATs for the detection of the MTC and drug resistance

There are several commercially available NAATs for the detection of *M. tuberculosis* with simultaneous detection of drug

Table 2.1. Commercially available NAATs for the detection of the MTC (Ling *et al.*, 2008a; Parsons *et al.*, 2011; WHO, 2011a; Chang *et al.*, 2012).

| NAAT name | Manufacturer | Amplification method | Sensitivity range (%) | | Specificity range (%) |
			Smear-positive samples	Smear-negative samples	
Amplicor MTB test	Roche Molecular Systems	PCR	90–100	50–95.9	91.3–100
Amplified MTD test	Gen-Probe Inc	Transcription-mediated amplification	91.7–100	65.5–92.9	92.1–100
BD ProbeTec ET	Becton Dickinson	Strand displacement amplification	98.5–100	33.3–85.7	98.9–100
Loopamp® Tuberculosis Complex Detection Reagent Kit	Eiken Chemical Co	Loop-mediated isothermal amplification	97.7	48.8	99
Xpert MTB/RIF	Cepheid	PCR	95–100	43.4–84.6	92–100

resistance. These include the Xpert MTB/RIF assay (Cepheid Inc, Sunnydale, California, USA), which detects RIF resistance, and LPAs (discussed in a separate section) for the detection of resistance to first-line drugs – MTBDR*plus* (Hain Lifesciences, GmbH, Nehren, Germany) and INNO-LiPA (Innogenetics, Gent, Belgium); and second-line drugs – MTBDR*sl* (Hain Lifesciences). Array-based assays are also available to test for a wider panel of resistance-determining mutations; these include QIAPlex (Qiagen, Valencia, California, USA), TruArray MDR-TB (Akonni Biosystems, Maryland, USA) and INFINTI MDR-TB (Autogenomics, California, USA) tests. Many in-house NAATs have also been published for the detection of resistance to both first- and second-line tuberculosis drugs (Parsons *et al.*, 2011). These are most commonly real-time PCR methods with resistance mutations detected by fluorescent probes (TaqMan probes or molecular beacons) or melting curve analysis (fluorescence resonance energy transfer (FRET) probe melting curve analysis or high-resolution melting (HRM) curve analysis) (Lin *et al.*, 2004; Wada *et al.*, 2004; Yesilkaya *et al.*, 2006; Ramirez *et al.*, 2010). More recently, several new probe-based melting curve analysis technologies have also been evaluated, with promising results (Chakravorty *et al.*, 2011; Luo *et al.*, 2011).

The Xpert MTB/RIF assay, recently developed by Cepheid Inc in collaboration with FIND, is the most promising molecular diagnostic technology for *M. tuberculosis*. This is a fully automated test for the simultaneous detection of MTC and RIF resistance directly from clinical samples. The assay utilizes a hemi-nested PCR to amplify an *M. tuberculosis* specific sequence of the *rpoB* gene (192 bp) and *M. tuberculosis* is detected by five overlapping molecular beacon probes that are complementary to the 81-bp RRDR (Lawn and Nicol, 2011). The Xpert MTB/RIF assay procedure has been described in detail elsewhere (Blakemore *et al.*, 2010; Helb *et al.*, 2010). Briefly, sputum samples or decontaminated sputum pellets are treated with a reagent to reduce *M. tuberculosis* viability and loaded manually into a cartridge, which is inserted into the GeneXpert instrument. All subsequent steps are performed automatically; each cartridge incorporates microfluidics technology and contains all the reagents required for bacterial lysis, nucleic acid extraction, amplification and amplicon detection (Lawn and Nicol, 2011). The results are generated automatically in a user-friendly format. Cartridges can be loaded and processed independently without the need for batching. The assay has a hands-on time of less than 15 min and can be performed by relatively low-skilled technicians, with minimal training, within 2 h (Lawn and Nicol, 2011). Safety studies have also proven the assay can be performed without the specialized bio-containment equipment that is usually required for handling viable *M. tuberculosis* (Banada *et al.*, 2010).

Two large multicentre, prospective evaluation studies have been carried out using reference laboratory facilities (Boehme *et al.*, 2010), and in district and subdistrict health facilities (Boehme *et al.*, 2011), and both have shown excellent performance. In the former, the sensitivity of a single Xpert MTB/RIF assay was 98.2% in smear-positive patients and 72.5% in smear-negative patients, with a specificity of 99.2% (Boehme *et al.*, 2010). For detection of RIF resistance, sensitivity was 97.6% and specificity was 98.1% (Boehme *et al.*, 2010). Importantly, performance data from the study at peripheral health facilities showed similar results, providing important data on the suitability of implementing the assay in low-resource settings (Boehme *et al.*, 2011). A number of other studies have evaluated the Xpert MTB/RIF assay in pulmonary tuberculosis (Helb *et al.*, 2010; Armand *et al.*, 2011; Marlowe *et al.*, 2011; Moure *et al.*, 2011; Rachow *et al.*, 2011) and a recent meta-analysis showed a pooled sensitivity of 90.4% and specificity of 98.4% for the detection of tuberculosis; and a pooled sensitivity of 94.1% and specificity of 97.0% for the detection of RIF resistance (Chang *et al.*, 2012). The Xpert MTB/RIF assay has also been shown to perform well in HIV-positive patients, with an overall sensitivity of 82.0% and specificity of 98.0% (Boehme *et al.*, 2010; Scott *et al.*, 2011; Chang *et al.*, 2012), outperforming other molecular tests in smear-negative patients (Scott *et al.*, 2011). There is potential for the Xpert MTB/RIF assay to be of great clinical value for tuberculosis screening in HIV treatment programmes (Lawn *et al.*, 2011). Tuberculosis is the one of the main causes of death early in antiretroviral treatment (ART), and pre-screening using the Xpert MTB/RIF assay prior to starting ART increased case detection by 45% compared to microscopy (Lawn *et al.*, 2011). The Xpert MTB/RIF assay has also been evaluated for use in paediatric tuberculosis, with promising results (Nicol *et al.*, 2011).

In December 2010, the WHO endorsed the use of Xpert MTB/RIF as the initial diagnostic test for individuals suspected of having MDR-TB or HIV-associated tuberculosis, and as a follow-on to microscopy in settings where MDR-TB and HIV are of lesser concern (WHO, 2010b), with the expectation for an initial phased implementation from 2011 onwards and a more rapid scale-up thereafter (WHO, 2010a; Lawn and Nicol, 2011).

Although the initial evaluation studies showed high specificity for RIF resistance, several subsequent studies have confirmed false positive RIF-resistance results, particularly in low-prevalence settings (Lawn *et al.*, 2011; Marlowe *et al.*, 2011; Van Rie *et al.*, 2012). Absolute numbers of these cases are small, but this has important implications if resistance data are to be used for treatment decisions. As such, the WHO recommends that RIF resistance detected by Xpert should be confirmed by culture-based methods (WHO, 2011c). This negates somewhat the use of the Xpert MTB/RIF assay for rapid resistance testing if additional facilities with the capacity for phenotypic drug sensitivity testing are required to validate the results. In response to this problem, Cepheid has made some minor changes to the Xpert MTB/RIF assay, including modifying one of the probes (FIND, 2011). The new G4 software and cartridge combination was released outside the USA in December 2011, and clinical data are required to determine if these modifications will result in more accurate RIF resistance detection.

Overall, the Xpert MTB system has been shown to provide excellent performance in a number of different patient groups, geo-graphical settings and health-care facilities, and is a major advance in tuberculosis diagnostic assay development. As for most molecular tests, the major drawback to implementing this technology in low- and middle-income countries is the high costs. FIND have negotiated substantial cost reductions, with the price of the instrument set at US$17,000 for a four-module instrument and a current cost per test of US$18, although this is expected to drop to US$10.70 following the WHO endorsement and increased sales (Lawn and Nicol, 2011; O'Grady *et al.*, 2011). The current costs are similar to those for culture identification and drug sensitivity testing, especially factoring in biosafety equipment costs, but higher than other molecular tests (Lawn and Nicol, 2011; Parsons *et al.*, 2011). There are also practical limitations associated with the use of specialized equipment and, together with the current need to confirm drug resistance by culture-based methods, this suggests the Xpert MTB/RIF assay has good potential for use in moderately equipped laboratories, but not in most peripheral settings where infrastructure and resources are limited (Van Rie *et al.*, 2010; Lawn and Nicol, 2011; O'Grady *et al.*, 2011). While there is no doubt this is currently the best available molecular diagnostic test for tuberculosis, it remains open for discussion if the high costs and logistical considerations required for an international roll-out programme would be better placed waiting for a real POC solution. Further studies into cost-effectiveness, impact on treatment and programme outcomes and tuberculosis transmission are needed to help answer these questions.

2.2.3 Array-based commercial tests for the detection of MTB and drug resistance

The recently developed QIAPlex test (Qiagen, Valencia, California, USA) uses a target-enriched multiplex PCR to amplify 24 mutations simultaneously in the *katG*, *inhA*, *rpoB*, *rrs*, *rpsL* and *embB* genes associated with resistance to INH, RIF, streptomycin (SM) and EMB (Gegia *et al.*, 2008; Parsons *et al.*, 2011). The PCR products are characterized using a suspension array for multiplex detection on the Luminex 100 instrument (Luminex, Austin, Texas, USA). One study in the Republic of Georgia showed good performance for INH and RIF detection, with sensitivity and specificity of 85.4% and 96.1%, 94.4% and 99.4%, respectively, and 86.7% and 100% for MDR-TB (Gegia *et al.*, 2008). Sensitivity and specificity was 69.6% and 99.2% for SM and 50% and 98.8% for EMB, reflecting the poor understanding of the molecular mechanisms of resistance to these drugs (Gegia *et al.*, 2008).

Two solid microarray detection systems, TruArray MDR-TB (Akonni Biosystems) and INFINTI MDR-TB (Autogenomics), are also available for MDR-TB detection (Akonni Biosystems, 2012; AutoGenomics, 2012). Both systems use multiplex PCR followed by detection on a microarray. The TruArray system uses gel element microfluidics array technology (Gryadunov *et al.*, 2011; Cooney *et al.*, 2012) to detect the most common mutations in the *rpoB*, *inhA* and *katG* genes and distinguish between MTC and *M. avium* by the detection of insertion sequences IS*6110* and IS*1245* (Akonni Biosystems, 2012). The INFINITI MDR-TB assay uses a novel film-based microarray (BioFilmChip) to evaluate INH, RIF and PZA resistance by the detection of 16 mutations in *rpoB*, *katG*, *inhA* and *pncA* genes, and can also identify *M. bovis* specifically (AutoGenomics, 2012). This test can be used directly from decontaminated sediment without the need for DNA extraction and can deliver results within 5 h. At present, both of these commercial tests are for experimental use only and published performance data are not yet available. However, the proprietary technology, TB-Biochip (used in the TruArray kits), is certified for diagnosis in the Russian Federation and has been evaluated in more than 20,000 clinical specimens. These studies have reported sensitivities between 89.5% and 96.9% for RIF resistance and between 82.1% and 89.3% for INH resistance, and specificities of 86.2–94.3% for RIF resistance and 80–95.1% for INH resistance (Gryadunov *et al.*, 2011). A similar microarray targeting mutations that determine fluoroquinolone resistance in the *gyrA* gene (TB-Biochip-2) is also available and

has reported sensitivity and specificity of 93% and 99%, respectively (Antonova *et al.*, 2008; Gryadunov *et al.*, 2011).

2.2.4 NAATs for differentiation of the MTC

Accurate differentiation of members of the MTC is necessary to perform epidemiological studies, to monitor whether tuberculosis transmission is human-to-human or zoonotic and to administer appropriate anti-*M. tuberculosis* drug treatment, as some members of the complex display inherent resistance to PZA (Reddington *et al.*, 2012). Differentiation of members of the MTC is difficult to achieve, as these species are 99% similar on a nucleotide sequence level (Brosch *et al.*, 2002; Mostowy *et al.*, 2002). Currently, there is only one commercially available diagnostic assay for differentiation of the MTC, namely the Genotype MTBC kit (Hain Lifesciences), which is an LPA (discussed in a separate section). There are also a number of in-house NAATs for MTC differentiation described in the literature (Parsons *et al.*, 2002; Huard *et al.*, 2003; Djelouadji *et al.*, 2008; Pinsky and Banaei, 2008; Halse *et al.*, 2011). The majority of these methods use regions of difference (RDs) as species-specific diagnostic targets. In mycobacteria, RDs represent regions of the genome present in *M. tuberculosis*, which are subsequently deleted in other members of the MTC (Brosch *et al.*, 1998; Behr *et al.*, 1999; Gordon *et al.*, 1999).

One of the first conventional PCR methods described for the accurate differentiation of the MTC was proposed by Parsons *et al.* (2002). In this study, six RDs (RD 1, 9, 10, 3, 5 and 11) were used to identify *M. tuberculosis*, *M. africanum*, *M. bovis*, *M. bovis* BCG and *M. microti* accurately (Parsons *et al.*, 2002). The method was tested on 88 well-characterized MTC strains and specificity was determined to be 100%, but the sensitivity of the method was not reported. Subsequently, 605 MTC clinical isolates were evaluated to demonstrate further the robustness of the method. However, since the addition of *M. caprae*, *M. canettii* and *M. pinnipedii* to the MTC, the species-specific diagnostic profile obtained using these six RDs is no longer valid.

In a study by Huard *et al.* (2003), a PCR-based method was developed using RDs to identify all members of the MTC accurately, with the exception of *M. pinnipedii*. In this study, seven genetic loci were used; a mycobacterial amplification control (16S rRNA), an MTC-specific target (Rv0577) and species-specific diagnostic targets (IS*1561*, Rv1510, Rv1970, Rv3877/8 and Rv3120) (Huard *et al.*, 2003). For each MTC member, seven individual amplification reactions were performed in parallel and the PCR products were visualized on an agarose gel. Depending on the profile observed, each individual species of the MTC could be identified accurately. A total of 71 MTC strains and 44 non-tuberculous mycobacteria (NTM) were evaluated and the specificity of the method was determined to be 100%, but the sensitivity of the method was not reported. However, in 2003, *M. pinnipedii* was elevated to rank species and added to the MTC (Cousins *et al.*, 2003). As it was not tested with this method, it was unknown if *M. pinnipedii* would give the same diagnostic profile as other MTC members. A limitation of this method is that it has not been evaluated directly on clinical samples.

Another conventional PCR approach for the differentiation of the MTC was proposed by Warren *et al.* in 2006. Two multiplex PCRs are performed sequentially to identify all eight members of the MTC accurately (Warren *et al.*, 2006). The first multiplex PCR targets areas of RDs 1, 4, 9 and 12 to identify *M. tuberculosis*, *M. canettii*, *M. bovis*, *M. caprae* and *M. bovis* BCG specifically, based on the amplification patterns observed when visualized on an agarose gel (Warren *et al.*, 2006). To differentiate between the remaining MTC members, namely *M. africanum*, *M. microti* and *M. pinnipedii*, RD1[mic] and RD2[seal] are targeted (Warren *et al.*, 2006). This method is highly specific (100%) and, as the reactions are multiplexed, less hands-on time and consumables are required; however, the sensitivity of the method has not been reported. This method was not evaluated directly on clinical samples, nor was an internal amplification control (IAC) incorporated.

More recently, multiplex real-time PCR assays have been developed for the differentiation of the MTC. One of the first such assays was described by Pinsky and Banaei in 2008. In this study, a two-stage multiplex real-time PCR method using melt curve analysis targeting RDs 9, 4 and 1 was developed. Based on the presence or absence of a melt peak at a certain temperature, *M. tuberculosis*, *M. bovis* and *M. bovis* BCG can be identified (Pinsky and Banaei, 2008). The test was optimized using 4 MTC and 10 NTM strains and tested subsequently with 80 MTC-positive clinical isolates. This method is rapid, specific (100%) and simple to perform; however, there are also a number of limitations. For example, if a sample is positive for RD9, it is assumed *M. tuberculosis* is present; however, this RD is also present in *M. canettii* (Brosch *et al.*, 2002). This method cannot identify *M. africanum*, *M. caprae*, *M. microti* or *M. pinnipedii* accurately and patient samples have not been tested directly.

Another multiplex real-time PCR method using melt curve analysis for accurate differentiation of the MTC was described recently by Pounder *et al.* (2010). In this assay, RDs 1, 4, 9, 10 and 12 are amplified and, based on the melting temperature (Tm) of the amplicon generated, the particular member of the MTC can be identified (Pounder *et al.*, 2010). This assay was validated against a panel of 129 MTC strains and 11 NTM and was highly specific for each MTC member (96%), rapid and simple to perform (Pounder *et al.*, 2010). However, as with previous studies described above, the sensitivity of the method was not reported. *M. canettii* and *M. pinnipedii* were not tested in this study and this method cannot differentiate unambiguously between *M. africanum* and *M. microti*. Again, as with the previous study, only cultured isolates were tested.

In a study by Halse *et al.*, a hydrolysis probe-based real-time PCR methodology (MTBC-RD real-time PCR) was developed for accurate differentiation between members of the MTC, both from cultured isolates and clinical specimens (Halse *et al.*, 2011). This multiplex assay targets RDs 1, 4, 9 and 12 and the external junction of RD9. This is among the most thoroughly evaluated methods described in the literature for differentiation of the MTC. The specificity of the method was tested against a panel of 727 positive mycobacterial growth indicator tubes (MGIT) and an additional 129 clinical specimens and found to be 100%. The analytical sensitivity of MTBC-RD real-time PCR was determined using DNA isolated from an *M. tuberculosis* strain known to contain one copy of IS*6110* and was determined to be 2.5 colony-forming units (CFU) in cultured isolates, and the limit of detection was 5 CFU in sputum specimens (Halse *et al.*, 2011). As culturing of specimens is not required, this method does allow for detection of the MTC and identification of the particular species in 1 working day. However, again, there were some limitations with this method; for example, *M. caprae* and *M. pinnipedii* were not evaluated in this study, therefore it was not known what RD PCR profile would be observed for these MTC members. Furthermore, there is no IAC included in this method. Incorporation of an IAC or, preferably, a process control is crucial when developing molecular-based diagnostics, particularly when working with clinical samples (Hoorfar *et al.*, 2003, 2004), to eliminate the reporting of false negatives due to PCR inhibition, thermocycler malfunction, reagent problems or errors in preparing mixes (Hoorfar *et al.*, 2004).

In a recent study by Reddington *et al.*, a two-stage internally controlled multiplex real-time PCR-based method, *Seek*TB, was described for the accurate detection and identification of all members of the MTC. Depending on which MTC species is present, the method takes between 1.5 and 3.5 h post-DNA extraction (Reddington *et al.*, 2012). The specificity of the method was determined to be 100% when evaluated against a panel of 180 well-characterized MTC, NTM and other bacteria strains and species. The method developed was also tested on 125 MGIT positive cultures and the results were compared to the Genotype MTBC kit (Hain Lifesciences) and were 100% concordant. The analytical sensitivity was <100 genome equivalents for each diagnostic assay (Reddington *et al.*, 2012). While *Seek*TB offers advantages over other methods described in the literature for the differentiation of the

MTC, a significant limitation is that it has not yet been evaluated directly on clinical samples.

2.3 Line Probe Assays

2.3.1 Line probe assays for the detection of the MTC and drug resistance

There are currently four commercially available LPAs for the detection of tuberculosis and drug-resistant *M. tuberculosis* (Table 2.2). Firstly, there is the GenoType Mycobacteria Direct assay (Hain Lifesciences), which detects the MTC and four common NTM directly from decontaminated pulmonary and extrapulmonary patient samples (Franco-Álvarez de Luna *et al.*, 2006). This test is broken into three phases, namely isolation of RNA using a magnetic bead capture method, nucleic acid sequence-based amplification (NASBA) and reverse hybridization of amplified products to a strip containing target-specific oligonucleotide probes (Syre *et al.*, 2009). This test procedure can be performed in approximately 5.5 h and has reported specificities and sensitivities of 90–100% and 92–93.7%, respectively, in smear-positive and smear-negative samples (Franco-Álvarez de Luna *et al.*, 2006; Neonakis *et al.*, 2009; Syre *et al.*, 2009).

The INNO-LiPA Rif. TB kit (Innogenetics) is a test for the detection of the MTC and determination of resistance to RIF and can be used on culture isolates or directly on patient samples (Rossau *et al.*, 1997). As over 90% of RIF-resistant isolates are also resistant to INH, this test can be useful in identifying potential cases of MDR-TB. Using this assay, the RIF-resistance determining region of the *rpoB* gene is amplified using conventional PCR. Subsequently, the amplified product is hybridized to a nitrocellulose strip containing ten specific probes. These probes include one MTC-specific probe, five wild-type sensitive probes and four probes for specific mutations in resistant strains (Rossau *et al.*, 1997). On completion of the hybridization, a colorimetric signal is observed on the strip and, based on the profile observed, it can be determined if an isolate is RIF resistant or

Table 2.2. Commercially available hybridization and line probe assays.

Molecular test	Manufacturer	Technology	Target sequence	IAC	Detects
GenoType Mycobacteria Direct	Hain Lifescience	NASBA + reverse hybridization	23S rRNA	Yes	MTC, *M. avium*, *M. intracellulare*, *M. kansasii*, *M. malmoense*
INNO-LiPA Rif. TB kit	Innogenetics	PCR + reverse hybridization	*rpoB*	No	MTC and resistance to RIF
GenoType MTBDR*plus*	Hain Lifescience	Multiplex PCR + reverse hybridization	*rpoB*, *inhA*, *katG*	Yes	MTC and resistance to RIF and INH
GenoType MTBDR*sl*	Hain Lifescience	Multiplex PCR + reverse hybridization	*gyrA*, *rrs*, *embB*	Yes	MTC and resistance to fluoroquinolones and aminoglycosides
GenoType MTBC	Hain Lifescience	Multiplex PCR + reverse hybridization	*gyrB*, RD1, 23S rRNA	Yes	MTC and some species
Accuprobe *Mycobacterium tuberculosis* complex culture identification test	Gen-probe	Hybridization	16S rRNA	No	MTC

sensitive. In a recent meta-analysis, it was determined that the specificity and sensitivity ranges of this test were 92–100% and 82–100%, respectively, when used on cultured isolates (Morgan *et al.*, 2005). The sensitivity may reduce to 80% when used directly on clinical samples (Morgan *et al.*, 2005).

The GenoType MTBDR*plus* test is also designed for the detection of the MTC and identification of MDR-TB. This second-generation test, which was endorsed for use by the WHO in 2008, allows for the identification of both RIF and INH resistance (WHO, 2008). This test can be used on bacterial cultures or smear-positive patient samples and takes approximately 5 h to perform (Neonakis *et al.*, 2009). The test procedure includes DNA extraction and conventional multiplex PCR, followed by reverse line hybridization (Hillemann *et al.*, 2007). It has been reported recently that the GenoType MTBDR*plus* test has a specificity of 96.8–99.7% and 95.4–99.8% and a sensitivity of 95.1–99.5% and 82.4–92.8% for the determination of RIF and INH resistance, respectively (Ling *et al.*, 2008b).

The GenoType MTBDR*sl* assay (Hain Lifesciences) was developed for the detection of the MTC and simultaneous detection of the most commonly reported resistances to fluoroquinolones, EMB and second-line aminoglycosides and cyclic peptide (Hillemann *et al.*, 2009). If a patient is reported to have MDR-TB, the GenoType MTBDR*sl* assay can be used to identify cases of extremely drug-resistant tuberculosis (XDR-TB) (Hillemann *et al.*, 2009; Brossier *et al.*, 2010). The test procedure is the same as the GenoType MTBDR*plus* and can be used on culture or sputum smear-positive samples. In recent evaluation studies, fluoroquinolone resistance detection was demonstrated to have a sensitivity of 87–90.2% and a specificity of 96–100%, EMB resistance detection was demonstrated to have a sensitivity of 57–77.3% and a specificity of 88.2–100% and for detection of resistance to the second-line injectable agents, a sensitivity of 42.7–100% and a specificity of 91–100% was reported (Hillemann *et al.*, 2009; Brossier *et al.*, 2010; Ignatyeva *et al.*, 2012).

2.3.2 Line probe assays for the differentiation of the MTC

The Genotype MTBC test (Hain Lifesciences) is currently the only commercially available molecular test for differentiation of the members of the MTC. Like the other two Hain kits, this test is based on the principle of DNA extraction and multiplex conventional PCR, followed by reverse-line hybridization (Richter *et al.*, 2004). This test procedure can be performed in approximately 5.5 h and can be used on culture or sputum smear-positive samples (Somoskovi *et al.*, 2008). This assay contains probes for a genus control, a conjugate control, the collective detection of the MTC and specific probes for *M. tuberculosis*, *M. africanum*, *M. bovis*, *M. caprae*, *M. bovis* BCG and *M. microti* (Richter *et al.*, 2004). However, it has been demonstrated that the *M. tuberculosis* probe can cross react with *M. canettii* and the *M. africanum* probe cross reacts with *M. pinnipedii* (Richter *et al.*, 2004; Kjeldsen *et al.*, 2009).

2.3.3 Direct hybridization assays for the detection of the MTC

An additional hybridization-based assay is the Accuprobe *Mycobacterium tuberculosis* complex culture identification test (Genprobe), which detects the presence of the MTC (Goto *et al.*, 1991). Unlike all other methods discussed above, there is no amplification step required in this procedure. This test takes approximately 1.5 h to perform and involves RNA extraction, hybridization and detection of 16S rRNA (Goto *et al.*, 1991). While the specificity of this method is almost 100% (Evans *et al.*, 1992), a significant limitation is that it is only suitable for use with positive cultures (Parsons *et al.*, 2011).

2.4 Sequencing-based Diagnostic Methods

DNA sequencing assays, which target variable genomic regions to identify species-specific sequence motifs, are rapid and accurate identification methods for myco-

bacteria; however, such methods are not yet practical for routine use in most resource-poor countries (Parsons *et al.*, 2011). Sequencing assays can be used for the identification of the MTC and NTMs (Kasai *et al.*, 2000; Cristea-Fernstrom *et al.*, 2007), molecular DST of first- and second-line anti-*M. tuberculosis* drugs (Isola *et al.*, 2005; Kontsevaya *et al.*, 2011) and MTC differentiation (Kahla *et al.*, 2011). One or more genes are targeted, depending on the required application.

Sequencing assays can be broken down into two types, namely conventional sequencing and pyrosequencing-based methods. Conventional sequencing methods are typically used on growth-positive cultures as culture confirmation tools. Pyrosequencing, a technique based on the real-time sequencing of short sequences during DNA synthesis (sequencing by synthesis), has been described as a promising new tool for the rapid identification of mycobacteria, not only in culture but also in smear-positive sputum specimens (Parsons *et al.*, 2011). Although this method is faster, simpler and less expensive than conventional sequencing, it produces sequence reads <100 bp, which have less discriminatory power than the 500-bp reads obtained using conventional sequencing. One of the most promising applications of sequencing assays in tuberculosis diagnosis is the use of pyrosequencing assays for molecular DST (Isola *et al.*, 2005; Kontsevaya *et al.*, 2011). Several target regions can be tested and all mutations in the target regions can be detected, including mutations not previously characterized. However, a better understanding of the molecular resistance mechanisms of some first- and second-line anti-*M. tuberculosis* drugs is required in order to identify the appropriate molecular targets and achieve high accuracy compared to phenotypic DST.

2.5 Next-generation Technologies for Tuberculosis Diagnosis

The potential of POC diagnostic technology to benefit health care is widely recognized (Mauk *et al.*, 2011). POC devices facilitate individualized medicine and more immediate diagnostic tools at doctors' offices, clinics and hospital bedsides. Perhaps the greatest impact of POC tests will be in developing nations by bringing affordable diagnostic tools to resource-poor settings for diseases such as tuberculosis and pneumonia (Mauk *et al.*, 2011). In recent years, the need for a POC tuberculosis test has been increasingly recognized and some support for research and development has become available, mainly through philanthropic organizations such as the Bill and Melinda Gates Foundation (Batz *et al.*, 2011). However, despite the effort and resources invested, POC diagnosis for tuberculosis has not yet materialized. The ideal POC tuberculosis test and its characteristics have recently been defined by Médecins Sans Frontières (MSF) and partner organizations (Table 2.3; Batz *et al.*, 2011). The Xpert MTB/RIF assay is currently the only tuberculosis diagnostic test that matches a significant number of these criteria, even though it is recognized as not being a true POC test.

Over the past two decades, many microfluidic lab-on-a-chip POC PCR-based devices have been described, some with performance characteristics better than existing PCR assays (Craw and Balachandran, 2012). However, the precise and repeated heating cycles required for PCR necessitate complex, power-consuming designs and require additional engineering considerations, such as the thermal constants of the materials used and unwanted evaporation of water. These characteristics ultimately render PCR inappropriate for lab-on-a-chip diagnostic devices (Craw and Balachandran, 2012). In order to avoid such difficulties, recent diagnostic POC test research has focused on isothermal methods for nucleic acid amplification such as LAMP, NASBA and TMA. Isothermal methods use enzymes

Table 2.3. Characteristics for a good POC tuberculosis test.

POC test characteristic	Minimum required value
Sensitivity (in adult pulmonary tuberculosis)	95% for smear-positive, culture-positive patients
	60–80% for smear-negative, culture-positive patients
Specificity	95% compared to culture
Time to result	3 h
Throughput	20 tests/staff member/day
Specimen type	Urine, oral, breath, venous blood, sputum
Sample preparation	Three steps maximum
	Biosafety level 1
	No need for pipetting
	No time-sensitive processes
Readout	Easy 'yes' and 'no' answers
	Readable for 1 h
Waste disposal	Simple burning, no glass
Controls	Positive control in test kit
Storage/shelf life	Shelf life 24 months, including reagents
	Stable at 30°C and higher for short periods of time
	Stable in high humidity
Instrumentation	If instrument, no maintenance
	Works in tropical conditions
	Acceptable replacement costs
	Fits in backpack
	Shock resistant
Power requirement	Can work on battery
Training	1 day maximum
	Can be used by any health-care worker
Costs	<US$10/test

instead of heat to perform strand separation. These techniques offer a better solution than PCR for nucleic acid amplification on POC diagnostic platforms (Craw and Balachandran, 2012). While biosensors for direct detection of nucleic acids without amplification have been described in the literature, an integrated system with clinically relevant specificity and sensitivity direct from complex samples has yet to reach the market. Therefore, it is likely that some form of target and/or signal amplification must be performed, given existing detection technology (Craw and Balachandran, 2012). Hence, the future for the molecular diagnosis of tuberculosis is likely to be a POC sample-in, answer-out diagnostic platform that combines isothermal nucleic acid amplification and inexpensive lab-on-a-chip nanobiosensor technology.

A recently published example of such a biosensor uses thermophilic helicase-dependent isothermal amplification and dextrin-coated gold nanoparticles for the electrochemical detection of the IS*6110* gene of *M. tuberculosis* (Torres-Chavolla and Alocilja, 2011). Gold nanoparticles and magnetic particles are each functionalized with probes specific to opposite ends of a fragment (105 bp) of the IS*6110* gene, specific to the MTC. After hybridization, the gold–DNA–MP complex is separated magnetically from the solution and gold nanoparticles are detected electrochemically. The limit of detection of this method is 0.01 ng/μl of isothermally amplified target. This biosensor system potentially can be implemented at POC in peripheral laboratories with the use of a portable, hand-held potentiostat (Torres-Chavolla and Alocilja, 2011).

2.6 Advantages and Disadvantages of Molecular Diagnosis for Tuberculosis

The major advantage of the molecular diagnosis of tuberculosis and molecular DST is the turnaround time to results compared to culture. The major disadvantage is the reduced accuracy of molecular methods compared to culture, particularly in smear-negative tuberculosis and in molecular DST of many first- and second-line anti-*M.*

tuberculosis drugs. The recent development of sample-in, answer-out molecular diagnostic technology for tuberculosis has negated some of the problems associated previously with molecular methods, such as crossover contamination, high method complexity, the necessity for skilled labour and the requirement for dedicated molecular biology facilities. The majority of commercially available molecular methods, however, are not sample-in, answer-out based and continue to suffer such problems. Molecular methods are still relatively expensive compared to traditional methods and often require expensive instrumentation, which must be maintained and which requires a relatively high test volume to be cost-effective (Parrish and Carroll, 2011).

2.7 Conclusions

The tuberculosis diagnostics pipeline has grown rapidly in recent years with the development of several promising molecular diagnostic technologies. A simple, rapid, inexpensive POC test, however, is still not on the horizon (Wallis *et al.*, 2010). The next generation of nanobiosensor-based tuberculosis diagnostic tests, designed for POC use, are likely to be still >5 years from commercialization, but have the potential to revolutionize the diagnosis of tuberculosis. Accurate, rapid tests are also required for childhood tuberculosis and latent tuberculosis, and diagnostic assays must be developed that can be applied not only to sputum but also to multiple sample types.

References

Akonni Biosystems (2012) TruArray® MDRTB. Rapid, accurate identification of rifampin/isoniazid susceptibility (http://www.akonni.com/docs/Akonni_TruArray_MDR-TB_Datasheet.pdf, accessed 30 April 2012).

Allix-Béguec, C., Fauville-Dufaux, M., Stoffels, K., Ommeslag, D., Walravens, K., Saegerman, C., *et al.* (2010) Importance of identifying *Mycobacterium bovis* as a causative agent of human tuberculosis. *European Respiratory Journal* 35, 692–694.

Andersen, A.B., Thybo, S., Godfrey-Faussett, P. and Stoker, N.G. (1993) Polymerase chain reaction for detection of *Mycobacterium tuberculosis* in sputum. *European Journal of Clinical Microbiology and Infectious Diseases* 12, 922–927.

Antonova, O.V., Gryadunov, D.A., Lapa, S.A., Kuz'min, A.V., Larionova, E.E., Smirnova, T.G., *et al.* (2008) Detection of mutations in *Mycobacterium tuberculosis* genome determining resistance to fluoroquinolones by hybridization on biological microchips. *Bulletin of Experimental Biology and Medicine* 145, 108–113.

Armand, S., Vanhuls, P., Delcroix, G., Courcol, R. and Lemaitre, N. (2011) Comparison of the Xpert MTB/RIF test with an IS6110-TaqMan real-time PCR assay for direct detection of *Mycobacterium tuberculosis* in respiratory and non-respiratory specimens. *Journal of Clinical Microbiology* 49, 1772–1776.

AutoGenomics (2012) INFINITI MDR-TB (http://www.autogenomics.com/infectious_MTB.php, accessed 30 April 2012).

Banada, P.P., Sivasubramani, S.K., Blakemore, R., Boehme, C., Perkins, M.D., Fennelly, K., *et al.* (2010) Containment of bioaerosol infection risk by the Xpert MTB/RIF assay and its applicability to point-of-care settings. *Journal of Clinical Microbiology* 48, 3551–3557.

Batz, H., Cooke, G. and Reid, S. (2011) *Towards Lab-free Tuberculosis Diagnosis*. Treatment Action Group, Stop TB Partnership, Imperial College London and Médecins Sans Frontières, New York.

Behr, M.A., Wilson, M.A., Gill, W.P., Salamon, H., Schoolnik, G.K., Rane, S., *et al.* (1999) Comparative genomics of BCG vaccines by whole-genome DNA microarray. *Science* 284, 1520–1523.

Beige, J., Lokies, J., Schaberg, T., Finckh, U., Fischer, M., Mauch, H., *et al.* (1995) Clinical evaluation of a *Mycobacterium tuberculosis* PCR assay. *Journal of Clinical Microbiology* 33, 90–95.

Blakemore, R., Story, E., Helb, D., Kop, J., Banada, P., Owens, M.R., *et al.* (2010) Evaluation of the analytical performance of the Xpert(R) MTB/RIF assay. *Journal of Clinical Microbiology* 48, 2495–2501.

Boehme, C.C., Nabeta, P., Henostroza, G., Raqib, R., Rahim, Z., Gerhardt, M., *et al.* (2007) Operational feasibility of using loop-mediated isothermal amplification for diagnosis of pulmonary tuberculosis in microscopy centers of developing countries. *Journal of Clinical Microbiology* 45, 1936–1940.

Boehme, C.C., Nabeta, P., Hillemann, D., Nicol, M.P., Shenai, S., Krapp, F., *et al.* (2010) Rapid molecular detection of tuberculosis and rifampin resistance. *The New England Journal of Medicine* 363, 1005–1015.

Boehme, C.C., Nicol, M.P., Nabeta, P., Michael, J.S., Gotuzzo, E., Tahirli, R., *et al.* (2011) Feasibility, diagnostic accuracy, and effectiveness of decentralised use of the Xpert MTB/RIF test for diagnosis of tuberculosis and multidrug resistance: a multicentre implementation study. *The Lancet* 377, 1495–1505.

Brosch, R., Gordon, S.V., Billault, A., Garnier, T., Eiglmeier, K., Soravito, C., *et al.* (1998) Use of a *Mycobacterium tuberculosis* H37Rv bacterial artificial chromosome library for genome mapping, sequencing, and comparative genomics. *Infection and Immunity* 66, 2221–2229.

Brosch, R., Gordon, S., Marmiesse, M., Brodin, P., Buchrieser, C., Eiglmeier, K., *et al.* (2002) A new evolutionary scenario for the *Mycobacterium tuberculosis* complex. *Proceedings of the National Academy of Sciences* 99, 3684–3689.

Brossier, F., Veziris, N., Aubry, A., Jarlier, V. and Sougakoff, W. (2010) Detection by GenoType MTBDRsl test of complex mechanisms of resistance to second-line drugs and ethambutol in multidrug-resistant *Mycobacterium tuberculosis* complex isolates. *Journal of Clinical Microbiology* 48, 1683–1689.

Chakravorty, S., Aladegbami, B., Thoms, K., Lee, J.S., Lee, E.G., Rajan, V., *et al.* (2011) Rapid detection of fluoroquinolone-resistant and heteroresistant *Mycobacterium tuberculosis* by use of sloppy molecular beacons and dual melting-temperature codes in a real-time PCR assay. *Journal of Clinical Microbiology* 49, 932–940.

Chang, K., Lu, W., Wang, J., Zhang, K., Jia, S., Li, F., *et al.* (2012) Rapid and effective diagnosis of tuberculosis and rifampicin resistance with Xpert MTB/RIF assay: a meta-analysis. *Journal of Infection* 64(6), 580–588.

Cooney, C.G., Sipes, D., Thakore, N., Holmberg, R. and Belgrader, P. (2012) A plastic, disposable microfluidic flow cell for coupled on-chip PCR and microarray detection of infectious agents. *Biomedical Microdevices* 14, 45–53.

Cousins, D.V., Bastida, R., Cataldi, A., Quse, V., Redrobe, S., Dow, S., *et al.* (2003) Tuberculosis in seals caused by a novel member of the *Mycobacterium tuberculosis* complex: *Mycobacterium pinnipedii* sp. nov. *International Journal of Systemic Evolutionary Microbiology* 53, 1305–1314.

Craw, P. and Balachandran, W. (2012) Isothermal Nucleic Acid Amplification Technologies for

Point-of-Care Diagnostics: A Critical Review. *Lab on a Chip* 12(14), 2469–2486.

Cristea-Fernstrom, M., Olofsson, M., Chryssanthou, E., Jonasson, J. and Petrini, B. (2007) Pyro-sequencing of a short hypervariable 16S rDNA fragment for the identification of non-tuberculous mycobacteria – a comparison with conventional 16S rDNA sequencing and phenotyping. *APMIS* 115, 1252–1259.

Cui, Z., Wang, Y., Fang, L., Zheng, R., Huang, X., Liu, X., *et al.* (2012) Novel real-time simultaneous amplification and testing method to accurately and rapidly detect *Mycobacterium tuberculosis* complex. *Journal of Clinical Microbiology* 50, 646–650.

Davis, J.L., Huang, L., Worodria, W., Masur, H., Cattamanchi, A., Huber, C., *et al.* (2011) Nucleic acid amplification tests for diagnosis of smear-negative TB in a high HIV-prevalence setting: a prospective cohort study. *PLoS One* 6, e16321.

de la Rua-Domenech, R. (2006) Human *Mycobacterium bovis* infection in the United Kingdom: incidence, risks, control measures and review of the zoonotic aspects of bovine tuberculosis. *Tuberculosis* 86, 77–109.

De Wit, D., Steyn, L., Shoemaker, S. and Sogin, M. (1990) Direct detection of *Mycobacterium tuberculosis* in clinical specimens by DNA amplification. *Journal of Clinical Microbiology* 28, 2437–2441.

Del Portillo, P., Thomas, M.C., Martinez, E., Maranon, C., Valladares, B., Patarroyo, M.E., *et al.* (1996) Multiprimer PCR system for differential identification of mycobacteria in clinical samples. *Journal of Clinical Microbiology* 34, 324–328.

Djelouadji, Z., Raoult, D., Daffé, M. and Drancourt, M. (2008) A single-step sequencing method for the identification of *Mycobacterium tuberculosis* complex species. *PLoS Neglected Tropical Disease* 2, e253.

Eiken Chemical Co Ltd (year?) Eiken Genome Site. The Principle of LAMP method. Animation (http://loopamp.eiken.co.jp/e/lamp/anim.html, accessed 30 April 2012).

Evans, K.D., Nakasone, A.S., Sutherland, P.A., de la Maza, L.M. and Peterson, E.M. (1992) Identification of *Mycobacterium tuberculosis* and *Mycobacterium avium–M. intracellulare* directly from primary BACTEC cultures by using acridinium-ester-labeled DNA probes. *Journal of Clinical Microbiology* 30, 2427–2431.

Franco-Álvarez de Luna, F., Ruiz, P., Gutiérrez, J. and Casal, M. (2006) Evaluation of the GenoType mycobacteria direct assay for detection of *Mycobacterium tuberculosis* complex and four atypical mycobacterial species in clinical samples. *Journal of Clinical Microbiology* 44, 3025–3027.

FIND (2011) Performance of Xpert MTB/RIF Version G4 assay.

Flores, L.L., Pai, M., Colford, J.M. Jr and Riley, L.W. (2005) In-house nucleic acid amplification tests for the detection of *Mycobacterium tuberculosis* in sputum specimens: meta-analysis and meta-regression. *BMC Microbiology* 5, 55.

Francois, P., Tangomo, M., Hibbs, J., Bonetti, E.J., Boehme, C.C., Notomi, T., *et al.* (2011) Robustness of a loop-mediated isothermal amplification reaction for diagnostic applications. *FEMS Immunology and Medical Microbiology* 62, 41–48.

Gegia, M., Mdivani, N., Mendes, R.E., Li, H., Akhalaia, M., Han, J., *et al.* (2008) Prevalence of and molecular basis for tuberculosis drug resistance in the Republic of Georgia: validation of a QIAplex system for detection of drug resistance-related mutations. *Antimicrobial Agents and Chemotherapy* 52, 725–729.

Gordon, S.V., Brosch, R., Billault, A., Garnier, T., Eiglmeier, K. and Cole, S.T. (1999) Identification of variable regions in the genomes of tubercle bacilli using bacterial artificial chromosome arrays. *Molecular Microbiology* 32, 643–655.

Goto, M., Oka, S., Okuzumi, K., Kimura, S. and Shimada, K. (1991) Evaluation of acridinium-ester-labeled DNA probes for identification of *Mycobacterium tuberculosis* and *Mycobacterium avium–Mycobacterium intracellulare* complex in culture. *Journal of Clinical Microbiology* 29, 2473–2476.

Greco, S., Girardi, E., Navarra, A. and Saltini, C. (2006) Current evidence on diagnostic accuracy of commercially based nucleic acid amplification tests for the diagnosis of pulmonary tuberculosis. *Thorax* 61, 783–790.

Gryadunov, D., Dementieva, E., Mikhailovich, V., Nasedkina, T., Rubina, A., Savvateeva, E., *et al.* (2011) Gel-based microarrays in clinical diagnostics in Russia. *Expert Review of Molecular Diagnostics* 11, 839–853.

Halse, T.A., Escuyer, V.E. and Musser, K.A. (2011) Evaluation of a single-tube multiplex real-time PCR for differentiation of members of the *Mycobacterium tuberculosis* complex in clinical specimens. *Journal of Clinical Microbiology* 49, 2562–2567.

Helb, D., Jones, M., Story, E., Boehme, C., Wallace, E., Ho, K., *et al.* (2010) Rapid detection of *Mycobacterium tuberculosis* and rifampin resistance by use of on-demand, near-patient technology. *Journal of Clinical Microbiology* 48, 229–237.

Hillemann, D., Rüsch-Gerdes, S. and Richter, E.

(2007) Evaluation of the GenoType MTBDRplus assay for rifampin and isoniazid susceptibility testing of *Mycobacterium tuberculosis* strains and clinical specimens. *Journal of Clinical Microbiology* 45, 2635–2640.

Hillemann, D., Rüsch-Gerdes, S. and Richter, E. (2009) Feasibility of the GenoType MTBDRsl assay for fluoroquinolone, amikacin-capreomycin, and ethambutol resistance testing of *Mycobacterium tuberculosis* strains and clinical specimens. *Journal of Clinical Microbiology* 47, 1767–1772.

Hlavsa, M.C., Moonan, P.K., Cowan, L.S., Navin, T.R., Kammerer, J.S., Morlock, G.P., *et al.* (2008) Human tuberculosis due to *Mycobacterium bovis* in the United States, 1995–2005. *Clinical Infectious Diseases* 47, 168–175.

Hoorfar, J., Cook, N., Malorny, B., Wagner, M., De Medici, D., Abdulmawjood, A., *et al.* (2003) Making internal amplification control mandatory for diagnostic PCR. *Journal of Clinical Microbiology* 41, 5835.

Hoorfar, J., Malorny, B., Abdulmawjood, A., Cook, N., Wagner, M. and Fach, P. (2004) Practical considerations in design of internal amplification controls for diagnostic PCR assays. *Journal of Clinical Microbiology* 42, 1863–1868.

Huard, R., de Oliveira Lazzarini, L., Butler, W., van Soolingen, D. and Ho, J. (2003) PCR-based method to differentiate the subspecies of the *Mycobacterium tuberculosis* complex on the basis of genomic deletions. *Journal of Clinical Microbiology* 41, 1637–1650.

Ignatyeva, O., Kontsevaya, I., Kovalyov, A., Balabanova, Y., Nikolayevskyy, V., Toit, K., *et al.* (2012) Detection of resistance to second-line antituberculosis drugs by use of the Genotype MTBDRsl assay: a multicenter evaluation and feasibility study. *Journal of Clinical Microbiology* 50, 1593–1597.

Isola, D., Pardini, M., Varaine, F., Niemann, S., Rüsch-Gerdes, S., Fattorini, L., *et al.* (2005) A pyrosequencing assay for rapid recognition of SNPs in *Mycobacterium tuberculosis* embB306 region. *Journal of Microbiological Methods* 62, 113–120.

Iwamoto, T., Sonobe, T. and Hayashi, K. (2003) Loop-mediated isothermal amplification for direct detection of *Mycobacterium tuberculosis* complex, *M. avium*, and *M. intracellulare* in sputum samples. *Journal of Clinical Microbiology* 41, 2616–2622.

Kahla, I.B., Henry, M., Boukadida, J. and Drancourt, M. (2011) Pyrosequencing assay for rapid identification of *Mycobacterium tuberculosis* complex species. *BMC Research Notes* 4, 423.

Kallenius, G., Koivula, T., Ghebremichael, S.,

Hoffner, S.E., Norberg, R., Svensson, E., *et al.* (1999) Evolution and clonal traits of *Mycobacterium tuberculosis* complex in Guinea-Bissau. *Journal of Clinical Microbiology* 37, 3872–3878.

Kasai, H., Ezaki, T. and Harayama, S. (2000) Differentiation of phylogenetically related slowly growing mycobacteria by their gyrB sequences. *Journal of Clinical Microbiology* 38, 301–308.

Kim, J.H., Kim, Y.J., Ki, C.S., Kim, J.Y. and Lee, N.Y. (2011) Evaluation of Cobas TaqMan MTB PCR for detection of *Mycobacterium tuberculosis*. *Journal of Clinical Microbiology* 49, 173–176.

Kjeldsen, M.K., Bek, D., Rasmussen, E.M., Priemé, A. and Thomsen, V.Ø. (2009) Line probe assay for differentiation within *Mycobacterium tuberculosis* complex. Evaluation on clinical specimens and isolates including *Mycobacterium pinnipedii*. *Scandinavian Journal of Infectious Diseases* 41, 635–641.

Koeck, J.L., Fabre, M., Simon, F., Daffé, M., Garnotel, É., Matan, A.B., *et al.* (2010) Clinical characteristics of the smooth tubercle bacilli '*Mycobacterium canettii*' infection suggest the existence of an environmental reservoir. *Clinical Microbiology and Infection* 17, 1013–1019.

Kontsevaya, I., Mironova, S., Nikolayevskyy, V., Balabanova, Y., Mitchell, S. and Drobniewski, F. (2011) Evaluation of two molecular assays for rapid detection of *Mycobacterium tuberculosis* resistance to fluoroquinolones in high-tuberculosis and -multidrug-resistance settings. *Journal of Clinical Microbiology* 49, 2832–2837.

Lawn, S.D. and Nicol, M.P. (2011) Xpert(R) MTB/RIF assay: development, evaluation and implementation of a new rapid molecular diagnostic for tuberculosis and rifampicin resistance. *Future Microbiology* 6, 1067–1082.

Lawn, S.D., Brooks, S.V., Kranzer, K., Nicol, M.P., Whitelaw, A., Vogt, M., *et al.* (2011) Screening for HIV-associated tuberculosis and rifampicin resistance before antiretroviral therapy using the Xpert MTB/RIF assay: a prospective study. *PLoS Medicine* 8, e1001067.

Lin, S.Y., Probert, W., Lo, M. and Desmond, E. (2004) Rapid detection of isoniazid and rifampin resistance mutations in *Mycobacterium tuberculosis* complex from cultures or smear-positive sputa by use of molecular beacons. *Journal of Clinical Microbiology* 42, 4204–4208.

Ling, D.I., Flores, L.L., Riley, L.W. and Pai, M. (2008a) Commercial nucleic-acid amplification tests for diagnosis of pulmonary tuberculosis in respiratory specimens: meta-analysis and meta-regression. *PLoS One* 3, e1536.

Ling, D.I., Zwerling, A.A. and Pai, M. (2008b) GenoType MTBDR assays for the diagnosis of multidrug-resistant tuberculosis: a meta-analysis. *European Respiratory Journal* 32, 1165–1174.

Luo, T., Jiang, L., Sun, W., Fu, G., Mei, J. and Gao, Q. (2011) Multiplex real-time PCR melting curve assay to detect drug-resistant mutations of *Mycobacterium tuberculosis*. *Journal of Clinical Microbiology* 49, 3132–3138.

Marlowe, E.M., Novak-Weekley, S.M., Cumpio, J., Sharp, S.E., Momeny, M.A., Babst, A., *et al.* (2011) Evaluation of the Cepheid Xpert MTB/RIF assay for direct detection of *Mycobacterium tuberculosis* complex in respiratory specimens. *Journal of Clinical Microbiology* 49, 1621–1623.

Mauk, M.G., Liu, C.-C., Corstjens, P.L.A.M. and Bau, H.H. (2011) Streamlining POC microfluidic molecular diagnostics. *IVD Technology* (http://www.ivdtechnology.com/article/streamlining-poc-microfluidic-molecular-diagnostics, accessed 30 April 2012).

Migliori, G.B., Dheda, K., Centis, R., Mwaba, P., Bates, M., O'Grady, J., *et al.* (2010) Review of multidrug-resistant and extensively drug-resistant TB: global perspectives with a focus on sub-Saharan Africa. *Tropical Medicine and International Health* 15(9), 1052–1066.

Mitarai, S., Okumura, M., Toyota, E., Yoshiyama, T., Aono, A., Sejimo, A., *et al.* (2011) Evaluation of a simple loop-mediated isothermal amplification test kit for the diagnosis of tuberculosis. *The International Journal of Tuberculosis and Lung Disease* 15, 1211–1217, i.

Morgan, M., Kalantri, S., Flores, L. and Pai, M. (2005) A commercial line probe assay for the rapid detection of rifampicin resistance in *Mycobacterium tuberculosis*: a systematic review and meta-analysis. *BMC Infectious Diseases* 5, 62.

Mostowy, S., Cousins, D., Brinkman, J., Aranaz, A. and Behr, M. (2002) Genomic deletions suggest a phylogeny for the *Mycobacterium tuberculosis* complex. *Journal of Infectious Diseases* 186, 74–80.

Moure, R., Munoz, L., Torres, M., Santin, M., Martin, R. and Alcaide, F. (2011) Rapid detection of *Mycobacterium tuberculosis* complex and rifampin resistance in smear-negative clinical samples by use of an integrated real-time PCR method. *Journal of Clinical Microbiology* 49, 1137–1139.

Neonakis, I.K., Gitti, Z., Baritaki, S., Petinaki, E., Baritaki, M. and Spandidos, D.A. (2009) Evaluation of GenoType mycobacteria direct assay in comparison with Gen-Probe *Mycobacterium tuberculosis* amplified direct test and GenoType MTBDRplus for direct detection of *Mycobacterium tuberculosis* complex in clinical samples. *Journal of Clinical Microbiology* 47, 2601–2603.

Neonakis, I.K., Spandidos, D.A. and Petinaki, E. (2011) Use of loop-mediated isothermal amplification of DNA for the rapid detection of *Mycobacterium tuberculosis* in clinical specimens. *European Journal of Clinical Microbiology and Infectious Diseases* 30, 937–942.

Nicol, M.P., Workman, L., Isaacs, W., Munro, J., Black, F., Eley, B., *et al.* (2011) Accuracy of the Xpert MTB/RIF test for the diagnosis of pulmonary tuberculosis in children admitted to hospital in Cape Town, South Africa: a descriptive study. *The Lancet Infectious Diseases* 11, 819–824.

Notomi, T., Okayama, H., Masubuchi, H., Yonekawa, T., Watanabe, K., Amino, N., *et al.* (2000) Loop-mediated isothermal amplification of DNA. *Nucleic Acids Research* 28, E63.

Nyendak, M.R., Lewinsohn, D.A. and Lewinsohn, D.M. (2009) New diagnostic methods for tuberculosis. *Current Opinion in Infectious Diseases* 22, 174–182.

O'Grady, J., Maeurer, M., Mwaba, P., Kapata, N., Bates, M., Hoelscher, M., *et al.* (2011) New and improved diagnostics for detection of drug-resistant pulmonary tuberculosis. *Current Opinion in Pulmonary Medicine* 17, 134–141.

Palomino, J.C. (2009) Molecular detection, identification and drug resistance detection in *Mycobacterium tuberculosis*. *FEMS Immunology and Medical Microbiology* 56, 103–111.

Parsons, L.M., Brosch, R., Cole, S.T., Somoskovi, A., Loder, A., Bretzel, G., *et al.* (2002) Rapid and simple approach for identification of *Mycobacterium tuberculosis* complex isolates by PCR-based genomic deletion analysis. *Journal of Clinical Microbiology* 40, 2339–2345.

Parsons, L.M., Somoskovi, A., Gutierrez, C., Lee, E., Paramasivan, C.N., Abimiku, A., *et al.* (2011) Laboratory diagnosis of tuberculosis in resource-poor countries: challenges and opportunities. *Clinical Microbiology Reviews* 24, 314–350.

Piersimoni, C. and Scarparo, C. (2003) Relevance of commercial amplification methods for direct detection of *Mycobacterium tuberculosis* complex in clinical samples. *Journal of Clinical Microbiology* 41, 5355–5365.

Pinsky, B. and Banaei, N. (2008) Multiplex real-time PCR assay for rapid identification of *Mycobacterium tuberculosis* complex members to the species level. *Journal of Clinical Microbiology* 46, 2241–2246.

Pounder, J.I., Anderson, C.M., Voelkerding, K.V., Salfinger, M., Dormandy, J., Somoskovi, A., *et al.* (2010) *Mycobacterium tuberculosis* complex differentiation by genomic deletion patterns with multiplex polymerase chain reaction and melting analysis. *Diagnostic Microbiology and Infectious Disease* 67, 101–105.

Rachow, A., Zumla, A., Heinrich, N., Rojas-Ponce, G., Mtafya, B., Reither, K., *et al.* (2011) Rapid and accurate detection of *Mycobacterium tuberculosis* in sputum samples by Cepheid Xpert MTB/RIF assay – a clinical validation study. *PLoS One* 6, e20458.

Ramirez, M.V., Cowart, K.C., Campbell, P.J., Morlock, G.P., Sikes, D., Winchell, J.M., *et al.* (2010) Rapid detection of multidrug-resistant *Mycobacterium tuberculosis* by use of real-time PCR and high-resolution melt analysis. *Journal of Clinical Microbiology* 48, 4003–4009.

Reddington, K., O'Grady, J., Dorai-Raj, S., Maher, M., van Soolingen, D. and Barry, T. (2011) Novel multiplex real-time PCR diagnostic assay for identification and differentiation of *Mycobacterium tuberculosis*, *Mycobacterium canettii*, and *Mycobacterium tuberculosis* complex strains. *Journal of Clinical Microbiology* 49, 651–657.

Reddington, K., Zumla, A., Bates, M., van Soolingen, D., Niemann, S., Barry, T., *et al.* (2012) SeekTB – a two stage multiplex real-time PCR based method for the differentiation of the *Mycobacterium tuberculosis* complex. *Journal of Clinical Microbiology* 50(7), 2203–2206.

Richter, E., Weizenegger, M., Fahr, A.-M. and Rusch-Gerdes, S. (2004) Usefulness of the GenoType MTBC assay for differentiating species of the *Mycobacterium tuberculosis* complex in cultures obtained from clinical specimens. *Journal of Clinical Microbiology* 42, 4303–4306.

Rossau, R., Traore, H., De Beenhouwer, H., Mijs, W., Jannes, G., De Rijk, P., *et al.* (1997) Evaluation of the INNO-LiPA Rif. TB assay, a reverse hybridization assay for the simultaneous detection of *Mycobacterium tuberculosis* complex and its resistance to rifampin. *Antimicrobial Agents and Chemotherapy* 41, 2093–2098.

Sandgren, A., Strong, M., Muthukrishnan, P., Weiner, B.K., Church, G.M. and Murray, M.B. (2009) Tuberculosis drug resistance mutation database. *PLoS Medicine* 6, e1000002.

Scott, L.E., McCarthy, K., Gous, N., Nduna, M., Van Rie, A., Sanne, I., *et al.* (2011) Comparison of Xpert MTB/RIF with other nucleic acid technologies for diagnosing pulmonary tuberculosis in a high HIV prevalence setting: a prospective study. *PLoS Medicine* 8, e1001061.

Soini, H., Skurnik, M., Liippo, K., Tala, E. and Viljanen, M.K. (1992) Detection and identification of mycobacteria by amplification of a segment of the gene coding for the 32-kilodalton protein. *Journal of Clinical Microbiology* 30, 2025–2028.

Somoskovi, A., Dormandy, J., Rivenburg, J., Pedrosa, M., McBride, M. and Salfinger, M. (2008) Direct comparison of the Genotype MTBC and genomic deletion assays in terms of their ability to distinguish between members of the *Mycobacterium tuberculosis* complex in clinical isolates and in clinical specimens. *Journal of Clinical Microbiology* 46, 1854–1857.

Somoskovi, A., Dormandy, J., Mayrer, A.R., Carter, M., Hooper, N. and Salfinger, M. (2009) *Mycobacterium canettii* isolated from a human immunodeficiency virus-positive patient: first case recognized in the United States. *Journal of Clinical Microbiology* 47, 255–257.

Syre, H., Myneedu, V.P., Arora, V.K. and Grewal, H.M.S. (2009) Direct detection of mycobacterial species in pulmonary specimens by two rapid amplification tests, the Gen-Probe amplified *Mycobacterium tuberculosis* direct test and the GenoType mycobacteria direct test. *Journal of Clinical Microbiology* 47, 3635–3639.

Tomita, N., Mori, Y., Kanda, H. and Notomi, T. (2008) Loop-mediated isothermal amplification (LAMP) of gene sequences and simple visual detection of products. *Nature Protocols* 3, 877–882.

Torres-Chavolla, E. and Alocilja, E.C. (2011) Nanoparticle based DNA biosensor for tuberculosis detection using thermophilic helicase-dependent isothermal amplification. *Biosensors and Bioelectronics* 26, 4614–4618.

Van Rie, A., Page-Shipp, L., Scott, L., Sanne, I. and Stevens, W. (2010) Xpert(R) MTB/RIF for point-of-care diagnosis of TB in high-HIV burden, resource-limited countries: hype or hope? *Expert Review of Molecular Diagnostics* 10, 937–946.

Van Rie, A., Mellet, K., John, M.A., Scott, L., Page-Shipp, L., Dansey, H., *et al.* (2012) False-positive rifampicin resistance on Xpert(R) MTB/RIF: case report and clinical implications. *The International Journal of Tuberculosis and Lung Disease* 16, 206–208.

Verma, A., Rattan, A. and Tyagi, J.S. (1994) Development of a 23S rRNA-based PCR assay for the detection of mycobacteria. *Indian Journal of Biochemistry and Biophysics* 31, 288–294.

Wada, T., Maeda, S., Tamaru, A., Imai, S., Hase, A. and Kobayashi, K. (2004) Dual-probe assay for rapid detection of drug-resistant *Mycobacterium tuberculosis* by real-time PCR. *Journal of Clinical Microbiology* 42, 5277–5285.

Walker, D.A., Taylor, I.K., Mitchell, D.M. and Shaw, R.J. (1992a) Comparison of polymerase chain reaction amplification of two mycobacterial DNA sequences, IS6110 and the 65kDa antigen gene, in the diagnosis of tuberculosis. *Thorax* 47, 690–694.

Walker, G.T., Fraiser, M.S., Schram, J.L., Little, M.C., Nadeau, J.G. and Malinowski, D.P. (1992b) Strand displacement amplification – an isothermal, *in vitro* DNA amplification technique. *Nucleic Acids Research* 20, 1691–1696.

Wallis, R.S., Pai, M., Menzies, D., Doherty, T.M., Walzl, G., Perkins, M.D., *et al.* (2010) Biomarkers and diagnostics for tuberculosis: progress, needs, and translation into practice. *The Lancet* 375, 1920–1937.

Warren, R.M., Gey van Pittius, N.C., Barnard, M., Hesseling, A., Engelke, E., de Kock, M., *et al.* (2006) Differentiation of *Mycobacterium tuberculosis* complex by PCR amplification of genomic regions of difference. *International Journal of Tuberculosis and Lung Disease* 10, 818–822.

WHO [World Health Organization] (2008) *Molecular Line Probe Assays for Rapid Screening of Patients at Risk of Multidrug-resistant Tuberculosis (MDR-TB)*. World Health Organization, Geneva, Switzerland.

WHO (2010a) *Roadmap for Rolling Out Xpert MTB/ RIF for Rapid Diagnosis of TB and MDR-TB*. World Health Organization, Geneva, Switzerland.

WHO (2010b) *Tuberculosis Diagnostics Automated DNA Test. WHO Endorsement and Recommendations*. World Health Organization, Geneva, Switzerland.

WHO (2011a) *Automated Real-time Nucleic Acid Amplification Technology for Rapid and Simultaneous Detection of Tuberculosis and Rifampicin Resistance: Xpert MTB/RIF System*. World Health Organization, Geneva, Switzerland.

WHO (2011b) *Global Tuberculosis Control: WHO Report 2011*. World Health Organization, Geneva, Switzerland.

WHO (2011c) *Rapid Implementation of the Xpert MTB/RIF Dianognostic Test: Technicial and Operational 'How to': Practical Considerations*. World Health Organization, Geneva, Switzerland.

Yang, Y.C., Lu, P.L., Huang, S.C., Jenh, Y.S., Jou, R. and Chang, T.C. (2011) Evaluation of the Cobas TaqMan MTB test for direct detection of *Mycobacterium tuberculosis* complex in respiratory specimens. *Journal of Clinical Microbiology* 49, 797–801.

Yesilkaya, H., Meacci, F., Niemann, S., Hillemann, D., Rüsch-Gerdes, S., Group, L.D.S., *et al.* (2006) Evaluation of molecular-beacon, TaqMan, and fluorescence resonance energy transfer probes for detection of antibiotic resistance-conferring single nucleotide polymorphisms in mixed *Mycobacterium tuberculosis* DNA extracts. *Journal of Clinical Microbiology* 44, 3826–3829.

3 Improving on the LJ Slope – Automated Liquid Culture

Miguel Viveiros,[1,2] Diana Machado,[1,3] Isabel Couto[1,4] and Leonard Amaral[1,2,3]

[1]Unit of Mycobacteriology, Instituto de Higiene e Medicina Tropical, Universidade Nova de Lisboa (IHMT/UNL), Lisbon, Portugal; [2]Cost Action BM0701 (ATENS) of the Cost Action of the European Commission; [3]UPMM, IHMT/UNL; [4]Centro de Recursos Microbiológicos (CREM), Faculdade de Ciências e Tecnologia, UNL, Caparica, Portugal

3.1 Introduction

The major priority for tuberculosis control programmes is the rapid and accurate diagnosis and treatment of individuals with active tuberculosis. This approach is intended to cut the chain of transmission of the bacillus and provide appropriate therapy to the tuberculosis patient. In this context, the mycobacteriology laboratory has a crucial role in the definitive diagnosis and therapy of tuberculosis that is based on the isolation, identification and antibiotic susceptibility profile of the infecting organism. Prior to the emergence of drug-resistant strains, the role of the laboratory was not considered as important as it is today. At that time, the demonstration of acid-fast bacteria in the sputum, followed by the culture of the specimen and the identification of *Mycobacterium tuberculosis* was sufficient to support the clinical diagnosis of pulmonary tuberculosis, which, for all practical purposes, was already confidently established and supported by physical clinical findings (Salfinger, 1977). Nowadays, the examination of the International Classification of Tuberculosis and the guidelines recommended by the Center for Disease Control (CDC, USA) for the management of individual cases of active pulmonary tuberculosis that differ with respect to underlying medical conditions (pregnancy, chronic liver disease, diabetes, HIV/AIDS), status of infection, the management of patients who have had close contact with individuals known to be infected with multidrug-resistant strains of *M. tuberculosis* (preventive) and the management of patients with reactive tuberculosis indicate how complex the management of tuberculosis has become (ATS/CDC/IDSA, 2003; Griffith *et al.*, 2007; WHO, 2009). Underlying these recommendations is the need for the accurate isolation, identification and antibiotic sensitivity testing of *M. tuberculosis* from clinical specimens in the shortest time possible (Salfinger and Pfyffer, 1994; Ridderhof *et al.*, 2007; Tortoli and Marcelli, 2007).

New and more rapid techniques for the laboratory diagnosis of mycobacterial infections were, therefore, greatly needed if the clinical mycobacteriology laboratory was to serve a useful purpose in the management of tuberculosis patients, especially in areas of the world that had large numbers of coinfected HIV/AIDS patients (WHO, 2008). Despite all the technological advancements in the area, culture remains the gold standard for the detection of mycobacteria. Therefore, all clinical specimens suspected of containing mycobacteria should be inoculated on to culture media. The reasons for this procedure are related to three main aspects: first, culture is more sensitive than microscopy, being able to detect less than ten bacteria/ml in the clinical sample; second, the isolation of mycobacteria in culture is indispensable for proper identification of the species; and third, antibiotic susceptibility tests require viable microorganisms. However, culture is a slow and expensive method, since the majority of these microorganisms do not grow in common culture media, requiring the employment of specific media. The main disadvantage of the culture-based methods for isolation and identification of mycobacteria is related with the time that is required to obtain results. Mycobacteria are a slow-growing group of bacteria, with the generation time varying with species from 2 (*M. smegmatis*) to more than 20 h (*M. tuberculosis*). Regarding *M. ulcerans*, for example, the primary cultures are usually positive within 6–12 weeks of incubation at 29–33°C, but much longer incubation (9 months or more) may be necessary for some isolates (David, 1989; Griffith *et al.*, 2007; Palomino *et al.*, 2007).

Growth-based methods for mycobacterial isolation, identification and drug susceptibility have been in practice since the 1930s, when the mycobacteria selective egg-based Löwenstein–Jensen (LJ) medium was developed (Löwenstein, 1931; Kent and Kubica, 1985). The commercial preparation of LJ medium was pioneered by Becton Dickinson (Towson, USA) in 1952, followed by agar-based Middlebrook 7H10 (Middlebrook and Cohn, 1958). The 1980s were marked by the development of the broth-based BACTEC™ 460TB Radiometric System by Becton Dickinson using Middlebrook 7H12 (BACTEC 12B vials) for specimens other than blood and Middlebrook 7H13 (BACTEC 13A vials) for blood specimens (Strand *et al.*, 1989). The strict safety regulations concerning the use of radiometric labelled material led, in the

1990s, to the development of non-radiometric broth technologies, such as the fluorescent BACTEC™ 9000MB system (Becton Dickinson), the fluorescent mycobacterial growth indicator tubes manual system BACTEC™ MGIT™ (Becton Dickinson) and the colorimetric MB/BacT®(Organon Teknika, Boxtel, Netherlands), later upgraded to the BacT/ALERT®Systems (bioMérieux SA, Marcy-l'Etoile, France). Nevertheless, the Center for Disease Control and many reference laboratories around the world still maintain the recommendation that broth and agar media should be employed as a complement for the recovery of mycobacteria and further recommend the solid egg-based (LJ) and agar-based (7H10 or 7H11) media as gold standards (Kent and Kubica, 1985; David, 1989; Tortoli and Marcelli, 2007).

For the recovery and isolation of mycobacteria from biological samples, three main types of media can be employed: egg-based medium, medium with agar and liquid medium. The introduction of antimicrobial agents (selective media) may be very useful for contaminated samples, but this type of media should not be used alone due to the probability of inhibiting mycobacterial growth.

3.2 Types of Media for Culture and Isolation of Mycobacteria

There are two types of solid media for the recovery and isolation of mycobacteria: egg-based (e.g. LJ and Ogawa) and agar-based (Middlebrook 7H10 and 7H11) (Figs 3.1 and 3.2). Among the solid culture media used for growth of mycobacteria, the LJ medium is the one mostly used.

3.2.1 Solid media

Egg-based medium

Löwenstein–Jensen (LJ), an egg-based medium, is a modification of the original Löwenstein medium (Löwenstein, 1931) by Jensen (Jensen, 1932) (Fig. 3.1). In this version of the media firstly described by Lowestein, the Congo red dye was suppressed, the concentration of malachite green was increased and the contents of citrate and phosphate were altered. Overall, the medium contains sources of nitrogen and vitamins (asparagine and potato flour), enhancers of growth (monopotassium phosphate and magnesium sulfate), fatty acids and proteins (glycerol and eggs) necessary for mycobacterial metabolism; sodium citrate and malachite green are used as selective agents (Table 3.1). LJ is used for primary isolation of mycobacteria from sterile and non-sterile sources. Besides the application of this type of media for the isolation and cultivation of mycobacteria, it is also used as a base for the selection and differentiation of mycobacteria. Currently available modifications of the LJ medium include the LJ without glycerol but supplemented with pyruvate to improve the growth of *M. bovis* and *M. africanum*; the Gruft modified LJ medium, which contains penicillin and nalidixic acid for a more selective isolation of mycobacteria, the BBL™ Mycobactosel™ Löwenstein–Jensen Medium Slants (from Becton Dickinson) supplemented with cycloheximide, lincomycin and nalidixic acid for specimens particularly contaminated; the LJ medium with iron used for the determination of mycobacterial iron uptake, which allows the differentiation and identification of some species; the LJ medium with

5% of sodium chloride used to characterize some species of mycobacteria and the LJ medium deep tubes for catalase semi-quantitative assay. The Ogawa medium is another egg-based medium, which is comparable with LJ in its composition. It is a cheaper alternative to the LJ medium due to the substitution of the amino acid asparagine by sodium glutamate. The two media also differ in malachite green concentration, volume of egg homogenate and pH.

The two major advantages of the egg-based media are related to the fact that they allow the growth of a wide variety of mycobacterial species and that this growth can be used for biochemical tests, like niacin and catalase production testing, for species differentiation. Besides these advantages, the media are easy to prepare, are the least expensive of all media available for mycobacteria culture, may be stored in the refrigerator for several weeks and possess low rates of contamination due to the addition of malachite green, which suppresses the growth of other non-mycobacterial organisms. The major disadvantage of this type of medium is related to the time necessary for the cultures to become positive, especially for samples that contain few bacilli (either from paubacillary samples or as the result of an aggressive decontamination process). In addition, the contamination of the medium

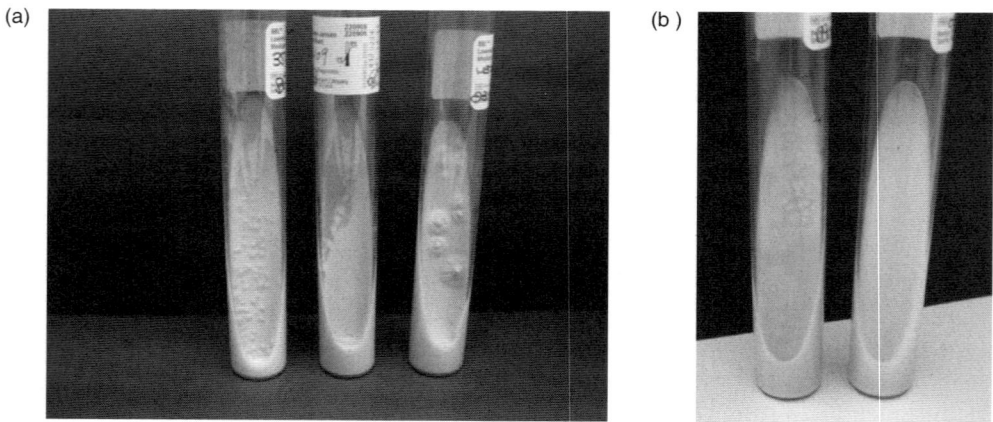

Fig. 3.1. Growth of different mycobacteria in Löwestein–Jensen media. (a) *Mycobacterium marinum, M. gordonae* and *M. tuberculosis*; (b) *M. tuberculosis* and *M. intracellulare*.

Table 3.1. Most commonly used commercially available media for cultivation of mycobacteria from clinical specimens.

Culture media	Composition
Liquid media	
Difco™ Middlebrook 7H9 Broth (Middlebrook 7H9)	Ammonium sulfate; L-glutamic acid; sodium citrate; pyridoxine; biotin; disodium phosphate; monopotassium phosphate; ferric ammonium citrate; magnesium sulfate; calcium chloride; zinc sulfate; copper sulfate
BBL MGIT Mycobacteria Growth Indicator Tube	Modified Middlebrook 7H9 broth base; tris 4, 7-diphenyl-1, 10-phenanthroline ruthenium chloride pentahydrate as a fluorescent indicator; casein peptone
BACTEC™ 12B (Middlebrook 7H12)	Middlebrook 7H9 broth base; casein hydrolysate; bovine serum albumin; 48,000 units of catalase; 1000 μCuries ^{14}C-substrate (palmitic acid)
BACTEC™ 13A (Middlebrook 7H13)	Middlebrook 7H9 broth base; casein hydrolysate; bovine serum albumin; sodium polyanetholesulfonate; polysorbate 80; 1440 units of catalase; 5 μCuries ^{14}C-substrate (palmitic acid)
Solid media	
BBL™ Löwenstein–Jensen Medium	Asparagine; monopotassium phosphate; magnesium sulfate; magnesium citrate; potato flour; malachite green; glycerol; whole egg
Difco™ Middlebrook 7H10 Agar (Middlebrook 7H10)	Ammonium sulfate; monopotassium phosphate; disodium phosphate; sodium citrate; magnesium sulfate; calcium chloride; zinc sulfate; copper sulfate; L-glutamic acid; ferric ammonium citrate; pyridoxine; biotin; malachite green; agar
Difco™ Mycobacteria 7H11 Agar (Middlebrook 7H11)	Magnesium sulfate; ferric ammonium citrate; sodium citrate; ammonium sulfate; disodium phosphate; monopotassium phosphate; agar; pyridoxine; biotin; malachite green; pancreatic digest of casein; L-glutamic acid

with other microorganisms may promote the liquefaction of the medium, which will lead to culture loss. Mycobacterial growth can be detected in less than 3 weeks, but requires an incubation of 8 weeks before the samples can be classified as negative. Their use for the determination of drug susceptibility of mycobacteria differs and requires careful adjustment of drug concentrations (Kent and Kubica, 1985; David, 1989).

Agar-based medium

In 1958, Middlebrook and Cohn described a medium based on agar that allowed a more rapid detection of the mycobacterial growth (Middlebrook and Cohn, 1958) (Fig. 3.2). These types of media are available in two formulations, the Middlebrook 7H10 and the Middlebrook 7H11 agar, and contain a variety of inorganic salts, vitamins, cofactors, glycerol, malachite green and agar (Table 3.1).

When combined with a supplement, Middlebrook enrichment medium (OADC), which consists of <u>o</u>leic <u>a</u>cid, bovine <u>a</u>lbumin, <u>d</u>extrose and <u>c</u>atalase, it can be used for the qualitative procedures of isolation and cultivation of mycobacteria. Middlebrook 7H11 agar is a modification of Middlebrook 7H10 agar enriched by the addition of 0.1% hydrolysed casein, which stimulates the growth of fastidious strains of *M. tuberculosis* and improves susceptibility testing. The use of agar-based media for the isolation of mycobacteria has significant advantages: it does not liquefy in the presence of proteolytic organisms and it is translucent, which allows the visualization of growth and colony morphology with a stereo microscope even in the presence of contaminating microorganisms within a few days of incubation (10–12 days). Besides this, susceptibility testing can be performed on agar-based medium without changing the concentration of the antibiotic,

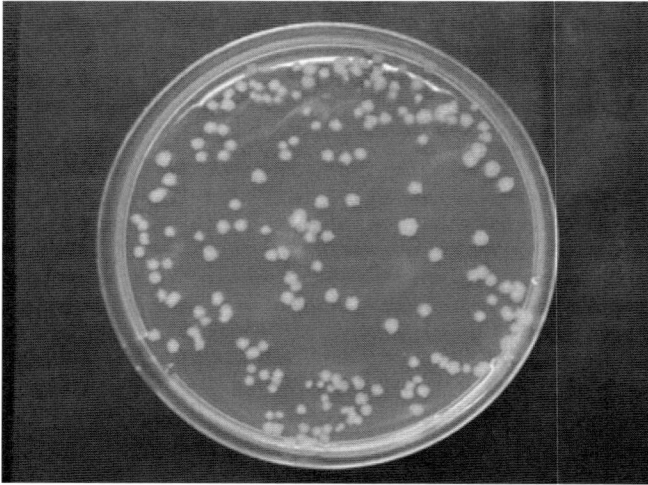

Fig. 3.2. Growth of *M. tuberculosis* in Middlebrook 7H11 medium after three weeks at 37°C.

as is the case with the egg-based media. It is important to note that this type of media is extremely sensitive, therefore it should be prepared in small quantities at a time to avoid loss of quality; exposure to daylight or heat results in the release of formaldehyde from the OADC supplement with a sufficiently high concentration to inhibit the growth of the mycobacteria. For this reason, it is important not to heat the OADC (stored at 4°C) but to allow it to warm to room temperature before adding to the agar. Also, the use of agar-based media is considerably more expensive than egg-based media. Several alternative solid media exist for specific research purposes, such as phage infection, Bacillus Calmette–Guérin (BCG) production or protein purification, namely the BCG, Top and Tryptic Soy Agar (Kent and Kubica, 1985; David, 1989; Parish and Stoker, 1998; Palomino *et al.*, 2007).

The time required for the detection of mycobacterial growth can be reduced by the use of liquid media for the recovery and primary isolation of mycobacteria, which provides a more rapid diagnosis.

3.2.2 Liquid media

While the LJ medium and the Middlebrook 7H10/7H11 agar are the solid media most widely used for culturing mycobacteria, as recommended by the International Union Against Tuberculosis and the WHO, liquid media have also been developed in order to hasten the growth of mycobacteria in culture. Examples such as the liquid Dubos's medium and Sauton's medium, for general growth purposes, or the Proskauer and Beck's medium, ideal for growth in high quantities and surface-pellicle formation, or M9 defined media for protein isolation have been widely used for specific research purposes (Parish and Stoker, 1998). These have been the source for further improvement of the original Middlebrook formulation, which later led to the commercial liquid-based systems for mycobacterial growth detection that are nowadays commonly used worldwide for the routine mycobacteria laboratory (Kent and Kubica, 1985; David, 1989; Palomino *et al.*, 2007).

The commercial liquid-based culture systems can be manual, semi-automated or automated using radiometric, colorimetric or fluorimetric detection methods. The liquid media generally used is the Middlebrook 7H9 or the Middlebrook 7H12/7H13 (Table 3.1), depending on the system and the source of the specimen. Examples of these systems include the BACTEC™ 460TB, BACTEC™ MB9000, BACTEC™ MGIT™ 960 or 320 and the manual MGIT, the Septi-Chek AFB™

systems (all from Becton Dickinson Instrument Systems, Sparks, Maryland, USA), the ESP® (Extra Sensing Power) Myco-ESPculture System II® (Trek Diagnostic Systems, USA) and the BacT/ALERT MB® (bioMérieux SA) (Salfinger and Pfyffer, 1994; Perkins, 2000; Watterson and Drobniewski, 2000; Fig. 3.3).

3.2.3 Manual culture systems

Septi-Chek™ AFB

The BBL™ Septi-Chek™ AFB is a biphasic culture system (Becton Dickinson Microbiology Systems) consisting of modified Middlebrook 7H9 broth and three specific solid media. The BBL™ Septi-Chek™ AFB Supplement and BBL™ Septi-Chek™ AFB slides are used in combination with the culture for the detection and isolation of mycobacteria. The system consists of a bottle of modified Middlebrook 7H9 media and a slide-plate containing chocolate agar (for isolation of bacteria other than mycobacteria), LJ and Middlebrook 7H11 media (for the growth of most mycobacteria). Prior to the

inoculation of the sample, an antibiotic and enrichment supplement are added and the bottle is subsequently inverted to inoculate the solid medium. Bacterial growth is detected by observing the surface of the solid media and the opacity of broth media. This system does not require specific instrumentation and is non-radioactive. However, it is a labour-intensive, manual method.

BBL™ MGIT™ mycobacterial growth indicator tube

This is a rapid and simple manual fluorimetric method to detect mycobacterial growth that uses BBL MGIT tubes with 4 ml of a modified Middlebrook 7H9 media and a gel with a fluorochrome (ruthenium) impregnated at the bottom. Using a Wood's lamp or other long-wave UV light source, tubes are read daily. Positive tests emit an intense orange fluorescent light at the bottom of the tube and at the meniscus; negative tests show slight or no fluorescence. This method does not require specific instrumentation or a dedicated incubator, does not use needles or radioactivity, uses plastic tubes that afford better security and

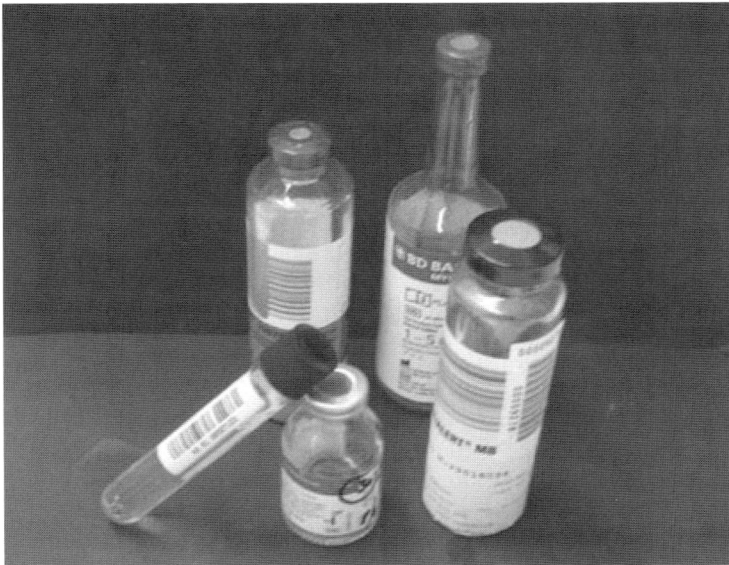

Fig. 3.3. Liquid media used for growth of mycobacteria.

represents an option for laboratories whose volume of work is small (Tortoli *et al.*, 1997; Watterson and Drobniewski, 2000).

3.2.4 Semi-automated culture systems

BACTEC™ 460TB system

The first semi-automated radiometric system to be developed was the BACTEC™ 460TB (Becton Dickinson) based on the works performed by Cummings *et al.* and Middlebrook *et al.* (Cummings *et al.*, 1975; Middlebrook *et al.*, 1977) and whose manufacture was discontinued in 2009. This system was used for isolation of mycobacteria, differentiation of the *M. tuberculosis* complex and susceptibility testing. Glass vials containing 4 ml of medium MB 7H12 or MB 7H13 (for blood samples) (BACTEC 12B or 13A bottles) were used for mycobacterial growth. The medium contained a radioactive substrate, palmitic acid labelled with ^{14}C, which was metabolized by mycobacteria. Growth was detected by measuring the release of radioactive CO_2 with the aid of a gas flow radio counter (Siddiqi *et al.*, 1981, 1985). The BACTEC™ 460TB system reads and records the radioactivity released by converting it into a growth index (GI), in a scale ranging from 0 to 999. Since the quantity of $^{14}CO_2$ released is a direct measure of respiration, it can be correlated with a growth standard curve when the values of radioactivity released are plotted against time (Siddiqi *et al.*, 1981, 1985). The bottles were incubated at 37°C and the $^{14}CO_2$ in the vial atmosphere sampled with an injection system with needles; the counts per minute of $^{14}CO_2$ were determined by the instrument and converted into GI units. The introduction of 5% CO_2 during each reading will enhance the growth of the mycobacteria present. To suppress the growth of microbial contaminants, an antimicrobial supplement BACTEC™ PANTA™ PLUS kit consisting of PANTA (polymyxin B, amphotericin B, nalidixic acid, trimethoprim and azlocillin) (Becton Dickinson) is added. In order to enhance the growth of mycobacteria, the growth promoter (POES, polyoxyethylene stearate) is incorporated in the dilution fluid supplement PANTA. The BACTEC™ 460 is a semi-automated system because the bottles incubated outside the instrument need to be placed into the BACTEC™ instrument, the instrument started, calibrated and the samples read daily and approximately at the same time by the operator. Once placed into the system, reading of the bottles is automated. This system enhances the probability of mycobacterial recovery and reduces the time required for mycobacterial growth when compared with conventional media used for isolation. With the BACTEC™ 460TB, mycobacterial growth can be detected in biological samples in less than 2 weeks. The disadvantages of this method are the costs associated with the acquisition of the instrument and the need for regular maintenance, the inability to observe colony morphology and detect mixed cultures, the overgrowth of contaminating bacteria, the risk associated with the use of radioactive materials and the safety measures necessary for their discard and the extensive use of needles. This system can be used to perform susceptibility testing of *M. tuberculosis* strains.

3.2.5 Automated culture systems

BACTEC™ MGIT™

This is a totally automated fluorimetric-culture system for isolation of mycobacteria and is currently the most widely used. The incubation and reading of cultures does not require the intervention of the operator. All the data obtained with the system can be stored and processed when equipped with EpiCenter software (Becton Dickinson). For mycobacterial growth, the previously described growth-indicator tubes (BBL MGIT, mycobacteria growth indicator tube) are used, now containing 7 ml of modified Middlebrook 7H9 media. Ruthenium gel, in the base of the tube, becomes increasingly fluorescent due to the reduction of the fluorochrome as oxygen levels dissolved in the media drop. Thus, fluorescence intensity is directly proportional to the amount of oxygen consumed. The MGIT tubes are usually incubated at 37°C in the system and the monitoring of growth by the detection of increased fluorescence is performed under UV light every 60 min and converted into growth units (GUs). A positive result is achieved at 75 GU. The time to detection (TTD, also known as time to positivity, TTP) for a positive culture that is obtained in the form of a report is provided by the system. Incubation and monitoring are carried out up to 45 days, after which cultures are reported as negative and discarded. Since it is a culture system based on liquid media, it is essential to add an antimicrobial supplement (MGIT PANTA™) to the primary culture to suppress the growth of other bacterial species. The system has significant advantages since it is totally automated, has a low rate of contamination, reduces TTD of mycobacterial growth to 1 week and can also be used to perform susceptibility testing of *M. tuberculosis* strains, both to first- and second-line antibiotics. The main disadvantage of this system is related to the high cost of the equipment, reagents and media necessary for the tests. The system is available in two models, both totally automated; the first to be developed is the BACTEC™ MGIT™ 960 and the new version is the BACTEC™ MGIT™ 320. The BACTEC™ 960TB system has become one of the most widely used systems for the determination of susceptibility of *M. tuberculosis* to antibiotics currently used to treat tuberculosis (Siddiqi and Rüsch-Gerdes, 2006). Based on the same principle of the original system, the BACTEC™ MGIT™ 320 could represent an option that is less expensive for laboratories with little volume of work and could be an alternative to the BACTEC™ MGIT™ 960 in low-income countries.

Myco-ESP Culture System II

The ESP® Culture System II (Trek Diagnostic Systems, USA) incorporates a unique and very sensitive technology which measures the pressure change inside the culture bottle. Each bottle is connected to a sensor and monitored continuously to detect any alteration in the pressure due to the metabolic activity by the growing microorganisms. Each bottle possesses a modified Middlebrook 7H9 broth and cellulose sponges. The sponges provide a growth support platform (Tortoli *et al.*, 1998). Prior to inoculation of the specimen, the medium in each bottle is supplemented with an antibiotic-containing reagent (PVNA; polymyxin B, vancomycin, nalidixic acid and amphotericin B) and a growth supplement. This is a non-radiometric method that eliminates the need for the treatment and discarding of radioactive material. The closed system design allows the safe handling of all specimens throughout the laboratory. The system is available with different capacities, that is, for 128, 256 or 384 unitary bottles, depending on the needs of each laboratory.

BacT/ALERT mycobacteria detection systems

The BacT/ALERT systems (bioMérieux SA), formerly MB/BacT (Organon Teknika, Boxtel, Netherlands), are automated microbiology systems which use a patented colorimetric sensor and constitute a non-isotopic alternative for the detection of mycobacteria. The Organon Teknika's BacT/Alert was the first system to use colorimetric technology. The system is based on the detection of a decrease in the pH of the medium by actively proliferating mycobacteria that metabolize the substrates present in the culture medium, resulting in the production of CO_2, which in turn acidifies the medium and causes a colour change in the sensor that is present at the base of each culture bottle. The sensor will change from dark green to yellow as microorganisms grow and this alteration is detected by a reflectometric unit in the instrument. The system automatically performs readings every 10 min using infrared rays. All data are transferred to and saved with the BacT/View software. This simplifies and reduces the errors associated with manual operations. Pre-processing is not required and specimen volumes can be inoculated directly into the culture bottle. The systems MB/Bact 240 (without shaking) and the BacT/ALERT 3D® (without shaking) use the BacT/ALERT MB (non-selective media for blood specimens) and MP culture bottles (for sterile body specimens other than blood, and from digested decontaminated samples) and can be used in combination with MB/BacT enrichment fluid or MB/BacT® antibiotic supplement. This is also a non-radiometric, needle-free, fully automated with continuous monitoring, 'walk-away' system introduced as an alternative to its counterpart, the BACTEC™ MGIT™ 960 system (Angeby *et al.*, 2003).

BACTEC™ 9000MB

The BACTEC™ 9000MB is an automated non-radiometric culture system for the isolation of mycobacteria (Becton Dickinson). This system uses the MYCO/F medium, a modified Middlebrook 7H9 media, which can be supplemented with an antimicrobial cocktail to suppress the growth of contaminating microorganisms (van Griethuysen *et al.*, 1996). The inoculated vials are inserted into the equipment for incubation and periodic reading (every 30 min) (Sharp *et al.*, 1997). The system responds to changes in oxygen concentration (van Griethuysen *et al.*, 1996). Each vial contains a silicon rubber disc, impregnated with ruthenium, which serves as an oxygen-specific sensor so that microorganism metabolism and growth are detected (van Griethuysen *et al.*, 1996; Sharp *et al.*, 1997). Oxygen consumption by microorganisms present in the medium can be detected by the increase in fluorescence and a positive reading indicates presumptive presence of viable microorganisms (van Griethuysen *et al.*, 1996; Sharp *et al.*, 1997). The BACTEC™ 9000MB system monitors fluorescence levels and detects the growth of microorganisms on the basis of software-based positivity algorithms and is a rapid, sensitive and efficient non-radiometric method suitable for isolation of mycobacteria in a clinical laboratory (van Griethuysen *et al.*, 1996).

Besides the recent improvement in the culture methods for mycobacteria, from solid to liquid and from manual to automated, all of them are more or less expensive and require more than 1–2 weeks to produce results. Methods that employ solid media for growth usually provide the detection of colonies after 3–8 weeks, under optimum conditions, depending on the species, but the use of liquid media decreases this period markedly to 1–2 weeks. Nevertheless, growth in solid media must be retained and used for certain mycobacterial species since the morphology and chromogenicity of the colonies continue to be important for the accurate identification of mycobacteria (Fig. 3.1; Leão *et al.*, 2004). Since each type of culture offers certain advantages, the combination of different culture media (solid medium plus liquid medium) is recommended for the recovery and primary isolation of mycobacteria.

3.3 Adaptation of Automated Liquid Culture Systems for the Qualitative and Quantitative Determination of Drug Susceptibility

With the increasing number of patients infected with drug-resistant strains of *M. tuberculosis*, in parallel with a significant increase of infections caused by non-tuberculous mycobacteria (NTM), especially in immunocompromised individuals, the determination of the antibiotic susceptibility profile of the isolated mycobacteria became mandatory and the new, fast culture methods quickly became the first choice to reduce the time between isolation and the determination of drug susceptibility (Perkins, 2000; Hazbón, 2004; Ridderhof *et al.*, 2007). For this purpose, the semi-automatic BACTEC™ 460TB and the BACTEC™ 960TB systems (Becton Dickinson Instrument Systems) were adapted for a quick and reliable susceptibility test that rapidly became the reference worldwide and replaced the labour-intensive proportion method in Middlebrook 7H11 (Cummings *et al.*, 1975; Salfinger, 1977; Siddiqi *et al.*, 1981). The adaptation of this susceptibility test is a direct extension of the method of detection of growth in the systems and the susceptibility of the microorganism to the critical concentration of the antibiotic to be tested is defined in terms of diminishing GUs when compared with the control (no antibiotic) (Siddiqi *et al.*,

1981). The criteria adopted for this method are based on the same principles of the proportion method. If there is a sufficient percentage of resistant bacilli (>1%) in the population to obtain a normal growth curve in vials containing the critical concentration of the antibiotic, then the strain is considered to be resistant. This interpretation is based on the growth curves recorded and the criteria defined in the operating manual (Lorian, 2005). Recently, this method has evolved for the quantitative drug susceptibility testing of *M. tuberculosis* using the BACTEC™ 960TB system EpiCenter software equipped with the TB eXiST module and has been created for determination of the minimum inhibitory concentration and evaluation of breakpoints for each antibiotic that might be used for therapeutic purposes against the clinical strain isolated (Springer *et al.*, 2009). This new feature of the BACTEC™ 960TB system allows personalized therapies implemented for each tuberculosis, multidrug-resistant tuberculosis (MDR-TB), extremely drug-resistant tuberculosis (XDR-TB) or NTM infected patient, adjusting the therapy and dosage to the susceptibility profile of the clinical isolate, providing the obvious advantages of increased efficacy and reduction of non-compliance. This technical improvement, although expensive, will have, in the future, a direct impact on the control of acquired resistance, as well as on the increase in the cure rate of XDR-TB infected patients. Furthermore, it will allow immunocompromised patients infected with NTM to receive efficient susceptibility testing for directed therapy as an alternative to the empiric therapeutic regimens implemented today against these infections (Viveiros *et al.*, 2010).

Acknowledgements

The authors would like to thank the Fundação Calouste Gulbenkian (Portugal) for its continuous support in the research and development of new approaches for the control of tuberculosis and drug-resistant tuberculosis.

References

American Thoracic Society, the Centers for Disease Control and Prevention and the Infectious Diseases Society of America (2003) ATS/CDC/IDSA statement: treatment of tuberculosis. *Morbidity and Mortality Weekly Report* 52, RR-11 (www.thoracic.org/sections/publications/statements/pages/mtpi/rr5211.html, accessed 21 December 2010).

Angeby, K.A., Werngren, J., Toro, J.C., Hedström, G., Petrini, B. and Hoffner, S.E. (2003) Evaluation of the BacT/ALERT 3D system for recovery and drug susceptibility testing of *Mycobacterium tuberculosis*. *Clinical Microbiology and Infection* 9, 1148–1152.

Cummings, D.M., Ristroph, D., Camargo, E.E., Larson, S.M. and Wagner, H.N. Jr (1975) Radiometric detection of the metabolic activity of *Mycobacterium tuberculosis*. *Journal of Nuclear Medicine* 16, 1189–1191.

David, H.L. (1989) *Méthodes de laboratoire pour mycobacteriologie clinique*. Institute Pasteur, Paris.

Griffith, D.E., Aksamit, T., Brown-Elliott, B.A., Catanzaro, A., Daley, C., Gordin, F., *et al.*; ATS Mycobacterial Diseases Subcommittee; American Thoracic Society; and Infectious Disease Society of America (2007) An official ATS/IDSA statement: diagnosis, treatment, and prevention of nontuberculous mycobacterial diseases. *American Journal of Respiratory and Critical Care Medicine* 175, 367–416.

Hazbón, M.H. (2004) Recent advances in molecular methods for early diagnosis of tuberculosis and drug-resistant tuberculosis. *Biomedica* 24(Suppl. 1), 149–162.

Jensen, K.A. (1932) Rinzuchtung und Typenbestimmung von Tuberkelbazillentamen. *Zentralblatt für Bakteriologie, Parasitenkunde, Infektionskrankheiten und Hygiene 1. Abt. Medizinisch-hygienische Bakteriologie, Virusforschung und Parasitologie. Originale* 125, 222.

Kent, P.T. and Kubica, G.P. (1985) *Mycobacteriology: A Guide for the Level III Laboratory*. US Dept of Health and Human Services, Public Health Service, Centers for Disease Control, Atlanta, Georgia.

Leão, S.C., Martin, A., Mejia, G.I., Palomino, J.C., Robledo, J., Telles, M.A.S., *et al.* (2004) Practical handbook for the phenotypic and genotypic identification of mycobacteria. Vanden Broele (ed.), Bruges, Belgium (www.esmycobacteriology.eu/PDF%20files/foreword.pdf, accessed 21 December 2010).

Lorian, V. (ed.) (2005) *Antibiotics in Laboratory Medicine*, 5th edn. Lippincott Williams and Wilkins, Philadelphia, Pennsylvania.

Löwenstein, E. (1931) Die Zacktung der Tuber kolbazillen aus dem stramenden Blute. *Zentralblatt für Bakteriologie, Parasitenkunde, Infektionskrankheiten und Hygiene 1. Abt. Medizinisch-hygienische Bakteriologie, Virusforschung und Parasitologie. Originale* 120, 127.

Middlebrook, G. and Cohn, M.L. (1958) Bacteriology of tuberculosis: laboratory methods. *American Journal of Public Health* 48, 844–853.

Middlebrook, G., Reggiardo, Z. and Tigertt, W.D. (1977) Automatable radiometric detection of growth of *Mycobacterium tuberculosis* in selective media. *American Review of Respiratory Disease* 115, 1067–1069.

Palomino, J.C., Leão, S.C. and Ritacco, V. (2007) *Tuberculosis 2007 – From Basic Science to Patient Care*, 1st edn. TuberculosisTextbook.com (www.tuberculosistextbook.com, accessed 21 December 2010).

Parish, T. and Stoker, N.G. (eds) (1998) *Mycobacteria Protocols*, Vol 101. Humana Press, Totowa, New Jersey.

Perkins, M.D. (2000) New diagnostic tools for tuberculosis. *International Journal of Tuberculosis and Lung Disease* 4, 182–188.

Ridderhof, J.C., van Deun, A., Kam, K.M., Narayanand, P.R. and Aziz, M.A. (2007) Roles of laboratories and laboratory systems in effective tuberculosis programmes. *Bulletin of the World Health Organization* 85, 354–359.

Salfinger, M. (1977) Diagnosis of tuberculosis and other diseases caused by mycobacteria. *Infection* 25, 60–62.

Salfinger, M. and Pfyffer, G.E. (1994) The new diagnostic mycobacteriology laboratory. *European Journal of Clinical Microbiology and Infectious Diseases* 13, 961–979.

Sharp, S.E., Lemes, M., Erlich S.S. and Poppiti, R.J. Jr (1997) A comparison of the Bactec 9000MB system and the Septi-Chek AFB system for the detection of mycobacteria. *Diagnostic Microbiology and Infectious Diseases* 28, 69–74.

Siddiqi, S.H. and Rüsch-Gerdes, S. (2006) *MGITTM Procedure Manual for BACTECTM MGIT 960TM TB System (also applicable for Manual MGIT) Mycobacteria Growth Indicator Tube (MGIT) Culture and Drug Susceptibility Demonstration Projects*. Foundation for Innovative New Diagnostics, 89 pp (http://www.finddiagnostics.org/export/sites/default/resource-centre/find_documentation/pdfs/mgit_manual_nov_2007.pdf, accessed 9 October 2012).

Siddiqi, S.H., Libonati, J.P. and Middlebrook, G. (1981) Evaluation of a rapid radiometric method for drug susceptibility testing of *Mycobacterium tuberculosis*. *Journal of Clinical Microbiology* 13, 908–912.

Siddiqi, S.H., Hawkins, J.E. and Laszlo, A. (1985) Inter-laboratory drug susceptibility testing of *Mycobacterium tuberculosis* by radiometric procedure and two conventional methods. *Journal of Clinical Microbiology* 22, 919–923.

Springer, B., Lucke, K., Calligaris-Maibach, R., Ritter, C. and Böttger, E.C. (2009) Quantitative drug susceptibility testing of *Mycobacterium tuberculosis* using MGIT960 and the EpiCenter instrumentation. *Journal of Clinical Microbiology* 47, 1773–1780.

Strand, C.L., Epstein, C., Verzosa. S., Effatt, E., Hormozi, P. and Siddiqi, S.H. (1989) Evaluation of a new blood culture medium for mycobacteria. *American Journal of Clinical Pathology* 91, 316–318.

Tortoli, E. and Marcelli, F. (2007) Use of the INNO LiPA Rif. TB for detection of *Mycobacterium tuberculosis* DNA directly in clinical specimens and for simultaneous determination of rifampin susceptibility. *European Journal of Clinical Microbiology and Infectious Diseases* 26, 51–55.

Tortoli, E., Mandler, F., Tronci, M., Penati, V., Sbaraglia, G., Costa, D., et al. (1997) Multicenter evaluation of mycobacteria growth indicator tube (MGIT) compared with the BACTEC radiometric method, BBL biphasic growth medium and Löwenstein–Jensen medium. *Clinical Microbiology and Infection* 3, 468–473.

Tortoli, E., Cichero, P., Chirillo, M.G., Gismondo, M.R., Bono, L., Gesu, G., et al. (1998) Multicenter comparison of ESP Culture System II with BACTEC 460TB and with Löwenstein–Jensen medium for recovery of mycobacteria from different clinical specimens, including blood. *Journal of Clinical Microbiology* 36, 1378–1381.

van Griethuysen, A.J., Jansz, A.R. and Buiting, A.G. (1996) Comparison of fluorescent BACTEC 9000 MB system, Septi-Chek AFB system, and Löwenstein–Jensen medium for detection of mycobacteria. *Journal of Clinical Microbiology* 34, 2391–2394.

Viveiros, M., Martins, M., Couto, I., Rodrigues, L., Machado, D., Portugal, I., et al. (2010) Molecular tools for rapid identification and novel effective therapy against MDRTB/XDRTB infections. *Expert Review of Anti-infective Therapy* 8, 465–480.

Watterson S.A. and Drobniewski, F.A. (2000) Modern laboratory diagnosis of mycobacterial infections. *Journal of Clinical Pathology* 53, 727–732.

World Health Organization [WHO] (2008) The WHO/IUATLD Global Project on Anti-tuberculosis Drug Resistance Surveillance – Report No 4 (2002–2007). World Health Organization, Geneva, Switzerland, pp. 1–142.

WHO (2009) Global tuberculosis control – epidemiology, strategy, financing. WHO Report 2009. World Health Organization, Geneva, Switzerland, pp. 1–314.

4 Interferon-gamma Release Assays in the Diagnosis of Latent Tuberculosis Infection

Ajit Lalvani[1] and Manish Pareek[2]

[1]Tuberculosis Research Unit, Department of Respiratory Medicine, National Heart and Lung Institute, Imperial College London, UK; [2]Department of Infection, Immunity and Inflammation, University of Leicester, UK

4.1 Introduction

The failure to control the global tuberculosis epidemic adequately may partly reflect the slow progress that has been made, over the last century, in developing innovative diagnostic tools for tuberculosis (Lalvani, 2007). However, the potential now exists to advance tuberculosis control significantly with the development of novel diagnostic modalities for latent tuberculosis infection (LTBI).

4.1.1 Latent tuberculosis infection: worldwide burden

Estimates suggest that one-third of the world's population is latently infected with tubercle bacilli but do not have overt clinical disease (Dye *et al.*, 1999). Infection with *Mycobacterium tuberculosis* arises through a complex pathogenic process following exposure to droplet-containing bacilli which eventually concludes with containment of the infection through infiltration of CD4+ T lymphocytes and the release of interferon-γ, which activate bacilli-containing macrophages (Cooper and Flynn, 1995; Bean *et al.*, 1999; Murray, 1999). While a number of situations increase the chance of being infected with *M. tuberculosis*, those individuals in close contact with smear-positive infectious cases or with underlying immunosuppressive states are often considered to be at highest risk of acquiring infection (see Table 4.1).

Table 4.1. Risk factors for acquiring latent tuberculosis infection (American Thoracic Society [ATS] and Centers for Disease Control and Prevention [CDC], 2000; National Collaborating Centre for Chronic Conditions, 2006).

Risk factor
Close contact with smear-positive TB case
Immunosuppression
HIV infection
Diabetes mellitus
End-stage renal disease
Long-term steroid use
Immunosuppressive drugs
Silicosis
Malnutrition
Old age
Birth in high tuberculosis burden region
Health-care workers
Homeless
Prisoners
Travel to high-burden region
Smoking

Latently infected individuals are at risk of future progression to active tuberculosis disease if immune control fails (Dye *et al.*, 1999; Corbett *et al.*, 2003). However, evidence suggests only 5–10% of infected immuno-competent people actually go on to develop active disease over their lifetime (Comstock *et al.*, 1974; American Thoracic Society [ATS] and Centers for Disease Control and Prevention [CDC], 2000; Horsburgh, 2004). Certain factors (see Tables 4.2 and 4.3), such as increasing age or the presence of Human Immunodeficiency Virus (HIV) infection, increase the proportion of and rates at which latently infected individuals go on to develop active tuberculosis disease (Comstock *et al.*, 1974; Horsburgh, 2004).

As a result, there is an increasing recognition, both in high and low tuberculosis burden settings, of the importance of specifically diagnosing and treating LTBI in those individuals with the highest risk of progression from LTBI to active tuberculosis (MacPherson and Gushulak, 2006; Cain *et al.*, 2008). This is reflected in the importance accorded to tracing recent contacts of smear-positive individuals in low-burden settings (National Collaborating Centre for Chronic Conditions, 2006) and the WHO's policy of recommending isoniazid-preventive therapy

Table 4.2. Incidence of active tuberculosis in persons with a positive tuberculin test, by selected risk factors – from US and global studies (ATS and CDC, 2000).

Risk factor	Incidence (per 1000 person-years)
Immunosuppressive states	
HIV	35.0–162
Intravenous drug use and HIV positive	76.0
Intravenous drug use and HIV negative	10.0
Weight deviation	
Underweight by 15%	2.6
Underweight by 10–14%	2.0
Underweight by 5–9%	2.2
Weight within 5% of standard	1.1
Silicosis	68.0
Recent infection with tuberculosis	
<1 year ago	12.9
1–7 years ago	1.6

Table 4.3. Relative risk for developing active tuberculosis by selected clinical conditions – from US and global studies (ATS and CDC, 2000).

Risk factor	Relative risk
Diabetes mellitus	2.0–4.1
Silicosis	30.0
Smoking	2.3
End-stage renal disease	10.0–25.3
Gastrectomy	2–5
Jejunoileal bypass	27–63
Solid organ transplant	
Renal	37
Cardiac	20–74
Carcinoma of head or neck	16

in HIV-positive individuals in high-burden settings (World Health Organization [WHO], 1998). However, the successful, cost-effective implementation of these policies requires a diagnostic test of sufficient specificity and sensitivity.

4.2 Methods of Diagnosing Latent Tuberculosis Infection

Identifying LTBI accurately is difficult. The combination of a low bacterial load and weak humoral response means that diagnosis relies primarily on cellular immunological markers of infection (Lalvani, 2003). Therefore, for much of the last century, a positive tuberculin skin test (TST) in an individual exposed to *M. tuberculosis* with no other clinico-radiographic evidence of active disease was considered diagnostic of LTBI.

The TST measures a cutaneous delayed-type hypersensitivity response to intra-dermally injected purified protein derivative (PPD), a mixture of over 200 *M. tuberculosis* proteins (Lalvani and Pareek, 2009); the resulting size of TST response determines whether an individual has LTBI and quantifies the risk of progression to active tuberculosis (ATS and CDC, 2000). Although the TST is cheap and widely used, it is neither specific, as the antigens present in PPD cross react with Bacillus Calmette–Guérin (BCG) and environmental mycobacteria, nor sensitive, due to anergy in those individuals with a compromised immune system (such as HIV, iatrogenic immunosuppression and children) (Lalvani, 2003). Logistic drawbacks include the need for the test to be performed by a trained health-care professional and the requirement for a return visit to have the result read.

4.2.1 T-cell interferon-gamma release assays

The development of T-cell interferon-gamma release assays (IGRAs) as an alternative immunodiagnostic modality for *M. tuberculosis* (Lalvani *et al.*, 2001b; Mori *et al.*, 2004; Richeldi, 2006) stems from the identification

of a genomic segment (region of difference 1 – RD1) which encodes two antigens – early secretory antigen target-6 (ESAT-6) and culture filtrate protein-10 (CFP-10) – which are strong specific targets of Th1 T cells in *M. tuberculosis* infection but are also deleted from all strains of BCG (Mahairas *et al.*, 1996) and the majority of environmental mycobacteria (except *M. kansasi, M. szulgai, M. marinum, M. flavescens* and *M. gastrii*) (Harboe *et al.*, 1996). By eliciting specific T-cell responses to these antigens, the frequency of false positive TST results in BCG-vaccinated individuals is reduced (Lalvani, 2007; Lalvani and Millington, 2007, 2008b); this property forms the basis of the two *ex vivo* IGRAs that are currently available (see Table 4.4): the enzyme-linked immunosorbent spot (ELISpot), which directly counts the number of IFN-γ secreting T cells (commercially available as the T-SPOT™.TB (Oxford Immunotec, Abingdon, UK)) and the whole blood enzyme-linked immunosorbent assay (ELISA), which measures the concentration of IFN-γ secretion (commercialized as the QuantiFERON™-TB Gold In-Tube (Cellestis, Carnegie, Australia)).

4.3 Clinical Performance of IGRAs in Different Populations

In the absence of a gold standard reference test for LTBI, objective comparisons of the performance of TST and IGRAs are challenging. Consequently, proxy markers of LTBI must be used, including: (i) active tuberculosis as a surrogate for LTBI; (ii) degrees of contact with smear-positive infectious cases; and (iii) negative IGRA results in healthy BCG-vaccinated individuals at low risk of tuberculosis infection due to the absence of risk factors for tuberculosis exposure.

4.3.1 Performance of IGRAs in immunocompetent persons

Active tuberculosis as a surrogate for LTBI in immunocompetent patients

In the absence of a gold standard reference test for LTBI, a commonly used measure of

Table 4.4. The similarities and differences between the ELISpot (TSPOT.TB) and ELISA (QuantiFERON-TB Gold In-tube).

	ELISpot	ELISA
Antigens	ESAT-6 and CFP-10	ESAT-6, CFP-10 and TB 7.7
Positive internal control	Yes	Yes
Readout units	IFN-γ spot-forming cells (SFC)	International units (IU) of IFN-γ
Technological platform	ELISpot (enzyme-linked immunospot – modified form of sandwich ELISA)	ELISA
Test's substrate	Peripheral blood mononuclear cells (PBMC)	Whole blood
Outcome measure	Number of IFN-γ producing T-cells	Serum concentration of IFN-γ produced by T-cells
Readout system	Enumeration of spots by naked eye, magnifying lens or automated reader	Measurement of optical density values using an automated reader
Technical procedures in diagnostic laboratory	Separation and enumeration and dispensing of PBMC into ELISpot wells required before incubation	Tubes into which blood is drawn are incubated directly without further procedures

the diagnostic sensitivity of IGRAs is to evaluate their performance in individuals with active tuberculosis disease who, by definition, are infected with *M. tuberculosis*.

This was first shown for the ELISpot in a small, proof-of-principle study among culture-confirmed cases (*n* = 47) where the ELISpot had a sensitivity of 96% versus 69% for the TST (Lalvani *et al.*, 2001b). Subsequent studies have described the performance of the ELISpot among immunocompetent individuals in both high- and low-burden settings. One of the largest and most rigorously designed studies to date, conducted in routine clinical practice, was undertaken in the UK by Dosanjh *et al.*, who found that the standard ELISpot had a sensitivity of 85% in culture-confirmed/highly probable tuberculosis as compared to 83% with the TST (Dosanjh *et al.*, 2008). A similarly large study, conducted in Singapore, found that the ELISpot had a sensitivity in culture-confirmed adult tuberculosis patients of 94.1% (Chee *et al.*, 2008). A smaller study in South Korean adults found the ELISpot to have a similarly high sensitivity of 95% (Lee *et al.*, 2006). Conversely, in a mixed population of Turkish children and adults, Soysal and colleagues found that the ELISpot had a slightly lower sensitivity of 83% in those with culture-confirmed tuberculosis (Soysal *et al.*, 2008). In general, most studies comparing the ELISpot against the TST have shown that its sensitivity is superior to that of the TST, with values in the range of 58–100% versus 46–100%, respectively (Diel *et al.*, 2010b).

Numerous studies have also assessed the sensitivity of the ELISA in culture-confirmed active tuberculosis. The first proof-of-principle study was conducted in 118 Japanese patients with culture-confirmed tuberculosis where the overall sensitivity was 89% (Mori *et al.*, 2004). Since this first report in 2004, the evidence base for the ELISA has also expanded rapidly. Data are now available from high- and low-burden settings for both children and adults. While a South African study of children with tuberculosis found the sensitivity of the ELISA to be 76% (Tsiouris *et al.*, 2006b), a smaller study from the UK found a higher sensitivity of 87% in children with active tuberculosis (Kampmann *et al.*, 2009). In adults, Chee and colleagues have conducted the largest evaluation of the ELISA to date and found the sensitivity to be 83% in adult patients with tuberculosis (Chee *et al.*, 2008); conversely, a Japanese study of 100 patients with active tuberculosis found that sensitivity in their population was higher at 93% (Harada *et al.*, 2008). In general, studies comparing the performance of the ELISA against the TST have found the sensitivity of the IGRA and the TST to be in the range of 56–93% and 63–100%, respectively (Diel et al., 2010b).

Two recent meta-analyses of the performance of the ELISpot and ELISA, where culture-confirmed tuberculosis was the reference gold standard, have come to slightly different calculations of the sensitivity of the IGRAs – although the overall conclusions are congruent. Pai et al. calculated a pooled sensitivity of the ELISpot of 90% (range 83–100%), which was significantly higher than the pooled sensitivities of the second-generation ELISA (78% – range 55–88%) and the latest-generation ELISA (QuantiFERON-Gold In-tube – pooled 70%, range 64–93%) (Pai et al., 2008). In contrast, Diel et al. calculated the pooled sensitivity of the ELISpot and latest-generation ELISA (Quanti-FERON-Gold In-tube) to be 88% (range 85–90%) and 81% (range 78–83%), respectively (Diel et al., 2010b).

Correlation of IGRA results with tuberculosis exposure in immunocompetent persons

Active tuberculosis, however, may not represent accurately the host–bacteria interaction that is present in LTBI. As a result, authors have suggested that an alternative method, namely correlation of IGRA responses with degree of exposure to tuberculosis, should be used to assess the performance of IGRAs. The rationale underpinning this is that as M. tuberculosis is transmitted by the airborne route, the risk of acquiring infection is determined by the frequency, duration and proximity of contact with an infectious source case (Houk et al., 1968; Grzybowski and Enarson, 1978; Stead, 1978; Kenyon et al., 1996) and therefore the logical sequelae is that if a new test is more sensitive and specific than the TST, it should correlate more closely with the level of exposure to M. tuberculosis while still remaining independent of BCG status (Lalvani et al., 2001a).

This was first demonstrated by Lalvani and colleagues, who showed that IGRA responses were correlated significantly (more

so than with the TST) with intensity of exposure and not affected by prior BCG vaccination (Lalvani et al., 2001a). Subsequently, many authors have used this principle to compare the diagnostic accuracy of IGRAs and the TST in outbreak and contact-tracing investigations – which often involve child contacts of infectious tuberculosis cases (Lalvani et al., 2001a; Ewer et al., 2003; Brock et al., 2004; Richeldi et al., 2004; Shams et al., 2005; Zellweger et al., 2005). One of the clearest demonstrations of this method was the outbreak investigation instigated as part of a large school outbreak comprising 535 students in the UK. This study found, uniquely, that the ELISpot correlated significantly more closely with M. tuberculosis exposure than the TST based on proximity and duration of exposure to the index case (Ewer et al., 2003). Other work from a variety of low-, intermediate- and high-prevalence settings has also confirmed that the ELISpot correlates significantly with tuberculosis exposure (Kang et al., 2005; Soysal et al., 2005; Hill et al., 2006, 2007; Detjen et al., 2007; Connell et al., 2008; Diel et al., 2008a; Dominguez et al., 2008; Nicol et al., 2009). In a Turkish community-based study of household contacts, positive ELISpot and TST results correlated significantly with the index patient being a parent and the number of cases of smear-positive pulmonary tuberculosis per household (Soysal et al., 2005). More recently, in a study of 243 children in South Africa, positive ELISpot and TST results in children were found to be associated significantly with the degree of exposure to smear-positive index cases (Nicol et al., 2009). Another recent study from a high-incidence setting (Zimbabwe) also confirmed that positive ELISpot results were associated with the degree of exposure to sputum smear-positive tuberculosis cases (Mutsvangwa et al., 2010).

For the ELISA platform, the first study to use degree of exposure as the reference standard was undertaken by Brock and colleagues in a contact-tracing study in Danish children. This study showed that the ELISA correlated with the degree of exposure and was unaffected by BCG status (Brock et *al.*, 2004). As with the ELISpot, the evidence base for studies correlating ELISA positivity with exposure to tuberculosis has since expanded rapidly (Connell *et al.*, 2006, 2008; Nakaoka *et al.*, 2006; Chun *et al.*, 2008; Okada *et al.*, 2008; Lighter *et al.*, 2009). The first study in a high tuberculosis burden setting (Nigeria) was a case control of child contacts of adult tuberculosis patients where there was a dose–response relationship, so that children who had been in contact with the most heavily smear-positive index cases, rather than smear-negative adults, were more likely to be TST and ELISA positive (Nakaoka *et al.*, 2006). Similar results have been found in recent work from Korea and Cambodia (Chun *et al.*, 2008; Okada *et al.*, 2008), However, in contrast, a study from a South African township of children at high risk of LTBI did not find any significant relationship between levels of exposure and ELISA positivity (Tsiouris *et al.*, 2006a). In a low tuberculosis burden setting, Lighter and colleagues undertook a study in US children and found that with increasing likelihood of exposure to *M. tuberculosis* (from minimal to high), the proportion of children with positive ELISA results also increased (Lighter *et al.*, 2009).

While the evidence base is currently more substantial for the ELISpot than the ELISA, the general consensus that can be drawn from these studies is that both IGRAs correlate either as well as, or better than, the TST with levels of exposure to tuberculosis, while also being independent of BCG status.

An important element of these studies is how concordant IGRAs and TSTs are when diagnosing individuals with suspected LTBI. Currently available data indicates that in BCG-vaccinated individuals the level of agreement is poor, as BCG confounds the TST but not IGRAs, and this is responsible for most TST+/IGRA− discordance. Where ELISpot and the TST have been investigated, concordance between the two tests has been moderate to high (Ewer *et al.*, 2003; Hill *et al.*, 2006; Connell *et al.*, 2008; Dominguez *et al.*, 2008; Lighter *et al.*, 2009). For example, a Gambian study of child contacts found a moderately high level of concordance (κ = 0.62) between the ELISpot and the ELISA/TST

(Hill *et al.*, 2006), which was similar to the level of agreement seen in an institutional outbreak in a low tuberculosis burden setting (κ = 0.72) (Ewer *et al.*, 2003). More recent work from South Africa and Australia has found moderate levels of agreement between the ELISpot and the TST (κ = 0.55 and 0.51, respectively) (Connell *et al.*, 2008; Nicol *et al.*, 2009).

In contrast, concordance between the ELISA and the TST appears to be more variable, with kappa values ranging from 0.19 to 0.87 (Brock *et al.*, 2004; Dogra *et al.*, 2007; Chun *et al.*, 2008; Connell *et al.*, 2008; Dominguez *et al.*, 2008; Okada *et al.*, 2008; Lighter *et al.*, 2009). While studies in high tuberculosis burden settings of hospitalized children in India (κ = 0.73) (Dogra *et al.*, 2007) and childhood contacts in Cambodia (κ = 0.63) (Okada *et al.*, 2008) found high concordance between the ELISA and the TST, other studies have found considerably lower levels of agreement. In a South Korean case-control study, the level of agreement between the ELISA and the TST was low (κ = 0.19) (Chun *et al.*, 2008). Similarly, in an Australian study, there was poor agreement between the ELISA and the TST (κ = 0.3) (Connell *et al.*, 2006); more importantly, in the 21 unvaccinated children who had a positive TST, only 4 were ELISA positive. Subsequently, over half of BCG-unvaccinated children with a positive TST had a negative ELISA (Dominguez *et al.*, 2008). These data may imply that the ELISA may have a lower sensitivity than the TST in diagnosing LTBI in children.

In the few studies which have compared the performance of the ELISA and the ELISpot (CDC, 2010; Diel *et al.*, 2010b), concordance between the two platforms has, in general, been good to very good (κ >0.6) (Detjen *et al.*, 2007; Dominguez *et al.*, 2008; Soysal *et al.*, 2008), although a notable exception is a Singaporean study by Chee *et al.* where concordance was only fair (κ = 0.26) (Chee *et al.*, 2008).

Ultimately, the significance of discordant results, whether they are TST/IGRA or ELISpot/ELISA, can only be clarified reliably through longitudinal studies with clinical outcomes.

4.3.2 Performance of IGRAs in immunocompromised persons

Individuals with impaired cell-mediated immunity such as those with HIV infection or immune-mediated inflammatory diseases (such as rheumatoid arthritis, Crohn's disease and ankylosing spondylitis) undergoing iatrogenic immunosuppression or anti-tumour necrosis factor (TNF) α therapy (Lalvani, 2003) are at increased risk of becoming latently infection with *M. tuberculosis* and progressing to active tuberculosis disease. Therefore, the evaluation of IGRAs as an accurate method of identifying LTBI in these high-risk groups is critical – especially as TST performance is recognized to be suboptimal (Lalvani and Millington, 2008b).

HIV-infected individuals

Since the first reports in 2002 (Chapman *et al.*, 2002) outlining the performance of IGRAs in HIV-positive individuals, the evidence base has expanded very rapidly, with both active tuberculosis and degree of exposure being used as the reference standard.

ACTIVE TUBERCULOSIS AS A SURROGATE FOR LTBI IN IMMUNOSUPPRESSED PATIENTS In general, fewer studies have used active tuberculosis as the reference standard when assessing the performance of IGRAs in HIV-positive individuals.

One of the first studies to evaluate the ELISpot in tuberculosis- and HIV-coinfected individuals was undertaken in Zambian adults, where the sensitivity of the IGRA was 90% (Chapman *et al.*, 2002). Subsequently, a large study of South African children with suspected tuberculosis found that the sensitivity of the ELISpot was 83% versus 63% for the TST and that IGRA responses were not affected adversely by the presence of HIV, malnutrition or extremes of age (under 3 years old) (Liebeschuetz *et al.*, 2004). In a small study of HIV-infected adults with untreated pulmonary tuberculosis in South Africa, the ELISpot performed better than the TST, with overall sensitivities for the two tests of 90% and 57%, respectively (Rangaka *et al.*, 2007a). In contrast to these studies from high

tuberculosis burden settings, relatively few studies have been conducted in HIV-positive subjects in low tuberculosis burden settings. Three studies from Europe have compared the ELISpot and the TST and found the sensitivity of the IGRA to be in the range of 84.6–90.3%, which is greater than that seen with the TST (range 46–50%) (Clark *et al.*, 2007; Goletti *et al.*, 2007; Vincenti *et al.*, 2007). The largest of these studies, which had 96 (48%) patients with a CD4 count <200 cell/μl, found that the ELISpot results were independent of CD4 cell counts in HIV-positive individuals (Clark *et al.*, 2007).

A few authors have assessed the performance of the ELISA in tuberculosis- and HIV-coinfected individuals. In a recent Zambian study, Raby and colleagues compared the relative performance of the ELISA and the TST in a cohort of HIV-positive and -negative subjects with active tuberculosis. Overall, the sensitivity of the ELISA in HIV-positive individuals (63%) was higher than the TST (55%) but significantly lower than in HIV-negative individuals (84%) (Raby *et al.*, 2008). In addition, the investigators found that ELISA performance was affected negatively by a falling CD4 count. Similar findings were seen in a study of culture-confirmed tuberculosis cases in Tanzania, where the subset of patients with HIV infection had a significantly lower ELISA sensitivity than those without HIV infection (65% and 81%, respectively), who were also affected adversely by a decreasing CD4 count (Aabye *et al.*, 2009). In a low-burden setting, Vincenti and colleagues found ELISA sensitivity to be 84.6% versus 46% for the TST (Vincenti *et al.*, 2007).

CORRELATION WITH DEGREE OF EXPOSURE IN IMMUNOSUPPRESSED PERSONS The alternative reference standard, correlation with exposure to *M. tuberculosis*, has also been used to assess the test performance of the ELISpot and ELISA.

Studies using this methodology to evaluate the ELISpot have, in general, found that in HIV-positive persons the diagnostic sensitivity of the ELISpot is higher than the TST, and consequently concordance between the two tests is only moderate at best. In a South African study of HIV-positive adults and children, the ELISpot had an overall positivity of 61% as compared to 41% for the TST – although there was no reference standard against which the results were compared. In this study, neither the ELISpot nor the TST correlated with exposure to *M. tuberculosis* (Mandalakas *et al.*, 2008). A larger study from South Africa confirmed that in HIV-infected individuals, the ELISpot had a higher positivity rate than the TST, was robust to changes in CD4 count and had a moderate level of agreement with the TST (κ = 0.52) (Rangaka *et al.*, 2007b). However, the ELISpot did not correlate with exposure to *M. tuberculosis*. In a recent study of HIV-positive individuals from a low-prevalence setting, the ELISpot was found to be more sensitive than the TST and also to correlate significantly with previous active tuberculosis disease, which was not the case for the ELISA or the TST (Stephan *et al.*, 2008). An additional finding that ELISpot responses were not affected by advancing immunosuppression, as evidenced by a falling CD4 count, has been confirmed by other studies (Dheda *et al.*, 2005). Most recently, Mutsvanga and colleagues undertook a study in Zimbabwe and found that ELISpot responses in recent household contacts (who were both HIV positive and negative) correlated significantly with sputum smear, and culture, positivity of the index case independently of contacts' HIV status; contacts' TST results were also associated with smear status of the index cases but were affected negatively by the contacts' HIV status (Mutsvangwa *et al.*, 2010).

Data from evaluations of the ELISA in HIV-positive populations are also beginning to accumulate. In a recent study from the USA, Talati and colleagues assessed the ELISA in HIV-positive clinic attenders. They found that the ELISA had a higher positivity rate than the TST, poor concordance with the TST (κ = 0.23) and, on multivariate analysis, was associated with a previous history of LTBI (Talati *et al.*, 2009). An earlier study from the USA also found a relatively low ELISA positivity rate of 4.9%, although the ELISA, but not the TST, was associated more closely with risk factors for tuberculosis exposure/LTBI (Jones *et al.*, 2007). In a cross-sectional study of HIV-infected individuals in a high-prevalence setting, the ELISA was found to have a lower rate of positivity than both the ELISpot and the TST, although the ELISA ESAT-6/CFP-10 responses in adults with known exposure to *M. tuberculosis* were significantly higher (Mandalakas *et al.*, 2008). In contrast, in HIV-positive Chilean adults, when compared to the TST, the ELISA had a higher sensitivity while also correlating with degree of exposure (Balcells *et al.*, 2008).

Although this Chilean study did not find that low CD4 counts affected ELISA results adversely, there is accumulating evidence that in HIV-positive individuals with advanced immunosuppression, and thus low CD4 cell counts, ELISA performance is affected adversely. In a study among a HIV cohort in San Francisco, Luetkemeyer and colleagues found that decreasing CD4 count affected the CD4 count adversely – particularly the rate of indeterminate results; when CD4 counts were less than 100, the odds ratio for an indeterminate result was 4.2 (Luetkemeyer *et al.*, 2007). Similar conclusions were drawn from a large Danish study of HIV-positive individuals; despite in-tube ELISA results being associated with risk factors for LTBI, there was also a significant association between low CD4 cell count and indeterminate ELISA results (Brock *et al.*, 2006). These findings have been confirmed by other authors, suggesting that in advanced immunosuppression, such as that seen in HIV, ELISA performance may be affected adversely (Jones *et al.*, 2007; Mandalakas *et al.*, 2008; Raby *et al.*, 2008).

Performance of IGRA in iatrogenically immunosuppressed subjects with immune-mediated inflammatory diseases

In individuals with immune-mediated inflammatory diseases (IMIDs), the evidence base for IGRAs as a diagnostic tool for LTBI has, until recently, been relatively limited. None the less, over the past 12–18 months there has been an increase in the number of authors evaluating IGRAs in individuals with IMID. As would be expected due to the rarity of finding individuals with both IMID and active tuberculosis, studies have not used active tuberculosis as a surrogate marker for LTBI; instead, the majority of the work has been cross-sectional in design and focused on the concordance between the TST and IGRAs and correlating IGRA responses with risk factors for LTBI (Lalvani and Millington, 2008b).

Evaluation of the ELISpot in individuals with IMID has found that concordance between the IGRA and the TST is, in general, poor or moderate. In a study of 70 Greek patients with a variety of rheumatological conditions who were being screened for LTBI pre anti-TNF therapy, overall concordance between the ELISpot and the TST was moderate; discordant TST positive/ELISpot negative results were associated with prior BCG vaccination (Vassilopoulos et al., 2008). In a US study, Behar and colleagues evaluated the ELISpot in 200 patients with rheumatoid arthritis and found poor concordance between the two tests; in addition, the ELISpot was not associated significantly with risk factors for LTBI (Behar et al., 2009). Fewer authors have correlated ELISpot response with risk factors for tuberculosis exposure. Recent work from Ireland found that in patients with inflammatory arthritides there was a significant association between ELISpot positivity and risk factors for LTBI (Martin et al., 2009). Laffitte and colleagues compared the ELISpot and the TST in 50 patients with psoriasis and found that the ELISpot, but not the TST, was associated significantly with risk factors for LTBI (Laffitte et al., 2009). Similar conclusions that ELISpot results correlate with risk factors for LTBI can be drawn from an Italian study of a heterogeneous group of subjects awaiting anti-TNF therapy (Bocchino et al., 2008).

Compared to the ELISpot, the evidence base for ELISA performance in individuals with IMID is larger. Matulis and colleagues assessed the performance of the ELISA in subjects with inflammatory arthritides and found that concordance between the two tests was poor ($\kappa = 0.17$) (Matulis et al., 2008). Similarly, in a Turkish study of individuals with a range of inflammatory conditions, the ELISpot and the TST had a poor level of agreement ($\kappa = 0.18$) (Cobanoglu et al., 2007). Schoepfer et al. studied patients with inflam-

matory bowel disease undergoing screening pre anti-TNF therapy and found that agreement between the ELISpot and the TST was poor ($\kappa = -0.02$); in addition, TST but not ELISpot results were affected adversely by severe iatrogenic immunosuppression (Schoepfer et al., 2008). Although numerous authors have confirmed these findings of poor/moderate levels of concordance between TST and IGRA (Cobanoglu et al., 2007; Sellam et al., 2007; Takahashi et al., 2007; Ponce de Leon et al., 2008; Gogus et al., 2009; Shovman et al., 2009; Qumseya et al., 2011), these findings are not universal. In a recent Italian study, the ELISA was used to screen individuals with IMID and found a relatively high concordance between the TST and the ELISA (87.5%, $\kappa = 0.55$), with a lower proportion of TST+/IGRA– discordant results, which was likely to relate to the low proportion of the population who had previously been BCG vaccinated (4.1%) (Bartalesi et al., 2009).

As with the ELISpot, relatively few authors have correlated ELISA results with risk factors for LTBI. Bartalesi et al. studied 398 Italian IMID patients and found that both ELISA and TST positivity were associated significantly with being close contacts of patients with sputum smear-positive tuberculosis (Bartalesi et al., 2009). Two separate studies from Switzerland and Ireland in IMID patients undergoing pre anti-TNF screening found that ELISA positivity was associated significantly with risk factors for LTBI (Matulis et al., 2008; Martin et al., 2009).

The general consensus that can be drawn from the published evidence on the performance of the ELISpot and the ELISA is that in individuals with IMID on immunosuppressive therapy, IGRAs maintain their diagnostic sensitivity better than the TST, but false negative results are not uncommon and, therefore, given the need for a high index of suspicion and a low threshold for treatment initiation in this vulnerable population, an IGRA and TST should be used when screening patients for LTBI prior to initiation of anti-TNF treatment and a positive result in either test be taken as existence of LTBI and thus an indication for chemoprophylaxis (Lalvani and Millington, 2008b).

4.3.3 Specificity of IGRAs

To quantify specificity of the IGRAs (in other words, the ability to identify correctly those individuals that are not latently infected), investigators have studied BCG-vaccinated individuals who live in low tuberculosis burden regions with no known risk factors for tuberculosis infection who would, therefore, be reasonably expected to be at low risk of being exposed to *M. tuberculosis* and hence acquiring LTBI.

Two meta-analyses have been published which address the issue of IGRA specificity. In the first, Pai *et al.* concluded that the specificity of the ELISA ranged from 89% to 100%, with a pooled specificity of 99% for the second-generation ELISA and 96% for the latest generation, in-tube ELISA (Pai *et al.*, 2008). For the ELISpot, the authors found a similarly high diagnostic specificity of 85–100%, with a pooled specificity of 93% (Pai *et al.*, 2008). However, a more recent meta-analysis, which had different study inclusion criteria, found slightly different estimates for the pooled specificity of the IGRAs: 99% (range 98–100%) for the in-tube ELISA and 86% (range 81–90%) for the ELISpot (Diel *et al.*, 2010b). Although the figures may differ slightly, the overall conclusion remains unchanged – IGRAs have a higher specificity than the TST, particularly in BCG-vaccinated populations.

4.3.4 Clinical experience with IGRAs: frequency of indeterminate results

As the IGRAs begin to be more widely used, it is important to consider their reliability in routine clinical use. Both IGRAs are known to suffer from indeterminate results (Lalvani, 2007), which usually occur either due to problems with the test/blood collection or underlying cellular immunosuppression. Indeterminate results seem to be associated particularly with extremes of age (<5 or >80) or, especially for the ELISA, with underlying immunosuppression due to HIV immunosuppressive medication (Kobashi *et al.*, 2009). Diel *et al.* have recently collated the numbers of indeterminate results for the

IGRAs and found that the proportions are very similar for both platforms: 2.14% (95% confidence interval 2.0–2.3%) for the in-tube ELISA and 3.8% (3.5–4.2%) for the ELISpot (Diel *et al.*, 2010b).

4.3.5 Predictive value of IGRAs for progression to active tuberculosis

Much of the preceding discussion has focused on the performance of the IGRAs in different populations. However, the question that remains is – what does a positive IGRA result at baseline imply for an individual's future risk of developing active tuberculosis? This is a critical point because providing chemoprophylaxis for IGRA-positive individuals (especially contacts) will only be of benefit if they are at increased risk of progressing to active tuberculosis compared to individuals/contacts who are IGRA negative. Data of this type from prospective studies have started to accumulate since 2008 (Bakir *et al.*, 2008; Diel *et al.*, 2008b); recent systematic reviews and meta-analyses have shown that IGRAs and TST are similarly predictive of progression to active tuberculosis, although IGRAs do reduce the number of individuals requiring unnecessary chemoprophylaxis through improved specificity (Sester *et al.*, 2011; Rangaka *et al.*, 2012).

Studies from a range of settings have evaluated the predictive power of the ELISpot and, on the whole, have found that a positive response is prognostic for the future development of active tuberculosis. A study from an intermediate burden setting (Turkey) with 908 child contacts in which 15 incident cases occurred found that ELISpot-positive contacts had a significantly increased risk of developing active tuberculosis as compared to ELISpot-negative contacts (Bakir *et al.*, 2008). Although the incidence of active tuberculosis was similar in contacts who were ELISpot-positive versus those who were TST-positive (although the prognostic value of the TST, unlike the ELISpot, did not remain statistically significant), the ELISpot predicted these from fewer contacts tested (Bakir *et al.*, 2008). However, in this study, a large proportion of the children, as per national guidelines, received isoniazid chemoprophylaxis, which was likely to have resulted in an under-estimation of the incidence rate ratios for both the TST and the ELISpot. A recent Senegalese study of 2679 household contacts, among whom 52 cases of tuberculosis occurred (40 of which were culture con-firmed), using an in-house ELISpot found that positive IGRA responses at baseline predicted progression to active tuberculosis disease – although on multivariate analysis this was only significant for progression to culture-confirmed tuberculosis; higher ELISpot responses at baseline were associated significantly with progressing to tuberculosis disease (Lienhardt *et al.*, 2010). In addition, contacts who had a positive ELISpot and TST were more likely to progress than those who were dual negative on these tests (Lienhardt *et al.*, 2010). In a Hong Kong study of 308 male silicotic patients, without recent tuberculosis exposure, who were followed up for 2.5 years, the ELISpot predicted progression to active tuberculosis; Leung *et al.* found that 15/204 (7.4%) ELISpot-positive and 13/203 (6.4%) TST-positive ($\geq$10 mm) individuals progressed to active tuberculosis as compared to only 2/104 (1.9%) of ELISpot-negative and 4/105 (3.8%) of TST-negative subjects (Leung *et al.*, 2010). A smaller study from Holland of 339 immigrant contacts, however, came to different conclusions. Over a 2-year follow-up, there were nine cases among the cohort; ELISpot-positive immigrant contacts had a higher risk of progression than those who were negative at baseline (Kik *et al.*, 2010). However, the ELISpot did not have a higher positive predictive value for progression to active tuberculosis than the TST, although the small numbers meant that it was not powered adequately to ascertain the superiority of one test over another (Kik *et al.*, 2010).

In contrast to the above studies, a prospective study of 2348 household contacts in a Gambian setting did not come to the same conclusions (Hill *et al.*, 2008). During the course of the study, active tuberculosis occurred in 11/649 ELISpot-positive subjects as compared to 14/843 TST-positive subjects; in those who were ELISpot-negative or TST-negative, 10/1087 and 11/1387, respectively, developed tuberculosis (Hill *et al.*, 2008). The

investigators concluded that either the TST or the ELISpot were equivalent in screening contacts for LTBI but that neither test predicted subsequent progression to tuberculosis disease. This lack of predictive power for both TST and ELISpot may relate to the endemic setting where a substantial pro-portion of incident tuberculosis cases occur through *de novo* community transmission outside the household setting (Verver *et al.*, 2004), although in Senegal, where endemicity is similar, the ELISpot was found to be significantly predictive (Lienhardt *et al.*, 2010).

Evidence for the prognostic power of the ELISA first came via a small German study which investigated the ELISA in 601 contacts and found that a significantly higher pro-portion of untreated ELISA-positive, com-pared to 5-mm TST-positive, household contacts progressed to tuberculosis disease; all 6 incident cases were ELISA positive at recruitment (Diel *et al.*, 2008b). These data have very recently been updated with a longer duration of follow-up. Among 903 untreated contacts, a significantly higher pro-portion of ELISA-positive subjects (19/147) developed active tuberculosis as compared to those subjects with a 10-mm positive TST (10/207); no ELISA-negative subjects de-veloped active tuberculosis (Diel *et al.*, 2010a). Supporting data for these results come from a recent Japanese study of 3102 household contacts; over 2 years, 20/419 (4.8%) ELISA-positive contacts developed tuberculosis disease as compared to only 19/2683 (0.7%) of ELISA-negative contacts. The authors did not undertake large-scale TST on the contacts (Yoshiyama *et al.*, 2010). Two unpublished studies have also reported their findings in recent conferences (Haldar *et al.*, 2009; Mahomed *et al.*, 2011). Haldar *et al.* followed up 1309 household contacts and over a 2-year follow-up period found that 20/204 ELISA-positive contacts developed active tubercu-losis as compared to 0/835 ELISA-negative contacts (Haldar *et al.*, 2009). A further study from South Africa, which is still under way, is evaluating the predictive power of the ELISA in a cohort of adolescents over a 2-year follow-up period. The investigators found that ELISpot-positive individuals were more likely to progress to active tuberculosis disease than ELISpot-negative contacts. However, when comparing the predictive power of the ELISA and the TST, they found that similar proportions of ELISA-positive and TST-positive adolescents progressed to tuberculosis disease (38/3235 versus 37/2405) (Mahomed *et al.*, 2011).

Most of the studies outlined above have explored the prognostic power of the IGRA in immunocompetent subjects – mainly household contacts. However, the group where evidence is needed more urgently is in the immunocompromised – particularly those with HIV infection. Recently, Aichelberg *et al.* explored the prognostic power of a positive ELISA (QuantiFERON-Gold In-tube) result in HIV-positive individuals without active tuberculosis at recruitment (Aichelburg *et al.*, 2009). The investigators found that over a median follow-up period of 19 months, 3/37 individuals with a positive ELISA at baseline went on to develop active tuberculosis, whereas 0/738 with a negative ELISA subsequently developed tuberculosis (Aichelburg *et al.*, 2009). This study, therefore, confirmed that the ELISA was prognostic for the future development of active tuberculosis in HIV-positive subjects.

These longitudinal clinical outcome studies provide the first evidence that the IGRAs predict the future development of tuberculosis in a range of populations including: recent contacts, remotely infected individuals, children/adults, HIV negative/positive and low/high tuberculosis burden settings. This supports the use of IGRAs to target preventive therapy, particularly for recent IGRA-positive contacts, as it enables prevention of a similar number of cases as when using the TST but necessitates treatment of significantly fewer contacts. However some current areas of uncertainty, which will be addressed by future studies, do remain:

1. It is not known how much more predictive IGRAs are than the TST and to what extent the number needed to treat will be reduced.
2. It is not known which IGRA platform is superior in predicting the future development of future tuberculosis disease.

3. At a population level, it is unknown whether chemoprophylaxis on the basis of IGRA results will decrease tuberculosis incidence more than on the basis of TST results.

4.3.6 Summary of clinical data

As the output of IGRA research accumulates, several general conclusions can be drawn from the data that are currently available (see Table 4.5). Published studies have demonstrated that IGRAs are not confounded by previous BCG vaccination and are more specific than the TST in the diagnosis of LTBI (Pai *et al.*, 2008; Diel *et al.*, 2010b). With active disease used as a surrogate marker for LTBI, both IGRAs are more sensitive than the TST, with the ELISpot having a higher sensitivity than the ELISA (Pai *et al.*, 2008; Diel *et al.*, 2010b). In children and those with HIV infection, both the ELISpot and the ELISA seem to be superior to the TST – although published data indicate that the ELISpot performs better than the ELISA. In individuals with IMID undergoing immunosuppressive therapy, there is still a lack of evidence but, on the basis of what has been published, the ELISpot and the ELISA seem to have comparable efficacy.

4.4 Incorporation of IGRAs into International Public Health Guidelines

As the evidence base for IGRAs has evolved and developed, they have gained regulatory approval in a number of countries and have also been incorporated into national tuberculosis control guidelines. Most European countries and Canada advise that IGRAs should be used in two situations (National Collaborating Centre for Chronic Conditions, 2006; Public Health Agency of Canada, 2007):

1. As a confirmatory test in individuals who have already tested positive with the TST.
2. As a direct replacement for the TST in those individuals in whom the TST is likely to be unreliable (immunocompromised individuals).

Table 4.5. Clinical utility of interferon-gamma release assays (IGRAs).

	Diagnosis of LTBI		Diagnosis of active tuberculosis			
	Does a positive test rule in?	Does a negative test rule out?	Does a positive test rule in?	Does a negative test rule out?	Treatment monitoring	Test of cure
Immunocompetent subjects						
Adults	Yes	Yes	No	No[b]	No	No
Children (under 5 years)	Yes	Yes[a]	No	No[b]	No	No
Immunocompromised subjects						
Pre anti-TNF	Yes	Yes[a]	No	No[b]	No	No
HIV positive	Yes	Yes[a]	No	No[b]	No	No
Future directions	Incorporating additional antigens improves sensitivity without reducing specificity; for example, Rv3879c for the ELISpot[PLUS] (Dosanjh et al., 2008). Alternative cytokines such as IP-10 (Lalvani and Millington, 2008c; Ruhwald et al., 2008).				IL-2 and IFN-γ measurement holds promise in this setting (Millington et al., 2007; Lalvani and Millington, 2008a).	

Notes: [a]With caution and preferably should be used adjunctively with the TST to maximize sensitivity, as the TST will detect LTBI in some patients with false negative IGRA results; [b]diagnostic sensitivity of currently available IGRAs not yet high enough to rule out tuberculosis. Use of the TST in parallel can detect some patients with false negative IGRA results (Dosanjh et al., 2008).

Conversely, in the USA and Japan, guidelines recommend that IGRAs should be used in place of (but not in addition to) the TST when diagnosing LTBI – in all groups of individuals (Mazurek et al., 2005; CDC, 2010).

Economic considerations have been an important determinant in the disparate recommendations made by different countries. While IGRAs have a greater unit cost than the TST (Lalvani, 2007), health economic analyses have shown that with their increased specificity they reduce the number of individuals being treated with chemoprophylaxis unnecessarily (with the associated clinical and laboratory monitoring), which makes them a cost-effective option (Wrighton-Smith and Zellweger, 2006; Diel et al., 2007). The UK National Institute of Health and Clinical Excellence (NICE) also undertook their own economic analyses and concluded that the two-step TST and confirmatory IGRA approach would be most cost-effective, forming the basis of the recommendation made by NICE and subsequently adopted by most other European countries (National Collaborating Centre for Chronic Conditions, 2006). Recent work has highlighted the cost effectiveness of using single step IGRA testing in diagnosing LTBI in migrants (Pareek et al., 2011).

The two-step TST and confirmatory approach recommended by Europe and Canada has the potential drawback that individuals with a negative TST who may have had a positive IGRA will not be diagnosed with LTBI and therefore not offered the appropriate chemoprophylaxis. In contrast, the US and Japanese recommendations could, potentially, result in overtreatment of individuals who are IGRA positive but TST negative – as the risk of subsequently progressing to active tuberculosis disease in this group with discordant results is not known (Fig. 4.1). Further research is urgently needed to quantify the risk of individuals with discordant IGRA/TST results progressing to active tuberculosis.

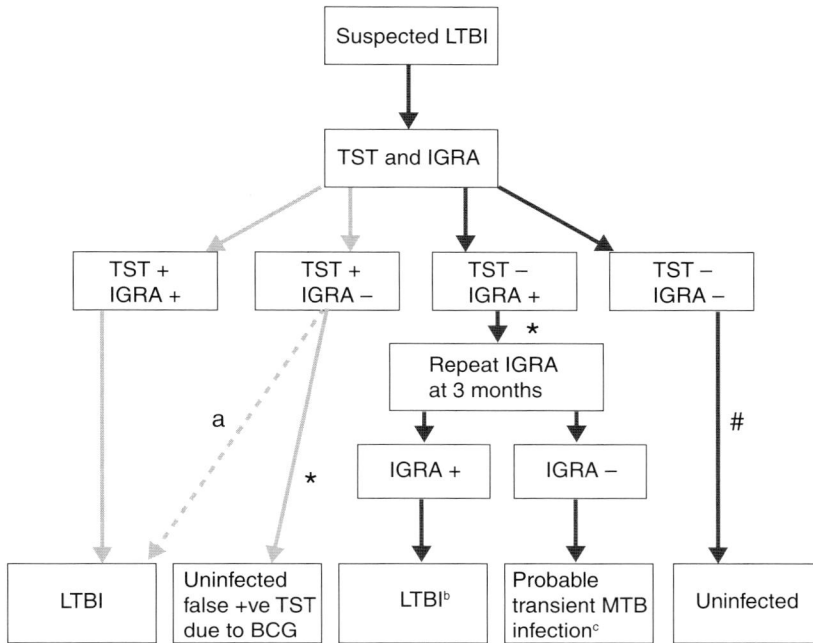

Fig. 4.1. Algorithm of all possible outcomes resulting from parallel IGRA and TST testing.*

┈┈▷ NICE guidance

──▶ Defines outcomes not captured by NICE guidance, which mandates undertaking the TST first followed by the IGRA in TST-positive individuals except in the immunosuppressed population, where IGRA only testing is recommended

Notes: Negative TST and IGRA indicates no infection. Positive TST and IGRA indicates LTBI. (a) With strong evidence for LTBI (e.g. >25-mm TST, ulcerating Mantoux, calcified lesions on chest x-ray), the possibility of false negative IGRA must be considered. (b) Risk of active tuberculosis development in this group is not yet known. (c) Longitudinal contact studies have defined a group of TST-negative individuals with transiently positive IGRAs, raising the possibility that some TST-negative contacts acquire and spontaneously clear transient *M. tuberculosis* infection. *A positive TST/IGRA must be evaluated carefully in immunocompromised patients in whom any positive result is significant. #Dual negative TST and IGRA results normally indicate the exclusion of tuberculosis infection but negative results should be evaluated carefully in immunocompromised patients.

This highlights the urgent need for more longitudinal data to quantify the predictive value of positive IGRA results and, in particular, the prognosis of contacts with discordant IGRA and TST results.

4.5 Treatment Monitoring and Future Directions

Although IGRAs have upgraded the TST, by which we can diagnose LTBI, they remain a work in progress with an evolving clinical and evidence base. This has meant that their limitations are becoming clearer. Neither IGRA can differentiate between active and latent tuberculosis and prospective studies which have undertake serial IGRA testing have highlighted the dynamic nature of IGRA responses during the course of treatment for active tuberculosis – which means that they cannot be used to monitor treatment response or as a test of cure (Lalvani, 2007). However, recent evidence that simultaneous profiling of IL-2 and IFN-γ secretion at the single T-cell level correlates with therapeutic response may be useful in disease monitoring (Millington *et al.*, 2007; Lalvani and Millington, 2008a).

Despite the current generation of IGRAs having higher sensitivity than the TST, research indicates that next-generation assays will have even higher sensitivity. This has been achieved by the next-generation ELISA and ELISpot including additional antigens (Liu *et al.*, 2004). Incorporating novel antigens, Rv2645 for the in-tube ELISA (Harada *et al.*, 2008) and RV3879c for the ELISpot[PLUS] (Dosanjh *et al.*, 2008), alongside ESAT-6 and CFP-10 has been shown in recent studies to improve sensitivity significantly without compromising specificity. Additionally, new mycobacterial antigens are being explored, such as heparin-binding haemagglutinin, which may help to distinguish active from latent tuberculosis (Place *et al.*, 2010).

Studies are also exploring whether measuring alternative, downstream chemokines secreted by IFN-γ-activated macrophages such as inducible protein 10 (IP-10), in combination with IFN-γ, may serve as a more amplified readout than IFN-γ alone, thereby resulting in higher sensitivity (Lalvani and Millington, 2008c; Ruhwald *et al.*, 2008).

A further area of ongoing research is focusing on whether IGRAs will be able to differentiate individuals who have been infected recently and remotely; the relevance of this being that those who are recently infected are more likely to progress to active tuberculosis and should, therefore, be given chemoprophylaxis. Evidence to date, however, suggests that IGRAs are unable to differentiate recent from remote infection (Hinks *et al.*, 2009).

4.6 Conclusions

With the recent development of IGRAs, the diagnosis of LTBI has moved on from the century-old TST. Evidence of their use in different settings and populations has expanded rapidly and IGRAs are an integral part of many national guidelines on LTBI diagnosis. However, further work is needed to understand the relevance of discordant IGRA and TST results and whether next-generation IGRAs will have improved sensitivity without compromising specificity.

Conflict of Interest Statement

Professor Lalvani is the inventor of several patents underpinning T-cell-based diagnosis. The ESAT-6/CFP-10 IFN-γ ELISpot was commercialized by an Oxford University spin-out company (T-SPOT.TB®, Oxford Immunotec Ltd, Abingdon, UK) in which Oxford University and Professor Lalvani have a minority share of equity and royalty entitlements.

References

Aabye, M.G., Ravn, P., Praygod, G., Jeremiah, K., Mugomela, A., Jepsen, M., *et al.* (2009) The impact of HIV infection and CD4 cell count on the performance of an interferon gamma release assay in patients with pulmonary tuberculosis. *PLoS ONE* 4, e4220.

Aichelburg, M.C., Rieger, A., Breitenecker, F., Pfistershammer, K., Tittes, J., Eltz, S., *et al.* (2009) Detection and prediction of active tuberculosis disease by a whole-blood interferon-gamma release assay in HIV-1-infected individuals. *Clinical Infectious Disease* 48, 954–962.

American Thoracic Society [ATS] and Centers for Disease Control and Prevention [CDC] (2000) Targeted tuberculin testing and treatment of latent tuberculosis infection. *American Journal of Respiratory and Critical Care Medicine* 161, 221S–247.

Bakir, M., Millington, K.A., Soysal, A., Deeks, J.J., Efee, S., Aslan, Y., *et al.* (2008) Prognostic value of a T-cell-based, interferon-gamma biomarker in children with tuberculosis contact. *Annuals of Internal Medicine* 149, 777–787.

Balcells, M.E., Perez, C.M., Chanqueo, L., Lasso, M., Villanueva, M., Espinoza, M., *et al.* (2008) A comparative study of two different methods for the detection of latent tuberculosis in HIV-positive individuals in Chile. *International Journal of Infectious Diseases* 12, 645–652.

Bartalesi, F., Vicidomini, S., Goletti, D., Fiorelli, C., Fiori, G., Melchiorre, D., *et al.* (2009) QuantiFERON-TB Gold and the TST are both useful for latent tuberculosis infection screening in autoimmune diseases. *European Respiratory Journal* 33, 586–593.

Bean, A.G., Roach, D.R., Briscoe, H., France, M.P., Korner, H., Sedgwick, J.D., *et al.* (1999) Structural deficiencies in granuloma formation in TNF gene-targeted mice underlie the heightened susceptibility to aerosol *Mycobacterium tuberculosis* infection, which is not compensated for by lymphotoxin. *Journal of Immunology* 162, 3504–3511.

Behar, S.M., Shin, D.S., Maier, A., Coblyn, J., Helfgott, S. and Weinblatt, M.E. (2009) Use of the T-SPOT.TB assay to detect latent tuberculosis infection among rheumatic disease patients on immunosuppressive therapy. *The Journal of Rheumatology* 36, 546–551.

Bocchino, M., Matarese, A., Bellofiore, B., Giacomelli, P., Santoro, G., Balato, N., *et al.* (2008) Performance of two commercial blood IFN-gamma release assays for the detection of *Mycobacterium tuberculosis* infection in patient candidates for anti-TNF-alpha treatment. *European Journal of Clinical Microbiology and Infectious Diseases* 27, 907–913.

Brock, I., Weldingh, K., Lillebaek, T., Follmann, F. and Andersen, P. (2004) Comparison of tuberculin skin test and new specific blood test in tuberculosis contacts. *American Journal of Respiratory and Critical Care Medicine* 170, 65–69.

Brock, I., Ruhwald, M., Lundgren, B., Westh, H., Mathiesen, L.R. and Ravn, P. (2006) Latent tuberculosis in HIV positive, diagnosed by the *M. tuberculosis* specific interferon-gamma test. *Respiratory Research* 7, 56.

Cain, K.P., Benoit, S.R., Winston, C.A. and MacKenzie, W.R. (2008) Tuberculosis among foreign-born persons in the United States. *JAMA* 300, 405–412.

Centers for Disease Control and Prevention [CDC] (2010) Updated guidelines for using interferon gamma release assays to detect *Mycobacterium tuberculosis* infection. *MMWR* 59, 1–25.

Chapman, A.L., Munkanta, M., Wilkinson, K.A., Pathan, A.A., Ewer, K., Ayles, H., *et al.* (2002) Rapid detection of active and latent tuberculosis infection in HIV-positive individuals by enumeration of *Mycobacterium tuberculosis*-specific T cells. *AIDS* 16, 2285–2293.

Chee, C.B.E., Gan, S.H., Khinmar, K.W., Barkham, T.M., Koh, C.K., Liang, S. and Wang, Y.T. (2008) Comparison of sensitivities of two commercial gamma interferon release assays for pulmonary tuberculosis. *Journal of Clinical Microbiology* 46, 1935–1940.

Chun, J.K., Kim, C.K., Kim, H.S., Jung, G.Y., Lee, T.J., Kim, K.H., *et al.* (2008) The role of a whole blood interferon-gamma assay for the detection of latent tuberculosis infection in Bacille Calmette–Guerin vaccinated children. *Diagnostic Microbiology and Infectious Disease* 62, 389–394.

Clark, S.A., Martin, S.L., Pozniak, A., Steel, A., Ward, B., Dunning, J., *et al.* (2007) Tuberculosis antigen-specific immune responses can be detected using enzyme-linked immunospot technology in human immunodeficiency virus (HIV)-1 patients with advanced disease. *Clinical and Experimental Immunology* 150, 238–244.

Cobanoglu, N., Ozcelik, U., Kalyoncu, U., Ozen, S., Kiraz, S., Gurcan, N., *et al.* (2007) Interferon-gamma assays for the diagnosis of tuberculosis infection before using tumour necrosis factor-alpha blockers. *The International Journal of Tuberculosis and Lung Disease* 11, 1177–1182.

Comstock, G.W., Livesay, V.T. and Woolpert, S.F. (1974) The prognosis of a positive tuberculin reaction in childhood and adolescence. *The American Journal of Epidemiology* 99, 131–138.

Connell, T.G., Curtis, N., Ranganathan, S.C. and Buttery, J.P. (2006) Performance of a whole blood interferon gamma assay for detecting latent infection with *Mycobacterium tuberculosis* in children. *Thorax* 61, 616–620.

Connell, T.G., Ritz, N., Paxton, G.A., Buttery, J.P., Curtis, N. and Ranganathan, S.C. (2008) A three-way comparison of tuberculin skin testing, QuantiFERON-TB Gold and T-SPOT.TB in children. *PLoS ONE* 3, e2624.

Cooper, A.M. and Flynn, J.L. (1995) The protective immune response to *Mycobacterium tuberculosis*. *Current Opinion in Immunology* 7, 512–516.

Corbett, E.L., Watt, C.J., Walker, N., Maher, D., Williams, B.G., Raviglione, M.C., *et al.* (2003) The growing burden of tuberculosis: global trends and interactions with the HIV epidemic. *Archives of Internal Medicine* 163, 1009–1021.

Detjen, A., Keil, T., Roll, S., Hauer, B., Mauch, H., Wahn, U., *et al.* (2007) Interferon-gamma release assays improve the diagnosis of tuberculosis and nontuberculous mycobacterial disease in children in a country with a low incidence of tuberculosis. *Clinical Infectious Disease* 45, 322–328.

Dheda, K., Lalvani, A., Miller, R.F., Scott, G., Booth, H., Johnson, M.A., *et al.* (2005) Performance of a T-cell-based diagnostic test for tuberculosis infection in HIV-infected individuals is independent of CD4 cell count. *AIDS* 19, 2038–2041.

Diel, R., Nienhaus, A. and Loddenkemper, R. (2007) Cost-effectiveness of interferon-{gamma} release assay screening for latent tuberculosis infection treatment in Germany. *Chest* 131, 1424–1434.

Diel, R., Loddenkemper, R., Meywald-Walter, K., Gottschalk, R. and Nienhaus, A. (2008a) Comparative performance of tuberculin skin test, QuantiFERON-TB-Gold in tube assay, and T-Spot.TB test in contact investigations for tuberculosis. *Chest* 135, 1010–1018.

Diel, R., Loddenkemper, R., Meywald-Walter, K., Niemann, S. and Nienhaus, A. (2008b) Predictive value of a whole blood IFN-gamma assay for the development of active tuberculosis disease after recent infection with *Mycobacterium tuberculosis*. *American Journal of Respiratory and Critical Care Medicine* 177, 1164–1170.

Diel, R., Loddenkemper, R., Niemann, S., Meywald-Walter, K. and Nienhaus, A. (2010a) Negative and positive predictive value of a whole-blood IGRA for developing active TB – an update. *American Journal of Respiratory and Critical Care Medicine* 183, 88–95.

Diel, R., Loddenkemper, R. and Nienhaus, A. (2010b) Evidence-based comparison of commercial interferon-gamma release assays for detecting active TB. *Chest* 137, 952–968.

Dogra, S., Narang, P., Mendiratta, D.K., Chaturvedi, P., Reingold, A.L., Colford, J.J.M., *et al.* (2007) Comparison of a whole blood interferon-gamma assay with tuberculin skin testing for the detection of tuberculosis infection in hospitalized children in rural India. *Journal of Infection* 54, 267–276.

Dominguez, J., Ruiz-Manzano, J., De Souza-Galvao, M., Latorre, I., Mila, C., Blanco, S., *et al.* (2008) Comparison of two commercially available gamma interferon blood tests for immunodiagnosis of tuberculosis. *Clinical and Vaccine Immunology* 15, 168–171.

Dosanjh, D.P., Hinks, T.S., Innes, J.A., Deeks, J.J., Pasvol, G., Hackforth, S., *et al.* (2008) Improved diagnostic evaluation of suspected tuberculosis. *Annals of Internal Medicine* 148, 325–336.

Dye, C., Scheele, S., Dolin, P., Pathania, V. and Raviglione, M.C. (1999) Consensus statement. Global burden of tuberculosis: estimated incidence, prevalence, and mortality by country. WHO Global Surveillance and Monitoring Project. *JAMA* 282, 677–686.

Ewer, K., Deeks, J., Alvarez, L., Bryant, G., Waller, S., Andersen, P., *et al.* (2003) Comparison of T-cell-based assay with tuberculin skin test for diagnosis of *Mycobacterium tuberculosis* infection in a school tuberculosis outbreak. *The Lancet* 361, 1168–1173.

Gogus, F., Gunendi, Z., Karakus, R., Erdogan, Z., Hizel, K. and Atalay, F. (2009) Comparison of tuberculin skin test and QuantiFERON-TB gold in tube test in patients with chronic inflammatory diseases living in a tuberculosis endemic population. *Clinical and Experimental Medicine* 10,173–177.

Goletti, D., Carrara, S., Vincenti, D. and Girardi, E. (2007) T cell responses to commercial *Mycobacterium tuberculosis* specific antigens in HIV-infected patients. *Clinical Infectious Diseases* 45, 1652–1654.

Grzybowski, S. and Enarson, D. (1978) Results in pulmonary tuberculosis patients under various treatment program conditions. *Bulletin International Union against Tuberculosis and Lung Disease* 53, 70–75.

Haldar, P., Thuraisingham, H., Hoskyns, W. and Woltmann, G. (2009) Contact screening with single-step TIGRA testing and risk of active TB infection: The Leicester Cohort Analysis. *Thorax* 64, A13.

Harada, N., Higuchi, K., Yoshiyama, T., Kawabe, Y., Fujita, A., Sasaki, Y., *et al.* (2008) Comparison of the sensitivity and specificity of two whole blood interferon-gamma assays for *M. tuberculosis* infection. *Journal of Infection* 56, 348–353.

Harboe, M., Oettinger, T., Wiker, H.G., Rosenkrands, I. and Andersen, P. (1996) Evidence for occurrence of the ESAT-6 protein in *Mycobacterium tuberculosis* and virulent *Mycobacterium bovis* and for its absence in *Mycobacterium bovis* BCG. *Infection and Immunity* 64, 16–22.

Hill, P.C., Brookes, R.H., Adetifa, I.M., Fox, A., Jackson-Sillah, D., Lugos, M.D., *et al.* (2006) Comparison of enzyme-linked immunospot assay and tuberculin skin test in healthy children exposed to *Mycobacterium tuberculosis*. *Pediatrics* 117, 1542–1548.

Hill, P.C., Brookes, R.H., Fox, A., Jackson-Sillah, D., Jeffries, D.J., Lugos, M.D., *et al.* (2007) Longitudinal assessment of an ELISPOT test for *Mycobacterium tuberculosis* infection. *PLoS Medicine* 4, e192.

Hill, P.C., Jackson-Sillah, D.J., Fox, A., Brookes, R.H., De Jong, B.C., Lugos, M.D., *et al.* (2008) Incidence of tuberculosis and the predictive value of ELISPOT and Mantoux tests in Gambian case contacts. *PLoS ONE* 3, e1379.

Hinks, T.S.C., Dosanjh, D.P.S., Innes, J.A., Pasvol, G., Hackforth, S., Varia, H., *et al.* (2009) Frequencies of region of difference 1 antigen-specific but not purified protein derivative-specific gamma interferon-secreting T cells correlate with the presence of tuberculosis disease but do not distinguish recent from remote latent infections. *Infection and Immunity* 77, 5486–5495.

Horsburgh, C.R. Jr (2004) Priorities for the treatment of latent tuberculosis infection in the

United States. *The New England Journal of Medicine* 350, 2060–2067.

Houk, V.N., Baker, J.H., Sorensen, K. and Kent, D.C. (1968) The epidemiology of tuberculosis infection in a closed environment. *Archives of Environmental Health* 16, 26–35.

Jones, S., De Gijsel, D., Wallach, F.R., Gurtman, A.C., Shi, Q. and Sacks, H. (2007) Utility of QuantiFERON-TB Gold in-tube testing for latent TB infection in HIV-infected individuals. *The International Journal of Tuberculosis and Lung Disease* 11, 1190–1195.

Kampmann, B., Whittaker, E., Williams, A., Walters, S., Gordon, A., Martinez-Alier, N., *et al.* (2009) Interferon-γ release assays do not identify more children with active tuberculosis than the tuberculin skin test. *European Respiratory Journal* 33, 1374–1382.

Kang, Y.A., Lee, H.W., Yoon, H.I., Cho, B., Han, S.K., Shim, Y.S., *et al.* (2005) Discrepancy between the tuberculin skin test and the whole-blood interferon gamma assay for the diagnosis of latent tuberculosis infection in an intermediate tuberculosis-burden country. *JAMA* 293, 2756–2761.

Kenyon, T.A., Valway, S.E., Ihle, W.W., Onorato, I.M. and Castro, K.G. (1996) Transmission of multidrug-resistant *Mycobacterium tuberculosis* during a long airplane flight. *The New England Journal of Medicine* 334, 993–938.

Kik, S.V., Franken, W.P.J., Mensen, M., Cobelens, F.G.J., Kamphorst, M., Arend, S.M., *et al.* (2010) Predictive value for progression to tuberculosis by IGRA and TST in immigrant contacts. *European Respiratory Journal* 35, 1346–1353.

Kobashi, Y., Sugiu, T., Mouri, K., Obase, Y., Miyashita, N. and Oka, M. (2009) Indeterminate results of QuantiFERON TB-2G test performed in routine clinical practice. *European Respiratory Journal* 33, 812–815.

Laffitte, E., Janssens, J.P., Roux-Lombard, P., Thielen, A.M., Barde, C., Marazza, G., *et al.* (2009) Tuberculosis screening in patients with psoriasis before antitumour necrosis factor therapy: comparison of an interferon-gamma release assay vs. tuberculin skin test. *British Journal of Dermatology* 161, 797–800.

Lalvani, A. (2003) Spotting latent infection: the path to better tuberculosis control. *Thorax* 58, 916–918.

Lalvani, A. (2007) Diagnosing tuberculosis infection in the 21st century: new tools to tackle an old enemy. *Chest* 131, 1898–1906.

Lalvani, A. and Millington, K.A. (2007) T cell-based diagnosis of childhood tuberculosis infection. *Current Opinion in Infectious Diseases* 20, 264–271.

Lalvani, A. and Millington, K.A. (2008a) T cells and tuberculosis: beyond interferon-gamma. *The Journal of Infectious Diseases* 197, 941–943.

Lalvani, A. and Millington, K.A. (2008b) Screening for tuberculosis infection prior to initiation of anti-TNF therapy. *Autoimmunity Reviews* 8, 147–152.

Lalvani, A. and Millington, K.A. (2008c) T-cell interferon-{gamma} release assays: can we do better? *European Respiratory Journal* 32, 1428–1430.

Lalvani, A. and Pareek, M. (2009) A 100 year update on diagnosis of tuberculosis infection. *British Medical Bulletin* 93, 69–84.

Lalvani, A., Pathan, A.A., Durkan, H., Wilkinson, K.A., Whelan, A., Deeks, J.J., *et al.* (2001a) Enhanced contact tracing and spatial tracking of *Mycobacterium tuberculosis* infection by enumeration of antigen-specific T cells. *The Lancet* 357, 2017–2021.

Lalvani, A., Pathan, A.A., McShane, H., Wilkinson, R.J., Latif, M., Conlon, C.P., *et al.* (2001b) Rapid detection of *Mycobacterium tuberculosis* infection by enumeration of antigen-specific T cells. *American Journal of Respiratory and Critical Care Medicine* 163, 824–828.

Lee, J.Y., Choi, H.J., Park, I.N., Hong, S.B., Oh, Y.M., Lim, C.M., *et al.* (2006) Comparison of two commercial interferon-gamma assays for diagnosing *Mycobacterium tuberculosis* infection. *European Respiratory Journal* 28, 24–30.

Leung, C.C., Yam, W.C., Yew, W.W., Ho, P.L., Tam, C.M., Law, W.S., *et al.* (2010) T-Spot.TB outperforms tuberculin skin test in predicting tuberculosis disease. *American Journal of Respiratory and Critical Care Medicine* 182, 834–840.

Liebeschuetz, S., Bamber, S., Ewer, K., Deeks, J., Pathan, A.A. and Lalvani, A. (2004) Diagnosis of tuberculosis in South African children with a T-cell-based assay: a prospective cohort study. *The Lancet* 364, 2196–2203.

Lienhardt, C., Fielding, K., Hane, A.A., Niang, A., Ndao, C.T., Karam, F., *et al.* (2010) Evaluation of the prognostic value of IFN-γ release assay and tuberculin skin test in household contacts of infectious tuberculosis cases in Senegal. *PLoS ONE* 5, e10508.

Lighter, J., Rigaud, M., Eduardo, R., Peng, C.H. and Pollack, H. (2009) Latent tuberculosis diagnosis in children by using the QuantiFERON-TB Gold in-tube test. *Pediatrics* 123, 30–37.

Liu, X.-Q., Dosanjh, D., Varia, H., Ewer, K., Cockle, P., Pasvol, G., *et al.* (2004) Evaluation of T-cell responses to novel RD1- and RD2-encoded *Mycobacterium tuberculosis* gene products for specific detection of human tuberculosis infection. *Infection and Immunity* 72, 2574–2581.

Luetkemeyer, A.F., Charlebois, E.D., Flores, L.L., Bangsberg, D.R., Deeks, S.G., Martin, J.N., *et al.* (2007) Comparison of an interferon-{gamma} release assay with tuberculin skin testing in HIV-infected individuals. *American Journal of Respiratory and Critical Care Medicine* 175, 737–742.

MacPherson, D.W. and Gushulak, B.D. (2006) Balancing prevention and screening among international migrants with tuberculosis: population mobility as the major epidemiological influence in low-incidence nations. *Public Health* 120, 712–723.

Mahairas, G.G., Sabo, P.J., Hickey, M.J., Singh, D.C. and Stover, C.K. (1996) Molecular analysis of genetic differences between *Mycobacterium bovis* BCG and virulent *M. bovis*. *Journal of Bacteriology* 178, 1274–1282.

Mahomed, H., Hawkridge, T., Verver, S., Abrahams, D., Geiter, L., Hatherill, M., *et al.* (2011) The tuberculin skin test versus QuantiFERON TB Gold® in predicting tuberculosis disease in an adolescent cohort study in South Africa. *PLoS ONE* 6(3), e17984.

Mandalakas, A.M., Hesseling, A.C., Chegou, N.N., Kirchner, H.L., Zhu, X., Marais, B.J., *et al.* (2008) High level of discordant IGRA results in HIV-infected adults and children. *The International Journal of Tuberculosis and Lung Disease* 12, 417–423.

Martin, J., Walsh, C., Gibbs, A., McDonnell, T., Fearon, U., Keane, J., *et al.* (2009) Comparison of interferon-{gamma}-release assays and conventional screening tests before tumour necrosis factor-{alpha} blockade in patients with inflammatory arthritis. *Annals of the Rheumatic Diseases* 69, 181–185.

Matulis, G., Juni, P., Villiger, P.M. and Gadola, S.D. (2008) Detection of latent tuberculosis in immunosuppressed patients with autoimmune diseases: performance of a *Mycobacterium tuberculosis* antigen-specific interferon gamma assay. *Annals of the Rheumatic Diseases* 67, 84–90.

Mazurek, G.H., Jereb, J., Lobue, P., Iademarco, M.F., Metchock, B., Vernon, A., *et al.* (2005) Guidelines for using the QuantiFERON-TB Gold test for detecting *Mycobacterium tuberculosis* infection, United States. *MMWR Recommendations and Reports* 54, 49–55.

Millington, K.A., Innes, J.A., Hackforth, S., Hinks, T.S., Deeks, J.J., Dosanjh, D.P., *et al.* (2007) Dynamic relationship between IFN-gamma and IL-2 profile of *Mycobacterium tuberculosis*-specific T cells and antigen load. *Journal of Immunology* 178, 5217–5226.

Mori, T., Sakatani, M., Yamagishi, F., Takashima, T., Kawabe, Y., Nagao, K., *et al.* (2004) Specific detection of tuberculosis infection: an interferon-gamma-based assay using new antigens. *American Journal of Respiratory and Critical Care Medicine* 170, 59–64.

Murray, P.J. (1999) Defining the requirements for immunological control of mycobacterial infections. *Trends in Microbiology* 7, 366–372.

Mutsvangwa, J., Millington, K.A., Chaka, K., Mavhudzi, T., Cheung, Y.-B., Mason, P.R., *et al.* (2010) Identifying recent *Mycobacterium tuberculosis* transmission in the setting of high HIV and TB burden. *Thorax* 65, 315–320.

Nakaoka, H., Lawson, L., Squire, S.B., Coulter, B., Ravn, P., Brock, I., *et al.* (2006) Risk for tuberculosis among children. *Emerging Infectious Diseases* 12, 1383–1388.

National Collaborating Centre for Chronic Conditions (2006) *Tuberculosis: Clinical Diagnosis and Management of Tuberculosis, and Measures for its Prevention and Control.* Royal College of Physicians, London.

Nicol, M.P., Davies, M.-A., Wood, K., Hatherill, M., Workman, L., Hawkridge, A., *et al.* (2009) Comparison of T-SPOT.TB assay and tuberculin skin test for the evaluation of young children at high risk for tuberculosis in a community setting. *Pediatrics* 123, 38–43.

Okada, K., Mao, T.E., Mori, T., Miura, T., Sugiyama, T., Yoshiyama, T., *et al.* (2008) Performance of an interferon-gamma release assay for diagnosing latent tuberculosis infection in children. *Epidemiology and Infection* 136, 1179–1187.

Pareek, M., Watson, J.P., Omerod, L.P., Kon, O.M., Woltmann, G., White, P.J., *et al.* (2011) Screening of immigration in the UK for imported latent tuberculosis: a multicentre cohort study and cost-effectiveness analysis. *Lancet Infectious Diseases* 11, 434–444.

Pai, M., Zwerling, A. and Menzies, D. (2008) Systematic review: T-cell-based assays for the diagnosis of latent tuberculosis infection: an update. *Annals of Internal Medicine* 149, 177–184.

Place, S., Verscheure, V., De San, N., Hougardy, J.-M., Schepers, K., Dirix, V., *et al.* (2010) Heparin-binding, hemagglutinin-specific IFN-{gamma} synthesis at the site of infection during active tuberculosis in humans. *American Journal of Respiratory and Critical Care Medicine* 182, 848–854.

Ponce de Leon, D., Acevedo-Vasquez, E., Alvizuri, S.G.C. and Cucho, M., *et al.* (2008) Comparison of an interferon-gamma assay with tuberculin skin testing for detection of tuberculosis (TB) infection in patients with rheumatoid arthritis in a TB-endemic population. *Journal of Rheumatology* 35, 776–781.

Public Health Agency of Canada (2007) Interferon gamma release assays for latent tuberculosis infection: an Advisory Committee Statement. *Canada Communicable Disease Report* 33, 1–18.

Qumseya, B.J., Ananthakrishnan, A.N., Skaros, S., Bonner, M., Issa, M., Zadvornova, Y., *et al.* (2011) QuantiFERON TB gold testing for tuberculosis screening in an inflammatory bowel disease cohort in the United States. *Inflammatory Bowel Diseases* 17, 77–83.

Raby, E., Moyo, M., Devendra, A., Banda, J., De Haas, P., Ayles, H., *et al.* (2008) The effects of HIV on the sensitivity of a whole blood IFN-γ release assay in Zambian adults with active tuberculosis. *PLoS ONE* 3, e2489.

Rangaka, M.X., Diwakar, L., Seldon, R., Van Cutsem, G., Meintjes, G.A., Morroni, C., *et al.* (2007a) Clinical, immunological, and epidemiological importance of antituberculosis T cell responses in HIV- infected Africans. *Clinical Infectious Diseases* 44, 1639–1646.

Rangaka, M.X., Wilkinson, K.A., Seldon, R., Van Cutsem, G., Meintjes, G.A., Morroni, C., *et al.* (2007b) Effect of HIV-1 infection on T-cell-based and skin test detection of tuberculosis infection. *American Journal of Respiratory and Critical Care Medicine* 175, 514–520.

Rangaka, M.X., Wilkinson, K.A., Glynn, J.R., Ling, D., Menzies, D., Mwansa-Kambafwile, J., *et al.* (2012) Predictive value of interferon-gamma release assays for incident active tuberculosis: a systematic review and meta-analysis. *The Lancet Infectious Diseases* 12, 45–55.

Richeldi, L. (2006) An update on the diagnosis of tuberculosis infection. *American Journal of Respiratory and Critical Care Medicine* 174, 736–742.

Richeldi, L., Ewer, K., Losi, M., Bergamini, B.M., Roversi, P., Deeks, J., *et al.* (2004) T cell-based tracking of multidrug resistant tuberculosis infection after brief exposure. *American Journal of Respiratory and Critical Care Medicine* 170, 288–295.

Ruhwald, M., Bodmer, T., Maier, C., Jepsen, M., Haaland, M.B., Eugen-Olsen, J., *et al.* (2008) Evaluating the potential of IP-10 and MCP-2 as biomarkers for the diagnosis of tuberculosis. *European Respiratory Journal* 32, 1607–1615.

Schoepfer, A.M., Flogerzi, B., Fallegger, S., Schaffer, T., Mueller, S., Nicod, L., *et al.* (2008) Comparison of interferon-gamma release assay versus tuberculin skin test for tuberculosis screening in inflammatory bowel disease. *The American Journal of Gastroenterology* 103, 2799–2806.

Sellam, J., Hamdi, H., Roy, C., Baron, G., Lemann, M., Puechal, X., *et al.* (2007) Comparison of *in vitro*-specific blood tests with tuberculin skin test for diagnosis of latent tuberculosis before anti-TNF therapy. *Annals of the Rheumatic Diseases* 66, 1610–1615.

Sester, M., Sotgiu, G., Lange, C., Giehl, C., Girardi, E., Migliori, G.B., *et al.* (2011) Interferon-γ release assays for the diagnosis of active tuberculosis: a systematic review and meta-analysis. *European Respiratory Journal* 37, 100–111.

Shams, H., Weis, S.E., Klucar, P., Lalvani, A., Moonan, P.K., Pogoda, J.M., *et al.* (2005) Enzyme-linked immunospot and tuberculin skin testing to detect latent tuberculosis infection. *American Journal of Respiratory and Critical Care Medicine* 172, 1161–1168.

Shovman, O., Anouk, M., Vinnitsky, N., Arad, U., Paran, D., Litinsky, I., *et al.* (2009) QuantiFERON-TB Gold in the identification of latent tuberculosis infection in rheumatoid arthritis: a pilot study. *International Journal of Tuberculosis and Lung Disease* 13, 1427–1432.

Soysal, A., Millington, K.A., Bakir, M., Dosanjh, D., Aslan, Y., Deeks, J.J., *et al.* (2005) Effect of BCG vaccination on risk of *Mycobacterium tuberculosis* infection in children with household tuberculosis contact: a prospective community-based study. *The Lancet* 366, 1443–1451.

Soysal, A., Torun, T., Efe, S., Gencer, H., Tahaoglu, K. and Bakir, M. (2008) Evaluation of cut-off values of interferon-gamma-based assays in the diagnosis of *M. tuberculosis* infection. *The International Journal of Tuberculosis and Lung Disease* 12, 50–56.

Stead, W.W. (1978) Undetected tuberculosis in prison. Source of infection for community at large. *JAMA* 240, 2544–2547.

Stephan, C., Wolf, T., Goetsch, U., Bellinger, O., Nisius, G., Oremek, G., *et al.* (2008) Comparing QuantiFERON-tuberculosis gold, T-SPOT tuberculosis and tuberculin skin test in HIV-infected individuals from a low prevalence tuberculosis country. *AIDS* 22, 2471–2479.

Takahashi, H., Shigehara, K., Yamamoto, M., Suzuki, C., Naishiro, Y., Tamura, Y., *et al.* (2007) Interferon gamma assay for detecting latent tuberculosis infection in rheumatoid arthritis patients during infliximab administration. *Rheumatology International* 27, 1143–1148.

Talati, N., Seybold, U., Humphrey, B., Aina, A., Tapia, J., Weinfurter, P., *et al.* (2009) Poor concordance between interferon-gamma release assays and tuberculin skin tests in diagnosis of latent tuberculosis infection among HIV-infected individuals. *BMC Infectious Diseases* 9, 15.

Tsiouris, S.J., Austin, J., Toro, P., Coetzee, D., Weyer, K., Stein, Z., *et al.* (2006a) Results of a tuberculosis-specific IFN-gamma assay in children at high risk for tuberculosis infection. *The International Journal of Tuberculosis and Lung Disease* 10, 939–941.

Tsiouris, S.J., Coetzee, D., Toro, P.L., Austin, J., Stein, Z. and El-Sadr, W. (2006b) Sensitivity analysis and potential uses of a novel gamma interferon release assay for diagnosis of tuberculosis. *Journal of Clinical Microbiology* 44, 2844–2850.

Vassilopoulos, D., Stamoulis, N., Hadziyannis, E. and Archimandritis, A.J. (2008) Usefulness of enzyme-linked immunosorbent assay (Elispot) compared to tuberculin skin testing for latent tuberculosis screening in rheumatic patients scheduled for anti-tumor necrosis factor treatment. *The Journal of Rheumatology* 35, 1271–1276.

Verver, S., Warren, R.M., Munch, Z., Richardson, M., Van der Spuy, G.D., Borgdorff, M.W., *et al.* (2004) Proportion of tuberculosis transmission that takes place in households in a high-incidence area. *The Lancet* 363, 212–214.

Vincenti, D., Carrara, S., Butera, O., Bizzoni, F., Casetti, R., Girardi, E., *et al.* (2007) Response to region of difference 1 (RD1) epitopes in human immunodeficiency virus (HIV)-infected individuals enrolled with suspected active tuberculosis: a pilot study. *Clinical and Experimental Immunology* 150, 91–98.

World Health Organization [WHO] (1998) *Policy Statement on Preventive Therapy Against Tuberculosis in People Living with HIV.* World Health Organization, Geneva, Switzerland.

Wrighton-Smith, P. and Zellweger, J.P. (2006) Direct costs of three models for the screening of latent tuberculosis infection. *European Respiratory Journal* 28, 45–50.

Yoshiyama, T., Harada, N., Higuchi, K., Sekiya, Y. and Uchimura, K. (2010) Use of the QuantiFERON-TB Gold test for screening tuberculosis contacts and predicting active disease. *The International Journal of Tuberculosis and Lung Disease* 14, 819–827.

Zellweger, J.P., Zellweger, A., Ansermet, S., De Senarclens, B. and Wrighton-Smith, P. (2005) Contact tracing using a new T-cell-based test: better correlation with tuberculosis exposure than the tuberculin skin test. *International Journal of Tuberculosis and Lung Disease* 9, 1242–1247.

5 Measuring Tuberculosis Immune Responses in the Lung – The Correct Target?

Ronan Breen[1] and Marc Lipman[2]

[1]Department of Respiratory Medicine, Guys' and St Thomas' NHS Trust, London, UK; [2]Centre for Respiratory Medicine, University College London, UK

5.1 Introduction. Why is the Lung Important?

Tuberculosis is associated with staggering global morbidity and mortality. Around 9 million people develop active disease and almost 2 million die each year. Tuberculosis immunology is highly relevant to disease control. It provides information on correlates of immune protection and failure against initial exposure to *Mycobacterium tuberculosis* infection as well as on the (possible) subsequent development of active disease. These data are of crucial importance to the development of an effective vaccine and also have a role in diagnosis and monitoring of treatment response. In this chapter, we discuss how the immune response in tuberculosis has been studied in the lung. We focus on tuberculosis pathogenesis as well as diagnosis; and evaluate the status of current research. Finally, we reflect on the value gained from lung-based work and review future directions in tuberculosis lung immunology programmes.

M. tuberculosis can cause disease in a variety of organs, although by far the most important of these clinically is the lung. Transmission of *M. tuberculosis* between individuals occurs via inhalation of cough-generated infected airborne droplets pro-duced during active pulmonary tuberculosis (Loudon *et al.*, 1969). Transmission dynamics are poorly understood but are likely to reflect physical factors such as aerosol velocity, distance between individuals at the time of coughing, sputum composition and how mycobacterial strains interact with the innate immune system and so alter virulence (Fennelly *et al.*, 2004; Reed *et al.*, 2004). This variation, along with the initial protection from infection provided by the physical barrier of the upper airway and the defence mechanisms of the innate immune system, probably explains why transmission from an infective source is usually only to close household contacts, with non-household transmission thought to require at least 8 h of contact in a poorly ventilated environment (Kenyon *et al.*, 1996). This may also explain why some individuals who experience multiple exposures show no evidence of infection (demonstrated by a repeatedly negative tuberculin skin test, TST) (Morrison *et al.*, 2008).

The physical parameters of airway angle and calibre determine where infected drop-lets are deposited within the lung (Murray, 2003). The typical site of deposition, as judged by the area in which a primary focus of infection is established, is in the periphery of the right lung base. It is here that initial infection can be established and the adaptive immune response begins to be employed. Adaptive immunity to M. tuberculosis both within the lung and elsewhere has been studied extensively and may be altered by the presence of states of lowered immunity such as HIV infection, the administration of immune-suppressing drugs or a previously primed response, as is postulated following Bacille Calmette–Guerin (BCG) vaccination in children. These factors are particularly important in understanding the rapid progression to clinical disease (which may be in the lung or associated draining lymph nodes; or disseminated via the bloodstream to cause miliary or central nervous system disease) that occurs in around 5% of infected cases compared to the establishment of a state of latent tuberculosis infection (LTBI) found in the other 95% of infected individuals. In the 5–10% of latently infected individuals in whom active disease develops at a later stage, the most common site is the lung (either in isolated form or together with active disease at a non-pulmonary site). This, plus its importance as the source of onward transmission, ensures the primacy of the lung and its local immune environment at all stages of tuberculosis.

The pathological response elicited by infection with M. tuberculosis is to produce inflammation characterized by granuloma formation. Granulomas are complex and immunologically active structures which serve to control M. tuberculosis through interactions mediated by multiple chemokines and cytokines such as interferon-gamma (IFN-γ), tumour necrosis factor-alpha (TNF-α) and interleukin-12 (IL-12), between lymphocytes and, perhaps most importantly, macrophages (Flynn et al., 2011). The function of the granuloma and how it can be disrupted is crucial to our understanding of how immunological control is maintained in those with long-term latent infection; and lost in the individuals who develop reactivation tuberculosis, for example in HIV infection with declining CD4+ lymphocyte numbers and function, or with therapeutic blockade of TNF-α (Keane et al., 2001; Diedrich and Flynn, 2011). In a disease such as tuberculosis, which is spread almost exclusively by aerosol

transmission from person to person, the lung has an intuitive appeal as a site of investigation. However, the fairly invasive nature of techniques that are required to sample either the peripheral lung or the associated lymph nodes means that reliance has been placed on the use of animal models to try to understand the pathogenesis of tuberculosis.

5.2 Animal Models

A useful animal model of tuberculosis should replicate relevant aspects of latent infection or active disease and be predictive of outcomes (with, for example, new drugs when these are given subsequently to humans). They should also be able to inform future work and not be so expensive to use that they become unfeasible economically in long-term studies. At present, no single model satisfies all of these criteria; and the reagents needed to work with the models are not necessarily available. However, one great advantage of tuberculosis animal systems is that tissue samples can be obtained with relative ease, although the detected tissue response may not correspond precisely to that found in humans. Further, one can generally standardize the model under test (something quite different to human research, which almost always involves participants with considerable genetic and phenotypic diversity). Animal models differ from each other and also from humans in both their innate and adaptive responses to mycobacteria, including M. tuberculosis. Thus, they may have clinical presentations and outcomes very different to ours, and extrapolation between animal systems and also to humans is not always straightforward or warranted (Rosenthal et al., 2007).

Successful animal models include the zebrafish, mouse, guinea pig, rabbit and non-human primates. In general, and largely depending on how closely an animal's immune response and clinical course map that of adult humans, these can be used to investigate specific aspects of human immunity to mycobacteria. For example, the (transparent) embryonic zebrafish when infected with M. marinum appears to have a predominant innate immune response, yet forms granulomas within days of infection (Lesley and Ramakrishnan, 2008). It therefore questions both the need for adaptive immunity in the initial generation of granulomas and whether these cell collections are beneficial to the host (as granuloma formation occurs when bacterial replication is maximal, rather than as a response to it), and thus has yielded important insights into the encounter at initial infection between microbe and immune system (Volkman et al., 2004).

The mouse, which has a granulomatous response different from that of humans when infected by aerosol (necrosis is not a recognized feature of most mouse models), has been used to model a wide variety of infection states, including acute primary infection and latent tuberculosis (Flynn, 2006). The rabbit and guinea pig can develop necrosis within granulomas, and are perhaps rather better models than the mouse. However, guinea pigs are almost too susceptible to disease (they get sick and die rapidly when infected with M. tuberculosis); and laboratory reagents are harder to obtain than for mice. Rabbits infected with M. bovis have similar pathology to human tuberculosis, though are a lot more expensive to house than guinea pigs (Dannenberg, 2001). Non-human primate models such as cynomolgus macaques have been used and may provide valuable data much more relevant to understanding human tuberculosis, though are very expensive (Green et al., 2010).

5.3 How Can the Lung be Sampled?

Large tissue samples in human tuberculosis are now obtained only rarely due to the efficacy of modern anti-tuberculosis therapy. Surgical resection is likely to be performed only in cases of very severe pulmonary disease, often with multidrug resistance, and so the findings may not be widely applicable. However, the study of a small number of resections has demonstrated heterogeneous activity in distinct parts of resected tissue and similar work may provide insights into the maintenance and loss of local immunological control (Kaplan et al., 2003). An alternative source for material might be patients with previous M. tuberculosis infection who are undergoing lung resection for other conditions such as malignancy in whom the ongoing successful granulomatous response can be evaluated.

A less invasive approach to lung biopsy can be performed via flexible, fibre-optic bronchoscopy. In many centres worldwide, bronchoscopy is used routinely to obtain diagnostic samples in individuals with suspected pulmonary tuberculosis in whom spontaneous sputum cannot be produced or is repeatedly acid-fast bacilli (AFB) smear negative. The physical flexibility and increasingly small diameter of modern bronchoscopes allows sampling to be directed to specific segments and even subsegments of the lung. The bronchoscope has a working channel down which biopsy forceps can be passed, and biopsies of the bronchial mucosa obtained, under direct vision. To sample alveolar tissue requires the forceps to be passed out well beyond the vision of the bronchoscopist (although radiological screening may be used as a guide). The use of the transbronchial biopsy technique for research is limited by the relatively frequent morbidity due to pneumothorax (4%), which is increased by the need for multiple biopsies to allow for the often small tissue samples obtained plus the patchy distribution of granulomas within the alveolar tissue (Milman et al., 1994).

The cell populations and their associated cytokines and chemokines within the alveolar space can be sampled less invasively via bronchoalveolar lavage (BAL) with saline. Here, the tip of the bronchoscope is wedged gently into a subsegmental bronchus, followed by the instillation of aliquots of normal saline (usually 30–60 mls up to a total volume of typically between 120 and 360 mls). Fluid can then be recovered into an appropriate container by applying gentle suction. The volume of lung wash obtained by BAL and the function of its contained cells is dependent on the skill of the operator in maintaining a correct wedged position and the use of minimal suction pressures (either with wall suction or manually via a syringe) to reduce airway collapse. BAL fluid returns can be as much as 75% of the instilled volume of saline, although this is often lower in severe infection or when airways disease is present (such as in smokers). It is affected also by which lung area has been sampled (there being smaller returns from the upper lobes). The ability to 'drive' the bronchoscope enables more than one segment or lobe to be sampled during a single procedure. Thus, useful information can be obtained from both affected and unaffected parts of the lung. Direct evaluations against lung biopsy specimens have suggested that the cell populations obtained from BAL, in which up to 1 million alveoli may be sampled, are similar to those within the interstitium in which granulomas reside (Law et al., 1996).

Limitations on the use of bronchoscopy do exist. The capital cost of equipment is high, and effective ongoing maintenance is vital to ensure adequate performance and to prevent cross-infection (Agerton et al., 1997). A high degree of technical competence is required to ensure consistent and high-volume returns of BAL fluid. Although only semi-invasive, many individuals undergoing bronchoscopy will require, in addition to topical anaesthesia, intravenous therapy if not conscious sedation for anxiolysis and to make the procedure tolerable (Rees et al., 1983). This adds both a small amount of extra risk and the need for more post-procedure monitoring, but may be particularly important if a repeat procedure is contemplated. Serious complications, however, are rare. Minor adverse effects such as post-procedure cough, sore throat, worsening of fever and breathlessness are common but short-lived. These limitations probably explain the relative paucity of studies using BAL to examine the immune response in human tuberculosis. When BAL is performed for diagnostic purposes, there is often 'surplus' fluid available for consented research. However, finding individuals who will undergo bronchoscopy purely as a research procedure is more difficult. Studies using this approach are not common and generally are of small size. It is not surprising, therefore, that longitudinal studies with repeat BAL are rare.

An alternative approach to fibre-optic bronchoscopy that simplifies lung sampling is the use of a 'blind' catheter, which is passed through the airway into the lung without direct visualization. This would reduce substantially the need for expensive equipment, but removes the directed nature of sampling and few data exist to support its use in practice (Ashton, 1992). Much better evaluated is sputum induction using inhalation of hypertonic saline. A number of studies have shown that this non-invasive method has a similar microbiological yield to BAL in tuberculosis diagnosis, yet at a substantially reduced cost and in a safe and more participant-friendly manner, which makes repeat sampling more feasible (McWilliams et al., 2002; Dunleavy et al., 2008). The technique involves the subject inhaling hypertonic saline (3–7%) delivered via an ultrasonic nebulizer. This is thought to modulate an increase in lung lining fluid through osmosis. The fluid and the cells contained within it are carried up by the mucociliary escalator before being expectorated. Sputum induction has been used for a number of years to observe changes in leucocyte populations and liquid phase markers of inflammation in airways disease such as asthma and chronic obstructive pulmonary disease (COPD) (Pin et al., 1992). Most data suggest that leucocyte populations in induced sputum differ when compared to BAL, especially in the proportion of neutrophils and macrophages present in the obtained sample (Pizzichini et al., 1998; Fireman et al., 1999). This may reflect that the cell populations arise from different levels of the bronchial tree rather than predominantly the alveolar space; and also that expectorated sputum comes from several areas of the lung rather than a single lung segment as with BAL. The heterogeneous origin of induced sputum may be of advantage when, for example, studying the immune protection produced within the lung by a candidate vaccine. Of interest, a study of subjects with the granulomatous condition sarcoidosis demonstrated similar results with both techniques with respect to lymphocyte number and subpopulations, but comparable data are not available for individuals with tuberculosis (Moodley et al., 2000; Tsiligianni et al., 2002). One feature of induced sputum which needs to be borne in mind is that the majority of cells expectorated are contained within mucus. In order to break down this mucus and so produce a liquid cell suspension and maximize cell numbers, the sample must be treated with the potent reducing agent dithiothreitol (DTT). This comes at the cost of reduced viable cell numbers, as assessed by immediate trypan blue staining, and variable effects on staining for cell surface markers using monoclonal antibodies (Efthimiadis *et al.*, 1997; Loppow *et al.*, 2000). The effects of DTT on specific molecules and novel bio-markers will require careful evaluation.

Finally, the Lung Flute™ has been developed to achieve successful sputum induction. This self-powered device requires the subject to blow into a plastic chamber, which contains a thin reed. Sound waves are generated that vibrate bronchial secretions, which can then be expectorated. This cheap plastic device requires no external power and has been shown to produce positive micro-biology efficiently in subjects with tubercu-losis, though detailed cellular data are awaited (Fujita *et al.*, 2009). It is important to stress that any technique which stimulates sputum production and cough can promote *M. tuberculosis* transmission. Stringent infec-tion control measures such as the use of negative pressure facilities are integral, there-fore, to such procedures.

5.4 Why Sample the Lung Rather Than Blood? – Human Studies

Obtaining peripheral blood samples is generally much easier than the methods described for lung sampling; and to justify this extra difficulty there must be clear differences in the cell composition and function of the two compartments. In healthy subjects, this is certainly the case, with BAL samples dominated by alveolar macrophages (90–95% of the total), while lymphocytes con-tribute 5–10%. This compares to peripheral blood where 50–70% are neutrophils, 15–45% lymphocytes and 0–10% monocytes (Schwander and Dheda, 2011). In subjects with active tuberculosis, the typical pulmon-ary immune profile observed has been a T-helper cell type 1 (Th1) cytokine and

chemokine response characterized by a CD4+ lymphocytosis in contrast to an immune-suppressed profile found in peripheral blood (Sadek *et al.*, 1998; Schwander *et al.*, 1998; Hirsch *et al.*, 1999).

Human studies have, to date, focused on this adaptive immune response, reflecting the generally better understanding of adaptive compared to innate immunity to *M. tuberculosis* provided by animal studies, the greater apparent relevance to clinical disease in situations such as advanced HIV infection and the ability to harness adaptive response for diagnosis. The initial response to the inhalation of aerosolized *M. tuberculosis* is its engulfment by macrophages found in large numbers in the bronchoalveolar compart-ment. It is in these cells that the organism is able to survive and multiply. An innate immune response, the understanding of which has accelerated in recent years through animal studies identifying pattern recognition receptors such as Toll-like receptors (TLRs), is then activated, which in turn appears to have a role in generating an adaptive immune response (Akira *et al.*, 2001; Saiga *et al.*, 2011). TLRs recognize a variety of mycobacterial components and signal via an adaptor molecule, MyD88, which is also part of the signalling pathway of IL-1 and IL-18. The *in vivo* importance of this molecule has been demonstrated by the susceptibility to acute infection of MyD88- deficient mice, despite being able to produce an adaptive immune response (Fremond *et al.*, 2004). Clear differ-ences exist between alveolar macrophages and peripheral blood-derived monocytes with respect to expression of TLRs (Juarez *et al.*, 2010). Production of IL-12 and IL-18 by macrophages and dendritic cells induces IFN-γ production by T-cells, natural killer (NK) cells and NK T-cells, which in turn activates macrophages and promotes intracellular killing of *M. tuberculosis*. The proinflammatory milieu that is produced facilitates chemokine attraction of further immune cells including γδ T-cells and neutrophils (Korbel *et al.*, 2008). *In vitro* human studies have demonstrated the ability of neutrophils to both phagocytose *M. tuberculosis* and restrict its growth via defensin peptides (Kisich *et al.*, 2002;

Martineau *et al.*, 2007). However, neutrophil-mediated inflammation may also be pathogenic and further work is needed on their role *in vivo* (Schneider *et al.*, 2010).

Non-TLR pattern recognition receptors, such as NOD-like receptors and C-type lectin receptors including DC-SIGN, have also been implicated in the recognition of *M. tuberculosis*. This can lead to the release of a number of locally active effector molecules such as nitric oxide and inducible nitric oxide synthase, and promoters of vitamin D activation and iron sequestration that restrict *M. tuberculosis* growth *in vitro* (Saiga *et al.*, 2011). Phagosome maturation and autophagy appear increasingly important in the innate response to human intracellular pathogens and further data on their role in tuberculosis are awaited with interest (Deretic, 2011). Our increasing understanding of the innate pulmonary immune response to *M. tuberculosis* will be of importance in the design of a protective inhaled vaccine against tuberculosis.

It is perhaps surprising to find a paucity of data evaluating the pulmonary immune response of individuals who by virtue of having been exposed to an infectious tuberculosis case though remain well, already appear able to generate protective immunity. To date, the best study of such adaptive immunity compared healthy household contacts of sputum smear-positive cases with community controls (Schwander *et al.*, 2000). This demonstrated a compartmentalized adaptive immune response to the antigen mixture purified protein derivative (PPD) and to *M. tuberculosis* Antigen 85, with enhanced response frequencies observed in BAL over peripheral blood mononuclear cells (PBMCs) in household contacts and increased responses to PPD among PBMCs compared to BAL cells in TST-positive community controls. Furthermore, *ex vivo* restriction of *M. tuberculosis* growth in alveolar macrophages was mediated by CD8+ T-cells from the household contacts but not the controls (Carranza *et al.*, 2005). Future work examining the cohorts of exposed individuals with clinical evidence of a protective immune phenotype will be valuable, though the need to increase participant accrual and evaluate

longitudinal responses may require simplified lung sampling through sputum induction rather than BAL.

An interesting attempt to model a protective response in the human lung has adapted the bronchoscopic challenge technique used to explore the Th2-like CD4+ predominant immune response found in asthma. This involves bronchoscopic instillation of antigen to specific subsegments, with subsequent BAL allowing analysis of the immune response generated. A pilot study used PPD as the stimulating antigen mixture in subjects who were TST positive or negative (Silver *et al.*, 2003). Here, PPD challenge was safe in all subjects and demonstrated a huge concentration of CD4+ lymphocytes expressing the CD45RO+, CCR7– phenotype of effector memory T-cells. PPD challenge produced significant increases in the IFN-γ inducible and CXCR3 ligands IP-10 and Mig, chemokines produced by the resident PPD-responsive CD4+ T-cells, with an enrichment of CD4+ cells expressing the α-4,β-1 integrin homing molecule (Walrath *et al.*, 2005; Walrath and Silver, 2011).

The majority of studies have sampled individuals with active tuberculosis in whom, by definition, the immune response has changed from that found during clinically latent tuberculosis infection. Pleural tuberculosis, especially in the setting of recently acquired infection, may provide a model of relative control. Here, CD4+ lymphocytes with a high frequency of mycobacterial antigen-specific responders predominate (Barnes *et al.*, 1993). BAL from subjects with miliary tuberculosis is also lymphocyte-predominate, with some work suggesting that an increase in the CD8+ proportion is associated with slow resolution of the disease (Ainslie *et al.*, 1992). This connection with CD8+ T-cells has also been observed in slow treatment responders who have pulmonary tuberculosis (Yu *et al.*, 1995). A lymphocyte-predominant alveolitis, with expression of proinflammatory Th1 cytokines and associated chemokines as shown by increased mRNA, cytokine concentrations in BAL fluid and *ex vivo* antigen stimulation assays, has often been reported in pulmonary tuberculosis (Robinson *et al.*, 1994). This lymphocytosis is associated with clinically less severe pulmonary tuberculosis characterized by infiltrates rather than cavitation, and this may be a compartmentalized response even within the lung as differences have been demonstrated when radiologically uninvolved and involved lung segments are compared (Ainslie *et al.*, 1992; Condos *et al.*, 1998). More advanced disease with increased cavitation is characterized by a macrophage and then neutrophil-dominated bronchoalveolar cell population, and a consequent reduction in both lymphocyte proportion and frequency of antigen-specific responders within the leucocyte population (Barry *et al.*, 2009). Whether this provides an insight on the failure or change occurring in the local immune response or is merely a reflection of the occurrence of cavitation is unclear. More relevant in this setting might be the demonstration of elevated concentrations of matrix metalloproteinase-1 in both BAL and induced sputum in active pulmonary tuberculosis compared to adult controls who had other pulmonary infections, and in tuberculosis cases with cavitation compared to those without (Elkington *et al.*, 2011).

The crucial importance of the adaptive immune response in tuberculosis mediated by CD4+ lymphocytes in conjunction with proinflammatory cytokines is shown by the loss of control of *M. tuberculosis* seen as CD4 counts fall in advancing HIV infection, the disseminated infections described in interferon-gamma knockout mouse models and humans with IFN-γ receptor deficiency and who use TNF-α blocking agents (Cooper *et al.*, 1993; Flynn *et al.*, 1993; Jones *et al.*, 1993; Keane *et al.*, 2001). This focus on the protective arm of the immune response despite the clinical picture of loss of protective control has perhaps distracted attention from the investigation of suppressive mechanisms, which might explain this conundrum. A number of studies have struggled to demonstrate significant concentrations of suppressive cytokines such as IL-4, IL-10 and TGF-β, though more recent work with induced sputum has shown high levels of both suppressive and proinflammatory mediators, and the further finding of a significant fall in relative suppressor activity

with treatment when subjects were resampled at day 30 (Almeida *et al.*, 2009). The data argue for more intensive longitudinal studies, which in BAL have demonstrated a trend to increased BAL lymphocytes and IFN-γ expression with decreased TNF-α expression during treatment (Condos *et al.*, 1998). Regulatory T-cells (CD4+CD25highFoxP3+) have been found at an increased frequency in the peripheral blood of individuals with active tuberculosis. Although identifiable in BAL, their importance in human tuberculosis has not been firmly established (Guyot-Revol *et al.*, 2006). In a non-human primate model, their frequency has been shown to be increased in animals with active tuberculosis. However, reported data have suggested this is a response to inflammation rather than a driver of disease itself (Green *et al.*, 2010).

5.5 Immune Diagnosis of Tuberculosis Using the Lung

The TST, which involves subcutaneous or intradermal injection of PPD, and subsequent assessment for local tissue immunity, utilizes the immune response to help diagnose *M. tuberculosis* infection. It has been available for over a century (von Pirquet, 1907). The concerns regarding sensitivity (especially in conditions of impaired immune function and active tuberculosis) and reduced specificity (largely due to BCG vaccination but also to cross-reactivity with non-tuberculous mycobacteria) are generally highlighted rather more than its manifest strengths. It has stood the test of time because it is cheap, easy to perform and evaluate, repeatable and can be undertaken without need of laboratory infrastructure or a reliable power supply. However, advances in the techniques available to measure antigen-specific cellular immune response, such as the development of the ELISpot assay and intracellular cytokine staining techniques with flow cytometry, alongside sequencing of the genomes of *M. tuberculosis* and BCG and recognition of the immunogenic proteins expressed by the former but not the latter, have facilitated the development of alternatives to the TST (Andersen *et al.*, 2000).

These assays, which measure IFN-γ synthesis following antigen stimulation, have been dubbed interferon-gamma release assays (IGRAs). The central importance of IFN-γ in the lymphocytic immune response to *M. tuberculosis* has been outlined above, but it is pertinent to remember that this cytokine is not essential for producing the delayed-type hypersensitivity response generated by the TST (Cooper *et al.*, 1993). Initial IGRAs used the same PPD antigen mixture as the TST, but soon changed to more *M. tuberculosis*-specific antigens such as early secretory antigen target-6 (ESAT-6) and culture-filtrate protein-10 (CFP-10), which are not expressed by BCG. Two commercially available assays are now widely available: Quantiferon™ assays use antigen stimulation of whole blood with IFN-γ measured by the ELISA method; T-Spot TB™ stimulates a fixed number of PBMCs and analysis is of IFN-γ secretion by single cells using the ELISpot technique. In the investigation of latent tuberculosis, they have shown superior specificity to the TST, especially in BCG-vaccinated individuals, but without great improvements in sensitivity (Pai *et al.*, 2008).

IGRA performance in investigating active tuberculosis has been more variable, with most studies reporting suboptimal sensitivity and specificity. Recent work using T-Spot TB™ showed improved sensitivity versus the TST (85% versus 79%), though few HIV-infected subjects were included (Dosanjh *et al.*, 2008). Given that active tuberculosis often is associated with failing immunity, it is no surprise that the sensitivity of IGRA is reduced in active tuberculosis in a similar manner to the TST (Hirsch *et al.*, 1999). This is even more the case if there is coexistent HIV infection characterized by progressive loss of the CD4+ lymphocyte population in which reside the antigen-specific effector cells that synthesize IFN-γ. Intuitively, therefore, sampling the lung in cases of active tuberculosis should provide sensitivity advantages over the use of blood, as the compartmentalized CD4+ lymphocyte-predominant response in the lung will yield many more antigen-specific cells for stimulation, as has been seen in household contacts of infectious cases (Schwander *et al.*, 2000).

An immune assay may be particularly useful to diagnose active tuberculosis when a rapid diagnosis cannot be made by simple smear for AFB. In pulmonary cases, sputum smear positivity is associated most commonly with the presence of radiologically advanced disease and cavitation. Here, neutrophils predominate with the potential for attenuated antigen-specific CD4+ lymphocyte responses. Sputum samples in these cases are likely to be least amenable to lung-based immune diagnostic tests. However, where spontaneous sputum is AFB smear negative or sputum cannot be expectorated (a fairly common clinical problem), an accurate rapid immune-assay would be of great value. Although obtaining a useful lung sample is more challenging than either performing a TST or taking blood for IGRA, this is already the standard of care in many clinical settings and thus a lung-orientated immune-assay could be performed efficiently in parallel to standard microbiology testing such as culture on a single split sample.

A pilot study of immune-competent subjects, 23 of whom received a final diagnosis of active tuberculosis and 13 with a variety of pulmonary conditions under investigation, analysed IFN-γ and TNF-α synthesis by CD3+ lymphocytes in whole blood and BAL after overnight stimulation with PPD (Barry *et al.*, 2003). Flow cytometry with intracellular cytokine staining was used, and a concentration of PPD-specific production of both cytokines was observed in the lung only in the active tuberculosis cases (predominantly among the CD4+ rather than CD8+ lymphocyte populations), with a 100-fold difference in the frequency of responding cells in BAL compared to blood. Interestingly, responses did not seem to differ between cases clinically classified as pulmonary and either disseminated or non-pulmonary. This may reflect the presence of subclinical pulmonary disease or that, regardless of organ involvement, all active tuberculosis produces a lymphocyte-homing response to the lung, as the original site of infection. HIV infection has been shown to impair Th1-cytokine responses significantly in BAL lymphocytes to both tuberculosis and other lung pathogen-related antigens and so, importantly, these findings have been extended to a cohort of 47 HIV-infected individuals with a median peripheral blood CD4 count of 131 cells/µl (Breen *et al.*, 2006; Kalsdorf *et al.*, 2009; Jambo *et al.*, 2011). No decline was observed in the proportion of IFN-γ synthetic lymphocytes among the CD4+ population in BAL as peripheral blood CD4 counts fell – suggesting an advantage to the analysis of proportions rather than absolute responder numbers in this group.

The utility of this BAL-based method was demonstrated in a cohort of 250 spontaneous sputum smear-negative or non-producing individuals, of whom 25% were HIV infected (median peripheral blood CD4 count 153 cells/µl) (Breen *et al.*, 2008). Again, PPD was the stimulating antigen, on the basis of the theoretical assumptions that the broader range of antigen responses elicited would be advantageous in conditions of immune suppression compared to more specific assays and that confounding by skin-based BCG vaccination would not be a problem in the lung, unlike peripheral blood. Using a diagnostic cut-off determined by receiver operating characteristic (ROC) curve analysis, the assay provided 95% sensitivity against a final clinical diagnosis of active tuberculosis (44% of the cohort; 75% culture confirmed). Sensitivity was not altered by HIV infection or site of tuberculosis, and was significantly superior to a commercial nucleic acid amplification assay (NAAT). In a subgroup with active tuberculosis in whom responses to ESAT-6 were also measured, no response at all could be detected in 19% of cases. What was less impressive in this single-centre study in a middle tuberculosis incidence setting (40/100,000 cases/annum) was a specificity of 76%, which was thought to reflect the presence of latent or healed disease rather than confounding by BCG or non-tuberculous mycobacteria. Comparison of responses in BAL with those in blood was not performed.

A multi-centre study from European centres in low-incidence settings analysed IFN-γ responses to ESAT-6 and CFP-10 using the T-Spot TB™ assay in 347 spontaneous sputum smear-negative or non-producing individuals with suspected tuberculosis

(Jafari *et al.*, 2009). A final diagnosis of active tuberculosis was made in 20% of cases (56% culture confirmed), while in the 'not tuberculosis' group, 46% were thought to be latently infected (positive T-Spot result from peripheral blood). Reported results for BAL were a sensitivity of 91% and specificity of 80%, while in PBMCs the sensitivity was nearly identical, though specificity was below 50%. The superiority of BAL extended to comparisons with the TST and NAAT in the complete cohort and, notably, BAL response was far less likely to be positive in subjects with previous but not current tuberculosis than was seen with PBMCs. Similar large studies in high-burden settings have yet to be performed. Evaluation of 85 tuberculosis suspects in South Africa using T-Spot TB™ with BAL (where 29% were HIV coinfected) demonstrated sensitivity and specificity of 89% and 94% when including those with definite diagnoses but not the 16% of subjects with diagnostic uncertainty or the 34% with inconclusive assays (Dheda *et al.*, 2009). Quantiferon-TB Gold In-Tube™ was much less sensitive than T-Spot TB™ and, perhaps surprisingly, so was a PPD-based assay. The superior specificity of BAL over PBMCs was in agreement with the European data. Replication of these findings in a larger cohort and a more technically consistent study would be welcome.

Where BAL is performed as part of the routine work-up of spontaneous sputum smear-negative or non-producing cases of suspected tuberculosis, its use as a one-off source of lung-derived cells for immune diagnosis of tuberculosis makes sense. What is needed now is to demonstrate how the assays may be used as part of a rapid, efficient and cost-effective algorithm that also incorporates AFB smear and NAAT prior to IGRA. However, even in resource-rich settings many centres routinely use sputum induction rather than BAL and any attempt at repeat sampling might be best served by a sputum-based method. A study of 42 subjects (38% HIV infected) of whom 27 were diagnosed with active tuberculosis, using flow cytometry and intracellular cytokine staining with PPD as the stimulating antigen, reported a fourfold reduction in lymphocyte percentage compared to previous BAL data (although the predominant effector memory phenotype of CD45RO+CCR7−CD27− was the same) and a fivefold fall in CD4+IFN-γ synthetic proportion (Breen et al., 2007). However, post hoc ROC analysis against final diagnosis of tuberculosis demonstrated 89% sensitivity and 80% specificity in this small group. Positive results using an ELISpot assay with the sputum-derived cells were also reported. These data have yet to be replicated and more work in this area is awaited with interest.

5.6 Conclusion

There are compelling reasons to support the use of lung- rather than blood-derived samples when investigating the immune response in tuberculosis. Whether these advantages overcome the increased expense and complexity compared to blood testing for both routine diagnostic work and also large-scale cross-sectional or longitudinal studies remains to be seen. It is clear that although comparative IGRA studies have shown superiority of BAL versus blood, diagnostic performance as an aid to clinical decision making is still inadequate. Specific questions that must be addressed include how to distinguish between different stages of tuberculosis (latent infection, active disease and previous treatment) and which markers robustly demonstrate an effective (and protective) immune response. More accurate diagnostic assays may use different antigens, though what will be of greater value is the ability to identify antigen-specific populations of cells which exist at lower frequency than those detected through synthesis of IFN-γ. Markers of full-effector T-cell differentiation such as CD27 and CD154 have shown promise using blood in discriminating latent from active tuberculosis (Streitz et al., 2007, 2011). Similarly, analysis of cell populations according to their ability to produce IFN-γ, IL-2 and/or TNF-γ alone or together may serve as biomarkers of disease states and treatment response (Millington et al., 2007; Caccamo et al., 2010). If this is the case, then future studies will need to analyse ever-smaller populations of cells. This will require increased use of both multi-colour flow cytometry and will re-enforce the advantages provided by the higher-frequency antigen-specific populations present in the lung in tuberculosis compared to blood.

References

Agerton, T., Valway, S., Gore, B., Pozsik, C., Olikaytis, B., Woodley, C., et al. (1997) Transmission of a highly drug-resistant strain (W1) of Mycobacterium tuberculosis. Community outbreak and nosocomial transmission via a contaminated bronchoscope. Journal of the American Medical Association 278, 1073–1077.

Ainslie, G.M., Solomon, J.A. and Bateman, E.D. (1992) Lymphocyte and lymphocyte subset numbers in blood and in bronchoalveolar lavage and pleural fluid in various forms of human pulmonary tuberculosis at presentation and during recovery. Thorax 47, 513–518.

Akira, A., Takeda, K. and Kaisho, T. (2001) Toll-like receptors: critical proteins linking innate and acquired immunity. Nature Immunology 8, 675–680.

Almeida, A.S., Lago, P.M., Boechat, N., Huard, R.C., Lazzarini, L.C., Santos, A.R., et al. (2009) Tuberculosis is associated with a down-modulatory lung immune response that impairs Th1-type immunity. Journal of Immunology 183, 718–731.

Andersen, P., Munk, M.E., Pollock, J.M. and Doherty, T.M. (2000) Specific immune-based diagnosis of tuberculosis. The Lancet 356, 1099–1104.

Ashton, M.R. (1992) 'Blind' bronchoalveolar lavage. The Lancet 340, 1104.

Barnes, P.F., Lu, S., Abrams, J.S., Wang, E., Yamamura, M. and Modlin, R. (1993) Cytokine production at the site of disease in human tuberculosis. Infection and Immunity 61, 3482–3489.

Barry, S.M., Lipman, M.C., Bannister, B., Johnson, M.A. and Janossy, G. (2003) Purified protein derivative-activated type 1 cytokine-producing CD4+ T lymphocytes in the lung: a characteristic feature of active pulmonary and non-pulmonary TB. Journal of Infectious Diseases 187, 243–250.

Barry, S., Breen, R., Lipman, M., Johnson, M. and Janossy, G. (2009) Impaired antigen-specific CD4(+) T lymphocyte responses in cavitary tuberculosis. Tuberculosis (Edinburgh) 89, 48–53.

Breen, R.A., Janossy, G., Barry, S.M., Cropley, I., Johnson, M.A. and Lipman, M.C. (2006) Detection of mycobacterial antigen responses in lung but not blood in HIV/tuberculosis co-infected subjects. *AIDS* 20, 1330–1332.

Breen, R.A., Hardy, G.A., Perrin, F.M., Lear, S., Kinloch, S., Smith, C.J., *et al.* (2007) Rapid diagnosis of smear-negative tuberculosis using immunology and microbiology with induced sputum in HIV-infected and uninfected individuals. *PLoS One* 2, e1335.

Breen, R.A., Barry, S.M., Smith, C.J., Shorten, R.J., Dilworth, J.P., Cropley, I., *et al.* (2008) Clinical application of a rapid lung-orientated immuno-assay in individuals with possible tuberculosis. *Thorax* 63, 67–71.

Caccamo, N., Guggino, G., Joosten, S.A., Gelsomino, G., Di Carlo, P., Titone, L., *et al.* (2010) Multifunctional CD4(+) T cells correlate with active *Mycobacterium tuberculosis* infection. *European Journal of Immunology* 40, 2211–2220.

Carranza, C., Juarez, E., Torres, M., Ellner, J.J., Sada, E. and Schwander, S.K. (2005) *Mycobacterium tuberculosis* growth control by lung macrophages and CD8 cells from patient contacts. *American Journal of Respiratory and Critical Care Medicine* 173, 238–245.

Condos, R., Rom, W.N., Liu, Y.M. and Schluger, N.W. (1998) Local immune responses correlate with presentation and outcome in tuberculosis. *American Journal of Respiratory and Critical Care Medicine* 157, 729–735.

Cooper, A.M., Dalton, D.K., Stewart, T.A., Griffin, J.P., Russell, D.G. and Orme, I.M. (1993) Disseminated tuberculosis in interferon gamma gene-disrupted mice. *Journal of Experimental Medicine* 178, 2243–2247.

Dannenberg, A.M. Jr (2001) Pathogenesis of pulmonary *Mycobacterium bovis* infection: basic principles established by the rabbit model. *Tuberculosis (Edinburgh)* 81, 87–96.

Deretic, V. (2011) Autophagy in immunity and cell-autonomous defense against intracellular microbes. *Immunological Reviews* 240, 92–104.

Dheda, K., van Zyl-Smit, R.N., Meldau, R., Meldau, S., Symons, G., Khalfey, H., *et al.* (2009) Quantitative lung T cell responses aid the rapid diagnosis of pulmonary tuberculosis. *Thorax* 64, 847–853.

Diedrich, C.R. and Flynn, J.L. (2011) HIV-1/*Mycobacterium tuberculosis* coinfection immunology: how does HIV-1 exacerbate tuberculosis? *Infection and Immunity* 79, 1407–1417.

Dosanjh, D.P., Hinks, T.S., Innes, J.A., Deeks, J.J., Pasvol, G., Hackforth, S., *et al.* (2008) Improved diagnostic evaluation of suspected tuberculosis. *Annals of Internal Medicine* 148, 325–336.

Dunleavy, A., Breen, R.A., Perrin, F. and Lipman, M.C. (2008) Is bronchodilation required routinely before diagnostic sputum induction? Evidence from studies with tuberculosis. *Thorax* 63, 473–474.

Efthimiadis, A., Pizzichini, M.M., Pizzichini, E., Dolovich, J. and Hargreave, F.E. (1997) Induced sputum cell and fluid-phase indices of inflammation: comparison of treatment with dithiothreitol vs phosphate-buffered saline. *European Respiratory Journal* 10, 1336–1340.

Elkington, P., Shiomi, T., Breen, R., Nuttall, R.K., Ugarte-Gil, C.A., Walker, N.F., *et al.* (2011) MMP-1 drives immunopathology in human tuberculosis and transgenic mice. *Journal of Clinical Investigation* 121, 1827–1833.

Fennelly, K.P., Martyny, J.W., Fulton, K.E., Orme, I.M., Cave, D.M. and Heifets, L.B. (2004) Cough-generated aerosols of *Mycobacterium tuberculosis*: a new method to study infectiousness. *American Journal of Respiratory and Critical Care Medicine* 169, 604–609.

Fireman, E., Topilsky, I., Greif, J., Lerman, Y., Schwarz, Y., Man, A., *et al.* (1999) Induced sputum compared to bronchoalveolar lavage for evaluating patients with sarcoidosis and non-granulomatous interstitial lung disease. *Respiratory Medicine* 93, 827–834.

Flynn, J.L. (2006) Lessons from experimental *Mycobacterium tuberculosis* infections. *Microbes and Infection* 8, 1179–1188.

Flynn, J.L., Chan, J., Triebold, K.J., Dalton, D.K., Stewart, T.A. and Bloom, B.R. (1993) An essential role for interferon gamma in resistance to *Mycobacterium tuberculosis* infection. *Journal of Experimental Medicine* 178, 2249–2254.

Flynn, J.L., Chan, J. and Lin, P.L. (2011) Macrophages and control of granulomatous inflammation in tuberculosis. *Mucosal Immunology* 4, 271–278.

Fremond, C.M., Yeremeev, V., Nicolle, D.M., Jacobs, M., Quesniaux, V.F. and Ryffel, B. (2004) Fatal *Mycobacterium tuberculosis* infection despite adaptive immune response in the absence of MyD88. *Journal of Clinical Investigation* 114, 1790–1799.

Fujita, A., Murata, K. and Takamori, M. (2009) Novel method for sputum induction using the Lung Flute in patients with suspected pulmonary tuberculosis. *Respirology* 14, 899–902.

Green, A.M., Mattila, J.T., Bigbee, C.L., Bongers, K.S., Lin, P.L. and Flynn, J.L. (2010) CD4+ regulatory T cells in a cynomolgus macaque model of *Mycobacterium tuberculosis* infection. *Journal of Infectious Diseases* 202, 533–541.

Guyot-Revol, V., Innes, J.A., Hackforth, S., Hinks, T. and Lalvani, A. (2006) Regulatory T cells are expanded in blood and disease sites in patients with tuberculosis. *American Journal of Respiratory and Critical Care Medicine* 173, 803–810.

Hirsch, C.S., Toosi, Z., Othieno, C., Johnson, J.L., Schwander, S.K., Robertson, S., *et al.* (1999) Depressed T-cell interferon- responses in pulmonary tuberculosis: analysis of underlying mechanisms and modulation with therapy. *Journal of Infectious Diseases* 180, 2069–2073.

Jafari, C., Thijsen, S., Sotgiu, G., Goletti, D., Domínguez Benítez, J.A., Losi, M., *et al.* (2009) Tuberculosis Network European Trials group. Bronchoalveolar lavage enzyme-linked immuno-spot for a rapid diagnosis of tuberculosis: a Tuberculosis Network European Trials group study. *American Journal of Respiratory and Critical Care Medicine* 180, 666–673.

Jambo, K.C., Sepako, E., Fullerton, D.G., Mzinza, D., Glennie, S., Wright, A.K., *et al.* (2011) Bronchoalveolar CD4+ T cell responses to respiratory antigens are impaired in HIV-infected adults. *Thorax* 66, 375–382.

Jones, B.E., Young, S.M., Antoniskis, D., Davidson, P.T., Kramer, F. and Barnes, P.F. (1993) Relation-ship of the manifestations of tuberculosis to CD4 cell counts in patients with human immunodeficiency virus infection. *American Review of Respiratory Disease* 148, 1292–1297.

Juarez, E., Nunez, C., Sada, E., Ellner, J.J., Schwander, S.K. and Torres, M. (2010) Differential expression of Toll-like receptors on human alveolar macrophages and autologous peripheral monocytes. *Respiratory Research* 11, 2.

Kalsdorf, B., Scriba, T.J., Wood, K., Day, C.L., Dheda, K., Dawson, R., *et al.* (2009) HIV-1 infection impairs the bronchoalveolar T-cell response to mycobacteria. *American Journal of Respiratory and Critical Care Medicine* 180, 1262–1270.

Kaplan, G., Post, F.A., Moreira, A.L., Wainwright, H., Kreiswirth, B.N., Tanverdi, M., *et al.* (2003) *Mycobacterium tuberculosis* growth at the cavity surface: a microenviroment with failed immunity. *Infection and Immunity* 71, 7099–7108.

Keane, J., Gershon, S., Wise, R.P., Mirabile-Levens, E., Kasznica, J., Schwieterman, W.D., *et al.* (2001) Tuberculosis associated with infliximab, a tumor necrosis factor alpha-neutralizing agent. *New England Journal of Medicine* 345, 1098–1104.

Kenyon, T.A., Valway, S.E., Ihle, W.W., Onorato, I.M. and Castro, K.G. (1996) Transmission of multidrug-resistant *Mycobacterium tuberculosis*

during a long airplane flight. *New England Journal of Medicine* 334, 933–938.

Kisich, K.O., Higgins, M., Diamond, G. and Heifets, L. (2002) Tumour necrosis factor alpha stimulates killing of *Mycobacterium tuberculosis* by human neutrophils. *Infection and Immunity* 70, 4591–4599.

Korbel, D.S., Schneider, B.E. and Schaible, U.E. (2008) Innate immunity in tuberculosis. Myths and truths. *Microbes and Infections* 10, 995–104.

Law, K.F., Jagirdar, J., Weiden, M.D., Bodkin, M. and Rom, W.N. (1996) Tuberculosis in HIV-positive patients: cellular response and immune activation in the lung. *American Journal of Respiratory and Critical Care Medicine* 153, 1377–1384.

Lesley, R. and Ramakrishnan, L. (2008) Insights into early mycobacterial pathogenesis from the zebrafish. *Current Opinion in Microbiology* 11, 277–283.

Loppow, D., Böttcher, M., Gercken, G., Magnussen, H. and Jörres, R.A. (2000) Flow cytometric analysis of the effect of dithiothreitol on leukocyte surface markers. *European Respiratory Journal* 16, 324–329.

Loudon, R.G., Bumgarner, L.R., Lacy, J. and Coffman, G.K. (1969) Aerial transmission of mycobacteria. *American Review of Respiratory Disease* 100, 165–171.

McWilliams, T., Wells, A.U., Harrison, A.C., Lindstrom, S., Cameron, R.J. and Foskin, E. (2002) Induced sputum and bronchoscopy in the diagnosis of pulmonary tuberculosis. *Thorax* 57, 1010–1014.

Martineau, A.R., Newton, S.M., Wilkinson, K.A., Kampmann, B., Hall, B.M., Nawroly, N., *et al.* (2007) Neutrophil-mediated innate immune resistance to mycobacteria. *Journal of Clinical Investigation* 117, 1988–1994.

Millington, K.A., Innes, J.A., Hackforth, S., Hinks, T.S., Deeks, J.J., Dosanjh, D.P., *et al.* (2007) Dynamic relationship between IFN-gamma and IL-2 profile of *Mycobacterium tuberculosis*-specific T cells and antigen load. *Journal of Immunology* 178, 5217–5226.

Milman, N., Faurschou, P., Munch, E.P. and Grode, G. (1994) Transbronchial lung biopsy through the fibre optic bronchoscope. Results and complications in 452 examinations. *Respiratory Medicine* 88, 749–753.

Moodley, Y.P., Dorasamy, T., Venketasamy, S., Naicker, V. and Lalloo, U.G. (2000) Correlation of CD4:CD8 ratio and tumour necrosis factor (TNF) alpha levels in induced sputum with bronchoalveolar lavage fluid in pulmonary sarcoidosis. *Thorax* 55, 696–699.

Morrison, J., Pai, M. and Hopewell, P.C. (2008) Tuberculosis and latent tuberculosis infection in close contacts of people with pulmonary tuberculosis in low-income and middle-income countries: a systemic review and meta-analysis. *The Lancet Infectious Diseases* 8, 359–368.

Murray, J.F. (2003) Bill Dock and the location of pulmonary tuberculosis. How bed rest might have helped consumption. *American Journal of Respiratory and Critical Care Medicine* 168, 1029–1033.

Pai, M., Zwerling, A. and Menzies, D. (2008) Systematic review: T-cell-based assays for the diagnosis of latent tuberculosis infection: an update. *Annals of Internal Medicine* 149, 177–184.

Pin, I., Gibson, P.G., Kolendowicz, R., Girgis-Gabardo, A., Denburg, J.A., Hargreave, F.E., *et al.* (1992) Use of induced sputum cell counts to investigate airway inflammation in asthma. *Thorax* 47, 25–29.

Pizzichini, E., Pizzichini, M.M., Kidney, J.C., Efthimiadis, A., Hussack, P., Popov, T., *et al.* (1998) Induced sputum, bronchoalveolar lavage and blood from mild asthmatics: inflammatory cells, lymphocyte subsets and soluble markers compared. *European Respiratory Journal* 11, 828–834.

Reed, M.B., Domenech, P., Manca, C., Su, H., Barczak, A.K., Kreiswirth, B.N., *et al.* (2004) A glycolipid of hypervirulent tuberculosis strains that inhibits the innate immune response. *Nature* 431, 84–87.

Rees, P.J., Hay, J.G. and Webb, J.R. (1983) Premedication for fibreoptic bronchscopy. *Thorax* 38, 624–627.

Robinson, D.S., Ying, S., Taylor, I.K., Wangoo, A., Mitchell, D.M., Kay, A.B., *et al.* (1994) Evidence for a Th1-like bronchoalveolar T-cell subset and predominance of interferon-gamma gene activation in pulmonary tuberculosis. *American Journal of Respiratory and Critical Care Medicine* 149, 989–993.

Rosenthal, I.M., Zhang, M., Williams, K.N., Peloquin, C.A., Tyagi, S., Vernon, A.A., *et al.* (2007) Daily dosing of rifapentine cures tuberculosis in three months or less in the murine model. *PLoS Medicine* 4, e344.

Sadek, M.I., Sada, E., Toosi, Z., Schwander, S.K. and Rich, E.A. (1998) Chemokines induced by infection of mononuclear phagocytes with mycobacteria and present in lung alveoli during active pulmonary tuberculosis. *American Journal of Respiratory, Cell and Molecular Biology* 19, 513–521.

Saiga, H., Shimada, Y. and Takeda, K. (2011) Innate immune effectors in mycobacterial infection. *Clinical and Developmental Immunology* 2011, 347594.

Schneider, B.E., Korbel, D., Hagens, K., Koch, M., Raupach, B., Enders, J., *et al.* (2010) A role for IL-18 in protective immunity against *Mycobacterium tuberculosis*. *European Journal of Immunology* 40, 396–405.

Schwander, S. and Dheda, K. (2011) Human lung immunity against *Mycobacterium tuberculosis*. Insights into pathogenesis and protection. *American Journal of Respiratory and Critical Care Medicine* 183, 696–707.

Schwander, S.K., Torres, M., Sada, E., Carranza, C., Ramos, E., Tary-Lehmann, M., *et al.* (1998) Enhanced responses to *Mycobacterium tuberculosis* antigens by human alveolar lymphocytes during active pulmonary tuberculosis. *Journal of Infectious Diseases* 178, 1434–1445.

Schwander, S.K., Torres, M., Carranza, C.C., Escobedo, D., Tary-Lehmann, M., Anderson, P., *et al.* (2000) Pulmonary mononuclear cell responses to antigens of *Mycobacterium tuberculosis* in healthy household contacts of patients with active tuberculosis and healthy controls from the community. *Journal of Immunology* 165, 1479–1485.

Silver, R.F., Zukowski, L., Kotake, S., Li, Q., Pozuelo, F., Krywiak, A., *et al.* (2003) Recruitment of antigen-specific Th1-like responses to the human lung following bronchoscopic segmental challenge with purified protein derivative of *Mycobacterium tuberculosis*. *American Journal of Respiratory, Cell and Molecular Biology* 29, 117–123.

Streitz, M., Tesfa, L., Yildirim, V., Yahyazadeh, A., Ulrichs, T., Lenkei, R., *et al.* (2007) Loss of receptor on tuberculin-reactive T-cells marks active pulmonary tuberculosis. *PLoS One* 2, e735.

Streitz, M., Fuhrmann, S., Powell, F., Quassem, A., Nomura, L., Maecker, H., *et al.* (2011) Tuberculin-specific T cells are reduced in active pulmonary tuberculosis compared to LTBI or status post BCG vaccination. *Journal of Infectious Diseases* 203, 378–382.

Tsiligianni, J., Tzanakis, N., Kyriakou, D., Chrysofakis, G., Siafakas, N. and Bouros, D. (2002) Comparison of sputum induction with broncho-alveolar lavage cell differential counts in patients with sarcoidosis. *Sarcoidosis, Vasculitis and Diffuse Lung Diseases* 19, 205–210.

Volkman, H.E., Clay, H., Beery, D., Chang, J.C., Sherman, D.R. and Ramakrishnan, L. (2004) Tuberculous granuloma formation is enhanced by a mycobacterium virulence determinant. *PLoS Biology* 2, 1946–1956.

von Pirquet, C. (1907) Frequency of tuberculosis in childhood. *Journal of the American Medical Association* 52, 675–678.

Walrath, J.R. and Silver, R.F. (2011) The α-4β1 integrin in localization of *Mycobacterium tuberculosis*-specific Th1 cells to the human lung. *American Journal of Respiratory, Cell and Molecular Biology* 45, 24–30.

Walrath, J., Zukowski, L., Krywiak, A. and Silver, R.F. (2005) Resident Th1-like effector memory cells in pulmonary recall responses to *Mycobacterium tuberculosis*. *American Journal of Respiratory, Cell and Molecular Biology* 33, 48–55.

Yu, C.-T., Wang, C.-H., Huang, T.-J., Lin, H.-C. and Kuo, H.-P. (1995) Relation of bronchoalveolar lavage T lymphocyte subpopulations to rate of regression of active pulmonary tuberculosis. *Thorax* 50, 869–874.

6   Sniffing Out Tuberculosis

Ruth McNerney[1] and Claire Turner[2]

[1]*Department of Pathogen Molecular Biology, London School of Hygiene and Tropical Medicine, London, UK;* [2]*Department of Life, Health and Chemical Sciences, The Open University, Milton Keynes, UK*

6.1 Introduction

Tuberculosis, or phthisis as it was previously known, is an ancient ailment that has perplexed health practitioners for millennia. One of the greatest challenges is diagnosing the disease. Unlike other infectious diseases such as malaria or HIV, the pathogen is rarely found in circulating body fluids and attempts to test for circulating antibodies have also proved unsatisfactory. *Mycobacterium tuberculosis* bacilli may be present in expectorated sputum in pulmonary forms of the disease but detecting the bacteria is not easy and specimens need to be processed in a laboratory. Poor access to diagnostic facilities in developing countries and the low sensitivity of current tests combine to frustrate efforts to identify patients. Case detection rates are low and millions of tuberculosis cases each year are not diagnosed and reported (McNerney and Daley, 2011). The need for rapid sensitive diagnostic tests that are affordable in the countries where tuberculosis is endemic has encouraged test developers to consider less traditional diagnostic strategies. In this chapter, we describe the analysis of volatile compounds for disease detection and review progress towards a diagnostic test for tuberculosis.

Volatile compounds are those that persist in a gaseous state. Compounds that exist exclusively as vapours at ambient temperatures and pressures are called gases. Compounds that are predominantly liquids at ambient temperatures but that partially evaporate to the gaseous state are described as volatile. Similarly, some solid substances have a capacity to sublime and enter the gaseous phase. Vapours so formed can condense back to their liquid state or deposit as the solid state. The propensity of a substance to convert to its gaseous form is indicated by its vapour pressure; being the pressure at which the gaseous and liquid or solid phases are at equilibrium. Compounds with a high vapour pressure at normal temperatures are more volatile than those with low vapour pressure. In reality, most atmospheres are mixtures of volatile compounds and gases and individual vapours contribute a partial vapour pressure to the mix. In general, the volatility of a compound and its ability to escape the liquid matrix increases with temperature. Eventually, boiling point will be reached, where the compound's vapour pressure equals ambient atmospheric pressure.

Volatile compounds and gases are produced by living organisms as a by-product of their metabolic processes, and volatile organic compounds (VOCs) are of particular interest to biologists and medical practitioners. Biological systems are water based and the solubility of a compound is another factor affecting its ability to vaporize. Humans and other animals have evolved an ability to recognize some compounds or mixtures of compounds via their olfactory systems (Firestein, 2001; Rouquier and Giorgi, 2007). Olfaction, or the 'sense of smell', is a vital attribute that informs basic behaviours such as food selection, territorial activity and mating. The olfactory systems in individual animal species have developed to smell selectively low concentrations of compounds which are in their interest to detect. This includes pheromones and semiochemicals which are present in very low concentrations for signalling between animals of the same species. It also includes rancid odours, which humans and other animals use to warn that food is not safe to eat, and faecal odours such as indole. Smells are also utilized in clinical situations, albeit informally at times (Palmer, 1993; Bomback, 2006).

6.1.1 Historical perspectives

The earliest description of an investigative test for tuberculosis comes from ancient Greece and the writings of Hippocrates, who recorded in his *Aphorisms*, 'In persons affected with phthisis, if the sputa which they cough up have a heavy smell when poured upon coals, and if the hairs of the head fall off, the case will prove fatal' (Hippocrates and Adams, 400 BC). A similar approach was recommended by the Roman, Caelius Aurelius (130 BC), who stated that a characteristic foul odour from phlegm over hot coals was indicative of physical decomposition (Drabkin, 1950). In more recent times, the sputa and breath of patients with phthisis has been reported to have a gangrenous odour (Bowditch, 1889). Fetid smells similar to rotten eggs have been reported that, on autopsy, were linked to the breakdown of tuberculous tissue, perforation of the lungs and the presence of purulent liquid in the thoracic cavity (Louis, 1844). In one case, a

woman's breath and sputum was found to become increasingly obnoxious during the month preceding her death. Less dramatic odours have also been described, sometimes as a 'sickly smell' (Shattuck, 1880; Louis, 1844), and Burney Yeo, a physician in 19th century London, reported to the British Medical Association 'a peculiar nauseating odour in the breath of many phthisical patients, even before the development of marked physical signs' (Yeo, 1877). An alternative approach concerned urine from patients with phthisis which, on storage, developed a smell reminiscent of rotten cheese or partially treated sewage (White, 1892). Though often reported, there are no published studies on the diagnostic value of the human olfactory system in the management of tuberculosis and evidence of its efficacy remains anecdotal. The majority of reports date from an era prior to chemotherapy, when tuberculosis was a common affliction and death rates were extremely high. Caseous necrosis of granulomatous and lung tissue is characteristic of tuberculosis disease and it would not be surprising if fetid odours were observed in the breath and sputum of patients with late-stage terminal disease. Of more interest to the diagnostician are the reports of patients on initial presentation and those with less advanced disease. It should be noted, however, that other conditions may also result in foul or sickly odours, particularly those bacterial or fungal infections that result in necrosis or pus formation. Thus, both the sensitivity and specificity of odour as a diagnostic tool for tuberculosis require further investigation.

6.2 Olfactory Detection

Human olfactory detection of tuberculosis is beset by two problems. The first is the intrinsic risk of contracting the disease, which spreads through the inhalation of tiny airborne droplet nuclei. The second is the relatively poor performance of the human olfactory system when compared to other creatures. Animals including dogs, pigs and rodents are believed to have olfactory senses superior to humans (Rouquier *et al.*, 2000). In addition, they can be trained using Pavlovian conditioning to respond physically to specific odours or smells, as is demonstrated by the use of dogs to detect illicit foods, narcotics and explosives (Johnston, 1999). The mammalian olfactory system is illustrated in Fig. 6.1. Vapours enter the nasal passages, where they interact with the olfactory epithelium. Molecules bind to receptors on highly specialized olfactory cells, triggering an electrical signal which transmits along neurons to the olfactory bulb, which is part of the central nervous system. Different receptors react with different classes of molecules, reporting to different parts of the olfactory bulb and forming a highly sophisticated neural network which, in conjunction with the brain, is capable of analysing complex mixtures of vapours. Pattern recognition combined with memory allows vapours to be differentiated and smells to be recognized.

Groundbreaking work on olfactory detection of tuberculosis has been performed in Tanzania, where giant African pouched rats (*Cricetomys gambianus*) have been trained to recognize samples of sputum from tuberculosis patients (Weetjens *et al.*, 2009). The animals are trained to sniff individual pots containing the samples and to pause for at least 5 s when they recognize a positive signal. Conditioning was undertaken using food rewards (banana). Though not as sensitive as other diagnostic techniques, a rat can test samples at a faster rate than a laboratory technician using conventional Ziehl–Neelsen (ZN) light microscopy. The yield of positives can be increased by exposing samples to multiple rats. In a recent study, 23,101 sputum samples from 10,523 patients collected during a routine diagnostic service were tested by the rats and results compared to the smear microscopy result.

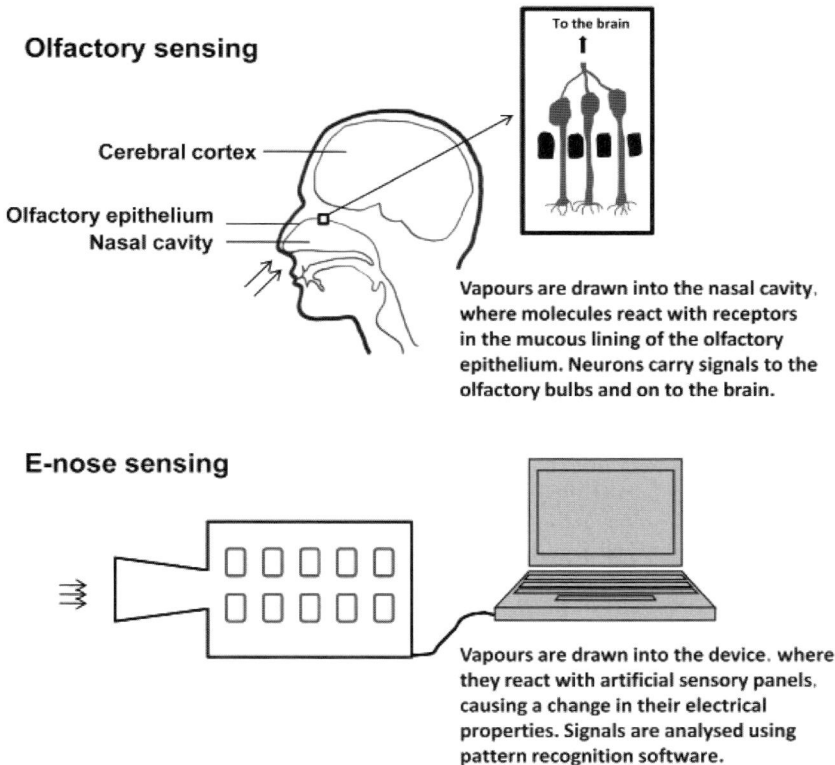

Olfactory sensing

To the brain

Cerebral cortex

Olfactory epithelium
Nasal cavity

Vapours are drawn into the nasal cavity, where molecules react with receptors in the mucous lining of the olfactory epithelium. Neurons carry signals to the olfactory bulbs and on to the brain.

E-nose sensing

Vapours are drawn into the device, where they react with artificial sensory panels, causing a change in their electrical properties. Signals are analysed using pattern recognition software.

Fig. 6.1. Olfactory and e-nose sensing.

Samples were first frozen and then sterilized by autoclaving before being presented to ten different rats (Poling *et al.*, 2010).

Any sample reported as negative by microscopy but positive by two or more rats was re-evaluated by smear microscopy in the laboratory performing the evaluation. Collectively, the rats identified 2274 (91%) of 2487 samples found positive by routine ZN. A further 3012 samples were found positive by the rats, of which 927 were found positive by smear microscopy when re-examined in the research laboratory. Thus, the ten rats gave an improved yield over a single routine smear result. A high proportion of the positive results (40%) did not correlate with a positive microscopy result, suggesting that specificity may not be sufficient and that confirmatory testing might be required. Unfortunately, further conclusions cannot be drawn as culture was not undertaken, preventing estimation of the actual sensitivity and specificity of the test. Despite the shortcomings of the study, the data presented indicate that differentiation of tuberculosis and non-tuberculosis patients may be achieved by assessing volatile compounds emitted by sputum samples. The authors did not speculate on the constituents of the olfactory signal recognized by the rats. Previous studies demonstrated that the animals could recognize positive sputum following training with cultured bacteria, suggesting that volatiles originating from the bacteria themselves may play a role (Weetjens *et al.*, 2009). Although these findings are highly interesting, it is unlikely that rats could provide rapid diagnosis at the point of care. The infrastructure to house and train them, the practical challenges of transporting live animals and the need for confirmatory testing suggest they would be more suited to referral laboratories. In addition, they and their handlers may suffer from fatigue and boredom, and careful management will be required to maintain high productivity and performance.

Some of the limitations of working with mammals may be overcome by using insects. Odour recognition is integral to an insect's life and they are constantly adapting, modifying and learning associations between odours and their environment. Insects such as the honeybee (*Apis mellifera*) can be conditioned to recognize specific odours by Pavlovian conditioning, where conditioned bees are stimulated to extend their proboscis when they encounter the olfactory signal (Bittermann *et al.*, 1983). Multiple receptors on the insect's antennae combine with advanced signal processing to provide highly sensitive identification of complex mixtures (Sandoz, 2003). Recognition of organic compounds occurs at a submolecular level and is influenced by carbon chain length and functional group (Guerrieri *et al.*, 2005). Preliminary work has suggested that honeybees might be trained to differentiate *M. bovis* BCG bacilli from environmental strains such as *M. smegmatis*, but further studies have yet to be undertaken (McNerney, unpublished data). Although large numbers of insects may be maintained at low cost, and training is more rapid than that for a dog or rat, they share some logistic challenges with the mammals. Maintenance of the hive and conditioning or training the bees requires specialist knowledge. In addition, insects are subject to environmental influences such as heat and humidity that affect their behaviour. Although an intriguing prospect, the application of insect-based diagnostic sensors for tuberculosis has yet to be demonstrated.

6.3 E-noses

The use of volatile biomarkers to diagnose patients will require robust and reliable means of measuring them. Two methodological strategies have been adopted. The first is to mimic olfaction, where the vapour under test is exposed to sensors that, on encountering target molecules, change their physical or electrical state, inducing a signal that can be measured. An instrument which does this is called an electronic nose, or e-nose. The second method is to determine the chemical composition of an odour and identify and quantify the compounds present in the mixture.

E-noses are devices containing an array of different sensors which each respond to a different degree to the chemicals in an odour. An e-nose will not identify the components of an odour but will compare odours and classify them, for example by positive or negative disease state. Some sensors may respond preferentially to water, for example, whereas others will respond to different chemical functional groups, recognizing other types of compounds such as alcohols, esters, aldehydes, ketones, amines, sulfides or carboxylic acids. If an odour is a complex mixture, containing many different compounds, then each sensor will have a different response, producing an output unique to that odour. The principle of an e-nose device is shown in Fig. 6.1. Sensors may be made from a variety of materials, but the most common are constructed from metal oxides or synthetic organic polymers called conducting polymers. Typically, the output of a sensor will be a change in an electrical property. For example, when compounds bind to a metal oxide sensor, there will be a proportional change in resistance and the absolute magnitude and duration of that change may be measured. The data collected are expressed as a curve, as shown in Fig. 6.2, where features such as amplitude, area and the rate of adsorption and desorption may be used to interpret sensor response.

With multiple sensors, more complex responses are obtained and interpreting the data requires significant computer processing. Similar or dissimilar responses can be clustered and, if associated with known compounds, a library of chemical smells may be established. For complex odours, pattern recognition software may be employed, where a comparison of positive and negative samples allows mapping of sensor responses. In this way, the e-nose mimics olfactory sensing, where animals or insects are trained to recognize and differentiate vapours. E-noses can be trained in the same way as people to recognize and distinguish smells without understanding which compounds are responsible for the odour.

The major difference between the e-nose and animal olfaction is in the sophistication of the olfactory system. Typically, an e-nose might house 30 sensors, whereas each human has approximately 5 million olfactory sensors. The neural system and brain also has far superior networking and processing capabilities to discern complex mixtures than the current e-nose technologies.

In the way that animals smell odours, an e-nose tests vapours directly without prior manipulation of the sample. The devices are simple to operate and, after doing the initial computation to classify sample types, are usually able to classify an unknown sample

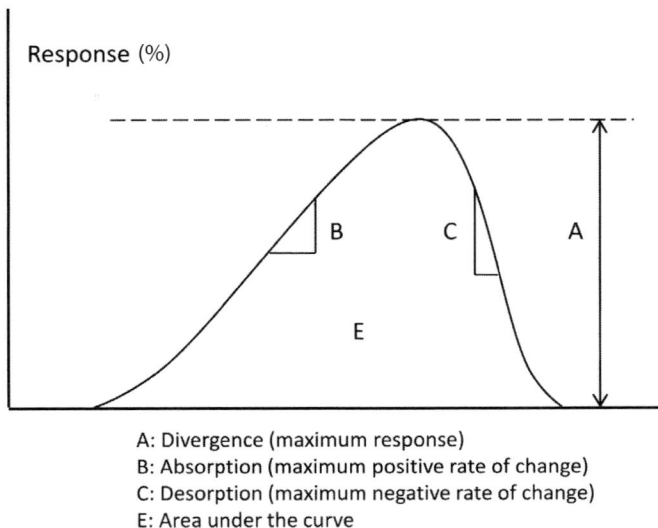

A: Divergence (maximum response)
B: Absorption (maximum positive rate of change)
C: Desorption (maximum negative rate of change)
E: Area under the curve

Fig. 6.2. Typical output from a metal oxide sensor.

in minutes. It is not a particularly sensitive technique, so if the odours indicative of disease are subtle, or if the natural variation between samples is great, then differentiation will be difficult (Nicolas and Romain, 2004; Rains *et al.*, 2004). Another factor to consider is the stability of the sensors, as both metal oxides and conducting polymers are prone to change their properties over time, causing a change or drift in their output (Li and Qian, 1993; Romain and Nicolas, 2010).

E-nose technology has been used to investigate samples from animals and humans infected with tuberculosis. A commercial electronic nose device (BH-114, Bloodhound Sensors, UK) with 14 conducting sensors based on polyaniline polymers was applied to samples from cattle and badgers infected with *M. bovis* and uninfected control animals (Fend *et al.*, 2005). Sera samples were stored frozen prior to dilution in saline and incubation at 37°C in sealed vials. Samples of headspace gas were extracted by inserting a needle through a septum in the cap of the vials. Data obtained from the e-nose were analysed using the multivariate data analysis techniques principal component analysis and linear discriminant function (LDF) analysis. The data obtained suggested that the e-nose could differentiate samples from infected and uninfected animals and the authors speculated that the technology had potential as a diagnostic test. Further work was performed on cultures of bacteria and showed that mycobacteria could be discriminated from *Pseudomonas aeruginosa* and that smaller but discernable differences were observed between *M. tuberculosis*, *M. avium* and *M. scrofulaceum* (Fend *et al.*, 2006). Differences were also observed when bacteria were added to sputum in spiking experiments. The application of neural networking to clinical samples (sputum) showed the e-nose could discriminate samples from patients infected with tuberculosis and from non-tuberculosis patients, and that it might be useful as a diagnostic tool for human tuberculosis. Unfortunately, subsequent studies have not supported these findings. Sensitivities of 68% and 75% and specificities of less than 70% were observed in a study of sputum samples performed in Tanzania (Kolk *et al.*, 2010).

Variations were seen between two e-nose instruments, the performance of which varied from day to day. The authors speculated that the accuracy of the test might have been affected by the sampling method used, as headspace vapours were taken directly from sputum containers with a smaller headspace rather than the sealed glass vials used previously. They also reported a small but significant instrument drift. Their conclusion that the commercial e-nose in its current state is not specific enough for tuberculosis diagnosis is supported by other studies (Knobloch *et al.*, 2009, 2010). Variation in performance across time and the undue influence of environmental factors such as temperature and moisture suggest these instruments lack the reliability required of a diagnostic device. In addition, the problem of making instruments behave reproducibly from day to day and the fact that no two instruments behave the same, even when manufactured at the same time, suggest the technology is not robust enough for field use. However, the fact that they are able to differentiate between positive and negative groups at the population level (if not at the individual level) indicates that there probably is an odour associated with tuberculosis and that other techniques may be able to identify the components of the odour and characterize the molecules associated with tuberculosis.

6.4 VOC Analysis

Although studies with e-noses suggest that there is an odour associated with tuberculosis, they are not able to identify the characteristic constituents of the odour. To develop a more robust test, it will be necessary to identify the components of the odour and to determine their significance as diagnostic markers for tuberculosis. There are five possible origins of VOCs in samples of body fluids of infected individuals. The most significant group of VOCs are those which are produced by the metabolic processes of the body. For example, acetone is an abundant VOC found in all body fluids including breath, blood and urine (Ashley *et al.*, 1994; Miekisch *et al.*, 2004). It originates through the regulation of blood sugar by insulin. If blood sugar is low, fat is broken down and keto-bodies are formed, leading to acetone production. Another example is ammonia, which is generated as a result of protein breakdown. These so-called endogenous VOCs are important indicators of the health of the person (Amann *et al.*, 2004). The second origin of VOCs is from the action of bacterial metabolism. Mostly, bacteria colonize the body in a symbiotic relationship, with several trillion living in the human gut, and these produce detectable VOCs (Amann *et al.*, 2004). However, bacteria that cause disease will also generate VOCs (Probert *et al.*, 2009) and, ideally, these VOCs are those that should be targeted as potential biomarkers. The third source of VOCs is from the modification of the VOCs produced by bacteria within the host organism. One compound may be converted chemically or enzymatically to another compound, which may be detectable. Fourth, the response of the host organism to infection is a potential source of VOC. When an animal is infected with a pathogen, the immune system modifies the metabolism, producing inflammatory markers and resulting in changes which can release VOC (Barker *et al.*, 2006; Chan *et al.*, 2009). The final source of VOCs is from exogenous compounds, which are those produced elsewhere and absorbed by the body. Exposure to any compound through inhalation, ingestion or injection could contaminate tissues of the body and subsequently be emitted as VOCs (Blount *et al.*, 2006). An example of this is the contamination of body tissues and fluids following an anaesthetic. Traces of the anaesthetic may remain in the body for weeks, and the time of removal will depend on the dose, its solubility and whether the body will metabolize the compound (Turner, unpublished results). Other examples are cigarette smoking and the consumption of ethanol (Ashley *et al.*, 1996).

6.5 Chromatography

Assessment of the concentration or relative abundance of the constituent volatile compounds in an odour requires separation of gaseous/volatile mixtures. Chromatographic methods are most frequently used for this, where compounds are separated according to their physical or chemical characteristics, such as size, ionic strength or polarity. The sensitivity of gas chromatography is dependent on the separation capacity of the columns used and the detection method employed. Highly sensitive instruments have been developed where, after separation, vapours are detected using novel sensing devices such as surface acoustic wave detectors (Watson *et al.*, 2003). Traditional gas chromatographs are sophisticated, laboratory-based instruments but rapid, portable versions have been developed that can be used in the field (Jia *et al.*, 2000; Staples and Viswanathan, 2008). The retention time, or the time at which the compound elutes from the chromatography column, may be compared to standard or reference compounds and so be used to infer the identity of a compound. However, it is possible that other compounds will elute at the same time and chromatography alone cannot be used to determine the identity of a compound. In order to be sure of a compound's identity, mass spectrometry is required.

6.6 Mass Spectrometry

Mass spectrometry may be used to identify compounds either as a detection method following chromatography or, with some simple mixtures, certain types of mass spectrometry may be used without pre-separation. In mass spectrometry, the VOCs or gases present are ionized using any one of a number of techniques and the ions are then separated according to the ratio of their mass to their charge (m/z ratio) by letting the ions enter a magnetic or electric field (depending on the type of mass spectrometry). Heavy ions (high m/z) are deflected less than light ions and so the ions are separated. The ions at each m/z value are then detected and a spectrum is produced as counts per second at each m/z value. Each compound will generally have its own unique spectrum and thus mass spectrometry can be used to identify compounds by comparing spectra obtained with library spectra. There are several configurations of the technology, with some instruments tailored to examine small gaseous molecules, while others are used to investigate larger semi-volatile compounds. In the latter case, instruments are usually connected to chromatography systems to separate the components.

Mass spectrometers are primarily research tools and are used for biomarker discovery, but portable versions have been developed (Yang *et al.*, 2008). An alternative detection technology, where gaseous ions are separated by shape and charge is differential mobility spectrometry (DMS) (Krylov *et al.*, 2007). This technology is amenable to miniaturization and portable devices have been developed that are being used as detectors for military and industrial applications (Zolotov, 2006). There is also interest in their use for medical purposes for testing breath (Molina *et al.*, 2008). However, DMS is not able to identify a compound with certainty, as it does not produce a unique spectrum, but may be of use if the compounds being detected are already known.

6.7 Volatile Biomarkers for Tuberculosis

Growing bacteria on various media enables the analysis of the VOCs produced by the bacteria as a result of their metabolism. These VOCs can be collected and analysed and it has been found that different bacteria, including mycobacteria, produce different combinations of VOCs (Scholler *et al.*, 1997; Pavlou *et al.*, 2004); however, these combinations vary in many cases with the type of growth media used. This is perhaps not surprising in the case of mycobacteria, as they have the ability to alter their metabolic process depending on the nutritive sources available (Wheeler and Radcliffe, 1994). This implies that when the bacteria then grow *in vivo*, having infected an animal or a human, they may produce yet a different set of biomarkers and this may also depend on the physiology of that animal. Mass spectrometry has led to the identification of a number of potential biomarkers produced by myco-

bacteria *in vitro* (Phillips *et al.*, 2007, 2010; Cunha *et al.*, 2008; Syhre and Chambers, 2008). Attempts to validate these biomarkers using clinical specimens have so far met with limited success. Syhre and colleagues examined samples of breath for derivatives of nicotinic acid (Syhre *et al.*, 2009). Breath was collected by asking volunteers to blow into 1 l bags and samples were concentrated using solid-phase microextraction (SPME: absorption on to activated fibres). Samples were then treated chemically (derivatized) prior to analysis by gas chromatography–mass spectrometry (GC-MS). Significant differences in the levels of the derivatives were observed in the breath of tuberculosis and non-tuberculosis patients (Syhre *et al.*, 2009). Levels were estimated to be in the femtomol/mol range, which is below the level at which they could be measured using current 'easy to use' VOC detection devices. A second and perhaps more difficult problem to be resolved is that nicotinic acid is not specific to tuberculosis and is present in some food and tobacco products. Smokers were excluded from their study, but such an approach does not offer a practical solution for the routine diagnostic clinic. A different approach was taken by Phillips, where samples of breath were collected on sorbent traps and transported to the laboratory. Following thermal desorption, the vapours released were analysed by GC-MS. Multivariate analysis (fuzzy logic and pattern recognition methods) of data from 134 volatile compounds suggested that tuberculosis patients could be differentiated from non-tuberculosis patients and healthy volunteers (Phillips *et al.*, 2007). Subsequent work from the same research group reported a sensitivity of 84% but a specificity of just 65% when testing microbiologically proven tuberculosis patients (Phillips *et al.*, 2010). In this study, several compounds were found to be associated with tuberculosis. Some were markers of oxidative stress, and these included alkanes. These are non-specific markers of illness and may not in themselves be able to distinguish between tuberculosis and other illnesses or ill health. However, the researchers also found other markers which might potentially be of use as specific biomarkers. These included those that might be produced directly by *M. tuberculosis*, namely cyclohexane and aromatic hydrocarbons. However, it should be noted that cyclohexane is frequently found in nature, so may not be specific to mycobacteria.

6.8 Multivariate Statistics

The ubiquitous nature of small, volatile compounds suggests that individual markers are unlikely to offer the specificity required for a diagnostic test.

The e-nose and olfactory data suggest that samples can be differentiated by the combination of biomarkers, or the pattern of VOCs, rather than by individual compounds, and it may be more appropriate to consider the 'VOC fingerprint' of an odour rather than its constituent molecules. It is conceivable that the markers that are responsible for the different patterns are a combination of those that are produced by the host's response to infection, such oxidative stress alkane markers and VOCs produced routinely by the body (e.g. ammonia, acetone, methanol, etc.) but present in different proportions. VOC originating from the *M. tuberculosis* bacilli growing in the body may also contribute, although current evidence suggests they may be present at very low and sometimes undetectable levels.

Multivariate statistics and bioinformatics provide us with the tools to discern patterns in large complex data sets. This approach was taken by Spooner and colleagues, who used selected ion flow tube mass spectrometry (SIFT-MS) to analyse the headspace above 250 samples of badger serum (Spooner *et al.*, 2009). They found that by using the method of partial least squares discriminant analysis on the raw MS data, they could distinguish between tuberculosis-positive and tuberculosis-negative badgers with 88% sensitivity. However, a false-positive rate of 38% was reported. The study was limited by inappropriate sample storage and low volumes of sample; nevertheless, the results were encouraging, again implying that there were patterns of VOCs that could distinguish tuberculosis-positive from tuberculosis-negative samples.

6.9 Conclusions: The Future of Odour Analysis for Tuberculosis Diagnosis

Current evidence suggests that odour analysis has the potential to identify tuberculosis disease in humans and animals either from their breath or by testing the headspace above clinical specimens such as sera or sputa. If unique biomarkers are present, the difficulty in detecting them implies that they are present at low concentration and distinguishing such endogenous markers from exogenous markers is extremely difficult. That different research groups report different markers suggests that samples need to be examined by a variety of techniques to 'rule in' or 'rule out' all potential biomarkers systematically. To validate such markers for diagnostic use, studies with a large number of subjects will be required. E-nose technology does not yet provide sufficient means of detection and more analytical approaches are required. Pattern recognition provides an attractive alternative, but the approach is dependent on knowledge of the patterns characteristic to the disease to aid the design of sensors of high sensitivity and specificity. Potential diagnostic biomarker patterns shall need to be verified with a large number of individuals with different backgrounds, lifestyles, ages, gender, health status, environment, diet and nutritional status. An additional problem is the collection of samples. Volatiles are, by their nature, unstable and samples need to be collected and stored in a manner to avoid loss of volatile material and to avoid contamination with VOC in the local environment. Analysis of body fluids potentially containing tuberculosis bacilli also requires careful health and safety assessment. Breath samples in particular need to be collected in a safe manner, as they may contain infectious droplet nuclei that could spread tuberculosis. Whether the ancient physicians will be proved correct in their assessment of odours as a tool to diagnose tuberculosis remains to be seen, but current evidence suggests this is a distinct possibility.

References

Amann, A., Poupart, G., Telser, S., Ledochowski, M., Schmid, A. and Mechtcheriakov, S. (2004) Applications of breath gas analysis in medicine. *International Journal of Mass Spectrometry* 239, 227–233.

Ashley, D.L., Bonin, M.A., Cardinali, F.L., McCraw, J.M. and Wooten, J.V. (1994) Blood-concentrations of volatile organic-compounds in a nonoccupationally exposed US population and in groups with suspected exposure. *Clinical Chemistry* 40, 1401–1404.

Ashley, D.L., Bonin, M.A., Cardinali, F.L., McCraw, J.M. and Wooten, J.V. (1996) Measurement of volatile organic compounds in human blood. *Environmental Health Perspectives* 104, 871–877.

Barker, M., Hengst, M., Schmid, J., Buers, H.J., Mittermaier, B., Klemp, D., *et al.* (2006) Volatile organic compounds in the exhaled breath of young patients with cystic fibrosis. *European Respiratory Journal* 27, 929–936.

Bittermann, M.E., Menzel, R., Fietz, A. and Schäfer, S. (1983) Classical conditioning of proboscis extension in honeybees (*Apis mellifera*). *Journal of Comparative Psychology* 97, 107–119.

Blount, B.C., Kobelski, R.J., McElprang, D.O., Ashley, D.L., Morrow, J.C., Chambers, D.M., *et al.* (2006) Quantification of 31 volatile organic compounds in whole blood using solid-phase microextraction and gas chromatography-mass spectrometry. *Journal of Chromatography B-Analytical Technologies in the Biomedical and Life Sciences* 832, 292–301.

Bomback, A. (2006) The physical exam and the sense of smell. *New England Journal of Medicine* 354, 327–329.

Bowditch, V.Y. (1889) Two cases of phthisis treated by intra-pulmonary injections. *Boston Medical and Surgical Journal* 120, 455–458.

Chan, H.P., Lewis, C. and Thomas, P.S. (2009) Exhaled breath analysis: novel approach for early detection of lung cancer. *Lung Cancer* 63, 164–168.

Cunha, M.G., Hoenigman, S., Kanchagar, C., Rearden, P., Sassetti, C.S., Trevejo, J.M., *et al.* (2008) Joint analysis of differential mobility spectrometer and mass spectrometer features for tuberculosis biomarkers. *2008 30th Annual International Conference of the Ieee Engineering in Medicine and Biology Society, Vols 1–8.* Engineering in Medicine and Biology Society, New Jersey, pp. 359–362.

Drabkin, I.E. (ed.) (1950) *Caelius Aurelianus, On Acute Diseases and on Chronic Diseases.* University of Chicago Press, Chicago, Illinois.

Fend, R., Geddes, R., Lesellier, S., Vordermeier, H.M., Corner, L.A., Gormley, E., *et al.* (2005) Use of an electronic nose to diagnose *Mycobacterium bovis* infection in badgers and cattle. *Journal of Clinical Microbiology* 43, 1745–1751.

Fend, R., Kolk, A.H., Bessant, C., Buijtels, P., Klatser, P.R. and Woodman, A.C. (2006) Prospects for clinical application of electronic-nose technology to early detection of *Mycobacterium tuberculosis* in culture and sputum. *Journal of Clinical Microbiology* 44, 2039–2045.

Firestein, S. (2001) How the olfactory system makes sense of scents. *Nature* 413, 211–218.

Guerrieri, F., Schubert, M., Sandoz, J.C. and Giurfa, M. (2005) Perceptual and neural olfactory similarity in honeybees. *PLoS Biology* 3, e60.

Hippocrates and Adams, T.B.F. (400 BC) *Aphorisms.* eBooks@Adelaide, Adelaide, Australia.

Jia, M.Y., Koziel, J. and Pawliszyn, J. (2000) Fast field sampling/sample preparation and quantification of volatile organic compounds in indoor air by solid-phase microextraction and portable gas chromatography. *Field Analytical Chemistry and Technology* 4, 73–84.

Johnston, J.M. (1999) Canine detection capabilities: operational implications of recent R & D findings (http://www.barksar.org/K-9_Detection_Capabilities.pdf, accessed March 2011).

Knobloch, H., Turner, C., Spooner, A. and Chambers, M. (2009) Methodological variation in headspace analysis of liquid samples using electronic nose. *Sensors and Actuators B-Chemical* 139, 353–360.

Knobloch, H., Schroedl, W., Turner, C., Chambers, M. and Reinhold, P. (2010) Electronic nose responses and acute phase proteins correlate in blood using a bovine model of respiratory infection. *Sensors and Actuators B-Chemical* 144, 81–87.

Kolk, A., Hoelscher, M., Maboko, L., Jung, J., Kuijper, S., Cauchi, M., *et al.* (2010) Electronic-nose technology in diagnosis of TB patients using sputum samples. *Journal of Clinical Microbiology* 48, 4235–4238.

Krylov, E.V., Nazarov, E.G. and Miller, R.A. (2007) Differential mobility spectrometer: model of operation. *International Journal of Mass Spectrometry* 266, 76–85.

Li, Y.F. and Qian, R.Y. (1993) Stability of conducting polymers from the electrochemical point-of-view. *Synthetic Metals* 53, 149–154.

Louis, P.C.A. (1844) Organs of respiration. Section 1: The lungs. In: Society, T.S. (ed.) *Researches on Phthisis: Anatomical, Pathological and Therapeutical*, 2nd edn. Translated by W.H. Walshe. C & J Adlard, London, pp. 1–35.

McNerney, R. and Daley, P. (2011) Towards a point-of-care test for active tuberculosis: obstacles and opportunities. *Nature Reviews Microbiology* 9, 204–213.

Miekisch, W., Schubert, J.K. and Noeldge-Schomburg, G.F.E. (2004) Diagnostic potential of breath analysis – focus on volatile organic compounds. *Clinica Chimica Acta* 347, 25–39.

Molina, M.A., Zhao, W., Sankaran, S., Schivo, M., Kenyon, N.J. and Davis, C.E. (2008) Design-of-experiment optimization of exhaled breath condensate analysis using a miniature differential mobility spectrometer (DMS). *Analytica Chimica Acta* 628, 155–161.

Nicolas, J. and Romain, A.C. (2004) Establishing the limit of detection and the resolution limits of odorous sources in the environment for an array of metal oxide gas sensors. *Sensors and Actuators B-Chemical* 99, 384–392.

Palmer, R. (1993) In bad odour: smell and its significance in medicine from antiquity to the seventeenth century. In: Bynum, W.F. and Porter, R. (eds) *Medicine and the Five Senses*. Cambridge University Press, Cambridge, UK.

Pavlou, A.K., Magan, N., Jones, J.M., Brown, J., Klatser, P. and Turner, A.R. (2004) Detection of *Mycobacterium tuberculosis* (TB) *in vitro* and *in situ* using an electronic nose in combination with a neural network system. *Biosensors and Bioelectronics* 20, 538–544.

Phillips, M., Cataneo, R.N., Condos, R., Ring Erickson, G.A., Greenberg, J., La Bombardi, V., *et al.* (2007) Volatile biomarkers of pulmonary tuberculosis in the breath. *Tuberculosis (Edinburgh)* 87, 44–52.

Phillips, M., Basa-Dalay, V., Bothamley, G., Cataneo, R.N., Lam, P.K., Natividad, M.P., *et al.* (2010) Breath biomarkers of active pulmonary tuberculosis. *Tuberculosis (Edinburgh)* 90, 145–151.

Poling, A., Weetjens, B.J., Cox, C., Mgode, G., Jubitana, M., Kazwala, R., *et al.* (2010) Using giant African pouched rats to detect tuberculosis in human sputum samples: 2009 findings. *American Journal of Tropical Medicine and Hygiene* 83, 1308–1310.

Probert, C.S.J., Ahmed, I., Khalid, T., Johnson, E., Smith, S. and Ratcliffe, N. (2009) Volatile organic compounds as diagnostic biomarkers in gastrointestinal and liver diseases. *Journal of Gastrointestinal and Liver Diseases* 18, 337–343.

Rains, G.C., Tomberlin, J.K., D'Alessandro, M. and Lewis, W.J. (2004) Limits of volatile chemical detection of a parasitoid wasp, *Microplitis croceipes*, and an electronic nose: a comparative study. *Transactions of the ASAE* 47, 2145–2152.

Romain, A.C. and Nicolas, J. (2010) Long-term stability of metal oxide-based gas sensors for e-nose environmental applications: an overview. *Sensors and Actuators B-Chemical* 146, 502–506.

Rouquier, S. and Giorgi, D. (2007) Olfactory receptor gene repertoires in mammals. *Mutation Research* 616, 95–102.

Rouquier, S., Blancher, A. and Giorgi, D. (2000) The olfactory receptor gene repertoire in primates and mouse: evidence for reduction of the functional fraction in primates. *Proceedings of the National Academy of Sciences* 97, 2870–2874.

Sandoz, J.C. (2003) Olfactory perception and learning in the honey bee (*Apis mellifera*): calcium imaging in the antenna lobe. *Journal de la Société de Biologie* 197, 277–282.

Scholler, C., Molin, S. and Wilkins, K. (1997) Volatile metabolites from some gram-negative bacteria. *Chemosphere* 35, 1487–1495.

Shattuck, F.C. (1880) Fibroid phthisis. *Boston Medical and Surgical Journal* 102, 241–243.

Spooner, A.D., Bessant, C., Turner, C., Knobloch, H. and Chambers, M. (2009) Evaluation of a combination of SIFT-MS and multivariate data analysis for the diagnosis of *Mycobacterium bovis* in wild badgers. *Analyst* 134, 1922–1927.

Staples, E.J. and Viswanathan, S. (2008) Detection of contrabands in cargo containers using a high-speed gas chromatograph with surface acoustic wave sensor. *Industrial and Engineering Chemistry Research* 47, 8361–8367.

Syhre, M. and Chambers, S.T. (2008) The scent of *Mycobacterium tuberculosis*. *Tuberculosis (Edinburgh)* 88, 317–323.

Syhre, M., Manning, L., Phuanukoonnon, S., Harino, P. and Chambers, S.T. (2009) The scent of *Mycobacterium tuberculosis* – part II breath. *Tuberculosis (Edinburgh)* 89, 263–266.

Watson, G.W., Staples, E.J. and Viswanathan, S. (2003) Performance evaluation of a surface acoustic wave analyzer to measure VOCs in air and water. *Environmental Progress* 22, 215–226.

Weetjens, B.J., Mgode, G.F., Machang'u, R.S., Kazwala, R., Mfinanga, G., Lwilla, F., *et al.* (2009) African pouched rats for the detection of pulmonary tuberculosis in sputum samples. *International Journal of Tuberculosis and Lung Disease* 13, 737–743.

Wheeler, P.R. and Radcliffe, C. (1994) Metabolism of *Mycobacterium tuberculosis*. In: Bloom, B.R. (ed.) *Tuberculosis: Pathogenesis, Protection,* and Control. American Society for Microbiology, Washington.

White, W.H. (1892) On a condition of the urine met with in phthisis. British Medical Journal 1, 1638.

Yang, M., Kim, T.Y., Hwang, H.C., Yi, S.K. and Kim, D.H. (2008) Development of a palm portable mass spectrometer. Journal of the American Society for Mass Spectrometry 19, 1442-1448.

Yeo, B.I. (1877) On the results of recent researches in the treatment of phthisis. British Medical Journal 1, 195–197.

Zolotov, Y.A. (2006) Ion mobility spectrometry. Journal of Analytical Chemistry 61, 519–519.

Part II

Measuring Resistance

7 Role of Phenotypic Methods for Drug Susceptibility Testing of *M. tuberculosis* Isolates in the Era of MDR and XDR Epidemics

Leonid Heifets

Mycobacteriology Reference Laboratory, National Jewish Health, Denver, Colorado, USA

7.1 Introduction

7.1.1 History lessons

The broad application of antimicrobial therapy of tuberculosis in the 1950s has not only changed the course of history of this disease but has also influenced social and political life in Europe and the USA. Continuing the broad application of anti-tuberculosis drugs resulted in the inevitability of emerging drug resistance of tubercle bacilli (Gupta *et al.*, 2004). The importance of this problem, in particular the role of patients with primary drug resistance as a source of infection with drug-resistant tuberculosis, has been underestimated for many years. Therefore, drug susceptibility testing of patients' isolates (particularly in new patients) was not considered a priority in the measures of control. Statements from leading national and international organizations illustrated this neglect. For example, the American Thoracic Society (ATS) and the Centers for Disease Control and Prevention (CDC) published the following joint statement, 'Given the low prevalence of drug-resistant *Mycobacterium tuberculosis* in most parts of the United States, the cost of routine testing of all initial isolates is difficult to justify' (ATS, 1990).

Severe outbreaks of drug-resistant tuberculosis in the USA in the late 1980s and early 1990s changed this attitude and testing of initial isolates for drug susceptibility became mandatory (Tenover *et al.*, 1993). For many years, this lesson did not influence attitudes outside the USA. Moreover, with the introduction of the directly observed therapy short-course (DOTS) strategy in 1994–1995, new arguments against the worldwide use of drug susceptibility testing emerged. One argument was that many countries could not afford the laboratory arrangement needed for such testing. Another reason was that, according to the original DOTS strategy, the focus was on using smear microscopy as the main diagnostic tool to detect most infectious patients. It did not matter that this testing was only able to detect less than 50% of the culture-positive patients, but culture isolation and drug susceptibility testing were not considered for broad implementation.

Table 7.1. Abbreviations of the drugs' names.

Isoniazid	INH or H
Rifampin	RMP, RIF or R
Pyrazinamide	PZA or Z
Streptomycin	SM or S
Ethambutol	EMB or E
Ethionamide	ETA
Amikacin	AK
Kanamycin	KM
Capreomycin	CM
Cycloserine	CS
Para-amino-salicylic acid	PAS
Levofloxacin	Levo
Moxifloxacin	Moxi
Ofloxacin	Oflox
Clofazimine	CF

The argument was that proper implementation of the DOTS strategy (including a
standard treatment regimen for all patients)
was supposed to prevent the spread of drug
resistance, and even make it 'virtually
impossible' for a patient to develop
multidrug-resistant tuberculosis (MDR-TB)
(World Health Organization [WHO], 1997).
A group of authors referring to their
experience in Peru stated, 'It is not true that
DOTS makes it virtually impossible to cause
a patient to develop MDR-TB' (Farmer *et al.*,
1998). They demonstrated how patients with
initial resistance to rifampin (RIF) or
isoniazid (INH) developed additional
resistance to other drugs through DOTS
treatment, a phenomenon they labelled as
'amplified effect of short-course therapy'.
Escalation of this phenomenon into the MDR
epidemics became unavoidable through
blindfolded application of either a standard
regimen or through the addition of any drug
to the failing treatment regimens, without
drug susceptibility results. In 1997, the WHO
guidelines for the management of drug-
resistant tuberculosis contained the following
statements, 'Susceptibility testing is not
recommended in all new cases of smear-
positive pulmonary tuberculosis… since it is
not practical, it is expensive, and it is useless'
and 'The level of resistance… is lower in
primary than in acquired resistance. This is

why primary resistance hardly affects the
outcome of treatment with a WHO standard
regimen …'.
   Have we learned lessons from this
approach?

7.1.2 The alarming situation today and new developments

Tuberculosis today is more widespread than
at any other time in the history of humankind.
A recent report by the WHO indicates that, in
2008, there were estimated 440,000 cases of
MDR-TB, resulting in the death of 150,000
patients (WHO, 2010). MDR-TB cases have
been reported in more than 50 countries, but
the WHO considered 27 of them as 'high MDR
burden countries'. For example, in seven areas
of the former Soviet Union, the proportion of
MDR-TB in new cases ranged between 12%
and 27% and between 50% and 60% in
previously treated cases. At the beginning of
2010, 58 countries had reported the emergence
of extremely drug-resistant tuberculosis
(XDR-TB). It is estimated that by 2015, we will
face nearly 1.6 million new cases of drug-
resistant tuberculosis annually, and it is hard
to predict what proportion of them will
represent MDR-TB and XDR-TB cases.
   There is a new important development
(compared to reports of previous years): the
WHO 2010 report states that, 'The laboratory
plays a central role in patient care and
surveillance' and 'Establishing reference
laboratory facilities to supervise DST (*sic*
Drug Susceptibility Testing) surveillance
activities in the country is a critical step in
MDR-TB control and care'. Yes, it is a 'critical
step' forward, but is this general statement
sufficient to address the issue of timely
detection of patients that harbour drug-
resistant bacteria? The report does say that
the WHO 'will promote new and rapid
technologies within appropriate laboratory
services through 2013 …'. It is not clear from
this report whether these new and rapid
technologies are planned for another surveillance programme only or if there is a plan
to implement these methods widely enough
to check all new patients in communities for
drug-resistant tubercle bacilli. The report

does not address the issue of the organization of laboratory services beyond having national reference laboratories. In other WHO documents, there were also recommendations on the enhancement of laboratory services, including drug susceptibility testing, but so far, there have been no specifics on this 'enhancement'.

In the USA, the Federal Tuberculosis Task Force published the 'Action Plan to Combat Extensively Drug-Resistant Tuberculosis' (CDC, 2009), in which two statements addressed the need for drug susceptibility testing: 'The laboratory plays a critical role in the diagnosis and management of drug-resistant TB' and 'To combat the growing problem of resistance to TB drugs, the most *current methods need to be applied to their fullest capacity* while better diagnostic tests are developed'. The reason for such an endorsement of the 'current methods' is an attempt to confront the widespread tendency of postponing broad implementation of drug susceptibility testing until the development and introduction of new rapid and affordable methods that would not require standard tuberculosis laboratory settings.

The phenotypic methods for drug susceptibility testing are among these 'current methods', with or without combination with molecular methods. Progress in molecular biotechnology makes it possible to detect MDR and XDR directly in raw specimens. Unfortunately, even the best of these methods are not sensitive enough to provide reliable results with smear-negative specimens. Therefore, for more than 50% of new patients having small contents of mycobacteria in their sputum (acid-fast bacilli smear-negative specimens), particularly among those with dual tuberculosis+HIV infection, these methods are not applicable. Therefore, there is a need for phenotypic cultural methods to test cultures grown from smear-negative specimens. A combination of molecular and phenotypic methods may provide the best results, combining rapidity for approximately half of the specimens and addressing specimens with low mycobacterial content. The choice of specific algorithm testing with a general goal of obtaining results in the shortest possible turnaround time of the

laboratory reports depends on the specific conditions of the laboratory.

7.2 Choices of the Phenotypic Methods

This overview is based on the update of our previous reports (Heifets, 1999, 2000; Heifets and Gangelosi, 1999, 2009). Based on the type of culture medium, solid or liquid, all drug susceptibility methods based on cultivation can be divided into two groups. Solid media include the following types: Löwenstein–Jensen (LJ) or Ogawa egg-based media, Middlebrook 7H10 or 7H11 agar media and HSTB agar medium. Liquid media are used in automated or semi-automated liquid medium systems, such as BACTEC 460 and BACTEC 960 (MGIT), MB/BacT and VersaTREK. The advantage of the solid media over the liquid systems is that they can be used for a direct drug susceptibility test with smear-positive sputum specimens, which provides a relatively short turnaround time of the laboratory reports. Although liquid media cannot be used for a direct test, it has the advantage of rapid growth detection. The advantages of solid media are that, historically, they have been in use for a longer period, with more experience and better validation of procedures using a large variety of drugs. The lower cost of solid media is another advantage compared to the liquid medium system. Liquid medium systems can be used not only for qualitative tests with critical concentrations but also for a quantitative determination of the MICs. These values can be compared with the pharmacokinetic parameters (for example with the C_{max}) as an option for interpretation of the drug susceptibility test results and the predictability of the patient's response to therapy.

Qualitative tests, either in solid or liquid media, are performed with the so-called critical drug concentrations that were proposed for distinguishing between 'resistant' and 'susceptible' isolates. These critical concentrations are not intended for comparison with the pharmacokinetic parameters, and they are different for various media (Tables 7.2–7.4). The concentrations shown in Tables

Table 7.2. Critical concentrations (µg/ml) for testing *M. tuberculosis* in solid media (National Jewish Health Mycobacteriology Laboratory, Denver, Colorado).

Drug	LJ	7H10 agar	7H11 agar	HSTB agar
Isoniazid	0.2	0.2, 1.0	0.2, 1.0	0.2, 1.0
Rifampin	40.0	1.0	1.0	1.0
Ethambutol	2.0	5.0, 10.0	7.5	12.0
Pyrazinamide	–	–	–	900.0
Streptomycin	4.0	2.0, 10.0	2.0, 4.0	5.0, 10.0
Amikacin	20.0	4.0	6.0	6.0
Kanamycin	20.0	5.0	6.0	6.0
Capreomycin	20.0	10.0	10.0	10.0
Ethionamide	20.0	5.0	10.0	10.0
Cycloserine	–	20.0	60.0	60.0
PAS	0.5	2.0	8.0	8.0
Levofloxacin	–	–	4.0	4.0
Moxifloxacin	–	–	4.0	4.0

Table 7.3. Critical concentrations (µg/ml) of first-line drugs for testing *M. tuberculosis* in liquid medium systems.

Drug	BACTEC 460 insert	BACTEC 460 (Heifets and Gangelosi, 2009)	BACTEC 960 (MGIT) insert	VersaTREK insert	MB/BacT Bemer *et al.*, 2004	MB/BacT Tortoli *et al.*, 2000	MB/BacT Heifets' proposal 2010
Isoniazid	0.1, 0.4	–	0.1	0.1, 0.4	0.09	1.0	0.1, 0.4
Rifampin	2.0	0.5, 2.0	1.0	1.0	0.9	1.0	2.0
Ethambutol	2.5, 7.5	5.0	5.0	5.0, 8.0	3.5	2.0	5.0
Streptomycin	2.0, 6.0	5.0	1.0	–	0.45	1.0	2.0
Pyrazinamide	100.0	300.0	100.0	300.0	200.0	50.0	300.0

Table 7.4. Suggested critical concentrations of second-line drugs for BACTEC 460 and BACTEC MGIT 960 systems.

Drug	Suggested for the BACTEC 460 system (Heifets, 1991)	Suggested for the BACTEC 460 system (Pfyffer *et al.*, 1999)	Suggested for the BACTEC MIGIT 960 system (Krüüner *et al.*, 2006)
Ethionamide	2.5	1.25	2.5, 5.0
Kanamycin	5.0	5.0	–
Amikacin	5.0	1.0	1.0
Capreomycin	5.0	1.25	1.25
Levofloxacin	4.0	–	–
Moxifloxacin	4.0	–	0.5, 1.0
Ofloxacin	4.0	2.0	1.0

7.2–7.4 are those incorporated into the media, not the concentrations actually interacting with the bacteria. Due to the various degrees of degradation and deterioration of the drugs in different media during their preparation, storage and incubation, the actual concentrations of the drugs interacting with the bacteria are variable and are not defined in the descriptions of the procedures.

The critical concentrations are rather empirical values and some of them have not been calibrated properly, even for traditional solid media such as 7H10 and 7H11 agar (Mitchison, 1998). The issue is even more problematic for the liquid medium systems (Tables 7.3 and 7.4).

There were problems with the definition of susceptible and resistant strains. Originally, the classical definition of the drug-resistant strain of *M. tuberculosis* was that it was significantly different by a degree of susceptibility from a wild strain that had never come into contact with the drug (Canetti *et al.*, 1969; Mitchison, 1969). In reality, over a period of many years, this definition became unreliable, particularly in determining critical concentrations.

The general idea of a correct critical concentration is that it should be somewhere between the highest MIC found for fully susceptible isolates ('wild' strains) and the lowest MIC for resistance to the particular drug strains. Unfortunately, this principle is rarely used for establishing the critical concentration for the new cultivation systems. Instead, some authors select these concentrations on the basis of comparison with other media or systems. The worst scenario, when based on MICs found for susceptible strains, is that a too low concentration is selected as a critical concentration. Use of such low concentrations often results in false resistance reports. It is known that resistance of tubercle bacilli to some drugs, if it is a true resistance, can be demonstrated at any high concentrations due to the loss of the genetic target through the mutation. Therefore, the possibility of false susceptible results is lower than that of false resistance. It seems that, currently, there is the possibility of addressing this issue by genetic testing for mutations as a basis for better choice of the correct critical

concentrations, as well as for selection of the quality control strains.

A quantitative test to determine the MIC as the lowest drug concentration that inhibits the bacterial growth completely has many advantages and fewer problems over the qualitative test with critical concentrations. So far, such a methodology has been developed for testing in 7H12 broth in the BACTEC 460 system (Heifets, 1988, 1991). There is no known significant deterioration/degradation of drugs in this simple medium, and there is the assumption that the drug concentrations incorporated into 7H12 broth are actually those that interact with the bacterial inoculum. Therefore, unlike testing in solid medium, the MIC determined in this system can be correlated with the concentrations attainable in blood. This approach was used for interpretation of the MICs shown in Table 7.5. Complete inhibition of growth by the lowest of the three concentrations is indicative of interpretation as 'susceptible'. No inhibition of growth by the highest concentration is reported as MIC equal or higher than this concentration and is interpreted as 'resistant'. Inhibition of growth by the highest and the middle concentrations without growth inhibition by the lowest concentration gives an MIC that is interpreted as 'moderately susceptible'.

7.2.1 Löwenstein–Jensen medium

This medium is the most traditional and oldest medium used for both cultivation and drug susceptibility testing of *M. tuberculosis*. Unfortunately, because of the strong attachment to the historically based tradition, this medium is often the only medium used for drug susceptibility testing in many parts of the world. The major problem is that cultivation on any egg-based medium (LJ or Ogawa) takes a longer period for growth recovery as compared to agar or liquid media. That is why the results obtained on this medium are often reported too late for a physician to make any adjustment to the treatment regimen. The situation is aggravated by the tendency to use this technology as an indirect rather than a direct test.

Table 7.5. Suggested guidelines for interpretation of MICs (µg/ml) determined in the BACTEC 460 system for *M. tuberculosis* isolates (in use at the National Jewish Health Mycobacteriology Reference Laboratory, Denver, Colorado).

Drug	Susceptible	Moderately susceptible	Resistant
Isoniazid	≤0.1	0.4	≥1.6
Rifampin	≤0.5	2.0	≥8.0
Rifabutin	≤0.12	0.25	≥0.5
Ethambutol	≤4.0	8.0	≥16.0
Ethionamide	≤1.25	2.5	≥5.0
Streptomycin	≤2.5	5.0	≥10.0
Amikacin	≤2.5	5.0	≥10.0
Kanamycin	≤2.5	5.0	≥10.0
Capreomycin	≤2.5	5.0	≥10.0
Ofloxacin	≤2.0	4.0	≥8.0
Levofloxacin	≤2.0	4.0	≥8.0
Moxifloxacin	≤2.0	4.0	≥8.0
Cycloserine	≤4.0	8.0	≥16.0
Clofazimine	≤0.12	0.25	≥0.5

Historically, three methods based on cultivation of *M. tuberculosis* on starch-free LJ medium have been proposed: (i) the proportion method; (ii) the resistance ratio (RR) method; and (iii) the absolute concentration method (Canetti *et al.*, 1963, 1969). Each of these methods can be used as either a direct or indirect test, but in reality a direct test is rarely used with this medium.

The proportion method in its simplified version has become the most popular among these three options. Both drug-free (controls) and drug-containing egg-based medium suspensions are coagulated in tubes in a slope position at 85°C for 50 min. This process alone inactivates a substantial proportion of some drugs in addition to their absorption by the medium. Therefore, the critical drug concentrations developed for this medium (Table 7.2) reflect the amounts of drugs added and not those that remain in the medium to interact with bacteria. Two sets of tubes with drug-containing and drug-free medium are inoculated with a bacterial suspension. There are various techniques to calibrate the inoculum, with a goal of being sufficient to produce a growth of 100–200 colonies on a

slant. The tubes are incubated at 37°C for 1–2 days in a slope position with caps slightly ajar. Afterwards, the caps are tightened and the tubes are incubated in an upright position. On the 28th day of incubation, the colonies are counted to calculate the proportion of colonies grown on drug-containing media to the number of colonies in the controls. Any proportion that exceeds 1% for INH, RIF and PAS (para-amino-salicylic acid), and 10% for other drugs, indicates 'resistant', and the results are final. If the proportion is less than 1%, then a second reading is required on the 42nd day of cultivation to confirm that the isolate is 'susceptible' to the specific drug.

The RR method is perhaps the most accurate and most labour-intensive and costly of the three methods. The RR is defined as a ratio of MIC for the patient's isolate to the MIC for the drug-susceptible reference strain ($H_{37}Rv$), both tested in the same experiment. MIC determination requires a large number of medium tubes containing a broad range of drug concentrations. For this method, the MIC is defined as the lowest drug concentration in the presence of which the number of colonies is less than 20 after 4 weeks of incubation. RR of 2 or less is an indication of 'susceptible' and RR of 8 or greater indicates 'resistant'.

The absolute concentration method is based on the comparison of growth intensity in the presence of critical concentrations (adjusted for each laboratory) and on drug-free controls. The original $H_{37}Rv$ strain preserved in aliquots at our laboratory is tested in parallel with the same drugs in multiple concentrations for QC of reproducibility. The results are determined after 4 weeks of incubation, or after 5–6 weeks if growth is insufficient at the 4-week reading. A 'susceptible' result is reported if the number of colonies in the presence of a drug is less than 20, while there are more than 100 colonies grown in drug-free controls.

7.2.2 Agar proportion method

The major advantage of performing drug susceptibility tests in agar plates is related to the transparency of the medium, which makes it possible to observe the growing colonies at the beginning of their formation. Therefore, final results can be reported within 3 weeks for most isolates, instead of 4–6 weeks or more when using egg-based media. There are at least three types of agar medium that can be used for either direct or indirect tests: 7H10, 7H11 and HSTB. A detailed description of their preparation and use can be found in the appropriate publications (David, 1971; Kent and Kubica, 1985; Heifets, 2000; Heifets and Sanchez, 2000, 2003). These media are made from commercially available 7H10 or 7H11 agar base. The HSTB agar is made from the 7H11 agar base with the addition of monosodium phosphate (0.6 g/100 ml of medium) to change the pH of the medium from 6.6 ± 0.2 to 6.2 ± 0.2.

To prepare agar media, one should follow the manufacturer's instruction marked on the label placed on each container of the base powder. The base powder is suspended in distilled water containing 0.5% glycerol, autoclaved at 121°C for 15 min, and then cooled in a water bath to 52–54°C. Afterwards, 10% enrichment supplement is added: the commercially available OADC (oleate-albumin-dextrose-catalase) for 7H10 or 7H11 medium, and calf or horse serum for HSTB agar. The appropriate drug solutions are added to ensure the intended critical concentrations (Table 7.2). The medium is distributed into plastic plates, usually into quadrant plates, approximately 5.0 ml/quadrant. It is now known that some isolates may have genetically predetermined low levels of resistance to INH (Madison et al., 2004). Therefore, two concentrations of INH are needed to distinguish between low and high levels of resistance to this drug. A higher concentration of streptomycin (SM) in addition to the critical concentration of this drug is usually employed in agar media for confirmation of resistance on some occasions when the presence of CO_2 in the incubator (for 7H10 and 7H11 agar) may have affected the activity of SM.

To detect MDR, only one quadrant plate of any of the agar medium type (with a drug-free quadrant) is needed for a test with RIF and two concentrations of INH. In the case of using HSTB agar, two quadrant agar plates can be used for a test with INH, rifampin (RMP), ethambutol (EMB) and pyrazinamide (PZA). Four quadrant plates of any agar type are needed for a test with ten drugs. For a direct test after processing the specimen, commonly described as the digestion–decontamination procedure, the concentrated sputum is inoculated on to plates, 0.1 ml/quadrant. For an indirect test, two sets of plates are used: one inoculated with 10^{-3}-fold and the other with 10^{-5}-fold dilutions of the bacterial suspension adjusted to the optical density of the McFarland No 1 standard. The plates are incubated at 35–37°C for 3 weeks, protected from light, in an atmosphere of 5–10% CO_2 for 7H10 and 7H11 agar plates and in a regular incubator (without CO2) for the HSTB agar. The plates are incubated in sealed plastic bags. After incubation, the plates are placed on the bench at room temperature for 3 h or overnight in an upside position (agar up) for elimination of the condensate. The colonies are counted and the results are reported as the percentage (proportion) based on comparison of the number of colonies on drug-containing and drug-free quadrants. The isolate is considered 'resistant' if this proportion is 1% or greater for all drugs except PZA. The established criterion for PZA is 10%. For 10–15% of isolates, the growth may not be sufficient at the 3-week reading. Then, the plates are re-examined at the 6-week reading, but in such cases only 'susceptible' results are considered valid. This is because growth at 6 weeks in drug-containing quadrants may be related to drug degradation during the prolonged incubation period rather than to the occurrence of true drug resistance.

7.2.3 Qualitative indirect test in liquid media

The need for expedited detection of drug resistance was first addressed in the 1980s by developing the drug susceptibility testing procedure for the semi-automated BACTEC 460 system introduced by Becton Dickinson, Sparks, Maryland, USA (Siddiqi *et al.*, 1981, 1985; Roberts *et al.*, 1983). The liquid medium for this system, 7H12 broth in 12B vials, contains ^{14}C-substrate, consumption of which by the growing bacteria results in the release of $^{14}CO_2$, measured by the instrument and expressed as the growth index (GI). The turnaround time for an indirect test in this system was 9.3 days, and the overall mean time for primary isolation plus indirect test was 18 days in a cooperative study by five institutions (Roberts *et al.*, 1983; Heifets, 1986). The major disadvantage of this system was the problem of disposal of radioactive materials (12B vials), which stimulated the development of new non-radiometric systems.

Three such systems, all fully automated and computerized, became commercially available: BACTEC MGIT 960 (Becton Dickinson Microbiology Systems, Sparks, Maryland, USA), MB/BacT (bioMérieux, Durham, North Carolina, USA) and VersaTREK, formerly the ESP-II Culture System by Difco (TREK Diagnostic Systems, Westlake, Ohio, USA).

In the BACTEC MGIT 960 system, the bacterial growth detection is based on the consumption of oxygen, which causes the indicator embedded in the bottom of tubes to fluoresce, and the instrument continuously monitors the increase of fluorescence. Comparison of these patterns in drug-containing and drug-free tubes is analysed automatically by the instrument and reported as 'susceptible' or 'resistant'.

In the MB/BacT system, a colorimetric sensor detecting the release of CO_2 by the growing bacteria is embedded in the bottom of the vial. The instrument continuously monitors and reports the colour as it changes from dark green to yellow. A 'susceptible' result is reported if no colour changes occur in the drug-containing vial or if a positive detection time in this vial is greater than in the drug-free control. A 'resistant' result is reported if growth is detected in the drug-containing vial or if the detection time for this vial is shorter than for the drug-free control.

In the VersaTREK system, growth monitoring is based on the reduction of pressure in the vials due to the consumption of oxygen by the growing bacteria. The conclusion is based on the comparison of drug-free controls and drug-containing vials after positive readings have occurred for 3 consecutive days in the drug-free vial. 'Susceptible' is reported if no growth is detected in the drug-containing vials and 'resistant' is reported if growth is detected in the drug-containing vials at this time point.

For all four liquid medium systems, critical concentrations have been either developed or suggested for four to five first-line drugs: INH, RIF, EMB, SM, PZA (4.3). Two concentrations of INH are needed to distinguish between low and high levels of resistance to this drug (Madison *et al.*, 2004). A lower concentration of EMB (2.5 µg/ml) by Becton Dickinson for the BACTEC 460 system appeared to cause false resistance results, and therefore the manufacturer suggested an additional higher concentration of 7.5 µg/ml. Instead, we introduced a concentration of 4.0 µg/ml and, later, 5.0 µg/ml, which appeared to be quite reliable in distinguishing between resistant and susceptible strains. For addressing the problem of false resistance to PZA, we replaced the concentration of 100.0 µg/ml suggested by the manufacturer with 300.0 µg/ml (Heifets, 1991, 2002).

Critical concentrations for the MB/BacT system shown in Table 7.3 include references to two publications to illustrate the diversity in the opinions of different authors regarding the critical concentrations needed (Tortoli *et al.*, 2000; Bemer *et al.*, 2004). Critical concentrations of various second-line drugs were suggested for the BACTEC 460 and BACTEC MGIT 960 systems (Table 7.4) (Heifets, 1991; Pfyffer *et al.*, 1999; Krüüner *et al.*, 2006). We are proposing now to use for this system the same concentrations as we are using for the BACTEC 460. There are debates about concentrations of quinolones to be defined as critical for testing *in vitro*. Unfortunately, there have been no clinical trails completed yet to indicate any possible correlation between resistance to various concentrations of quinolones *in vitro* and a patient's response to therapy with these drugs. Often, testing with very low concentrations results in false resistance reports. One should keep in mind that for these drugs, as is true for some other agents as well, loss of a genetic target due to mutation makes the isolate resistant to any drug concentration. Therefore, it is reasonable to use a drug concentration significantly higher (at least four- or eightfold higher) than the highest MIC found for wild strains obtained from patients never treated with the agent in question.

In addition to the qualitative tests, a quantitative MIC test was proposed for the BACTEC 460 system (Table 7.5), in which the category 'moderately susceptible' corresponded to the critical concentrations in Tables 7.3 and 7.4. The critical concentrations listed in the tables reflect the situation at the time of preparation of this paper. However, one should be aware that the manufacturers of liquid medium systems review and change these concentrations periodically according to the progress in their evaluation. Up-to-date suggestions are usually listed in the manufacturer's inserts. In addition, some authors have used their own 'critical concentrations'. Recommendations by the Clinical and Laboratory Standards Institute (NCCLS, 2003; CLSI, 2009) may not help to resolve inevitable controversies. Therefore, each laboratory should re-evaluate the protocol suggested by the manufacturer and, based on appropriate studies, consider different or additional concentrations than those suggested by the manufacturer or various authors.

The validity of results by non-radiometric systems has been analysed in some publications based on comparison with the BACTEC 460 system and/or with the agar proportion method. Both are used as reference methods. Unfortunately, even the agar proportion method has been criticized as having improperly calibrated critical concentrations (Mitchison, 1998). As mentioned above, critical concentrations for the BACTEC 460 system are also far from perfect. Therefore, acceptance of these two systems as reference methods may have a relative value. It would be more reasonable to use strains, resistant and susceptible, with an established genetic characterization for the development of critical concentrations in new systems. Such an approach would resolve conflicting results and suggestions from different laboratories.

A review of the literature regarding drug susceptibility testing in non-radiometric automated liquid medium systems suggests that each of the available systems provides an opportunity for relatively rapid turnaround time of the indirect drug susceptibility test, although time ranges reported by different authors have been broad, and that each of these methods has certain advantages and disadvantages (Piersimoni *et al.*, 2006). Authors of this review concluded that the BACTEC MGIT 960 system appears to be the most reliable option among the non-radiometric liquid medium systems for testing drug susceptibility to the first-line antituberculosis drugs in an indirect test.

7.3 Optimal Algorithms

Described below are various combinations of different procedures presented in the order of affordability/cost, from the simplest to the most complex.

The least expensive protocol, and still with concern for minimizing the turnaround time of the laboratory report, is the use of a single HSTB agar plate with four quadrant (segments) containing a drug-free control and three quadrants containing INH 0.2, INH

1.0 and RIF 1.0 µg/ml. Use of this type of plate is the simplest way to detect MDR. The costs of materials for such a plate is less than US$1.00 (USA costs, 2010), and it can be cultivated in a regular incubator (without CO_2). Instead of the HSTB agar, the test can be performed on 7H10 or 7H11 agar, if the laboratory is equipped with the CO_2 incubators and has a reliable supply of the OADC supplement. The turnaround time of the direct test with a smear-positive sputum specimen is 3 weeks for 80–85% of specimens. For culture isolation, parallel with or without (for smear-negative specimens) the direct test, the specimen should be inoculated on to an agar bi-plate consisting of plain and selective agar. The isolated culture is necessary for setting up an indirect test when the direct test fails, as well as for cultures isolated from smear-negative specimens. The total turnaround time of culture isolation plus an indirect test is 6 weeks for 80–85% of smear-negative specimens.

The next option is an expansion of the agar proportion method through testing not only against INH and RIF, but, with any of the other drugs listed in Table 7.1, under conditions that in each plate one quadrant is used as a control containing a drug-free medium. An agar proportion method, either a one-plate test as described above or its expanded version, should be recommended as a replacement for the LJ medium in countries where the traditional use of the egg-based medium is still in place. The advantages of the agar plates over the egg-based media are obvious in regard to the turnaround time, cost of materials and labour. Unlike with supplies sold by manufacturers for agar plates, the basic cost for egg-based media is the local cost of eggs. This is one of the reasons for the cost variability among countries for this type of medium. It is likely that such a cost may be significantly higher than the cost of an agar plate.

Incorporation of a liquid medium system into the laboratory protocol for both culture isolation and drug susceptibility testing shortens the turnaround time of the drug susceptibility reports for smear-negative specimens, but it also increases the cost significantly. Perhaps it is reasonable to combine the direct test on agar plates for the smear-positive specimens with culture isolation from all specimens in the liquid medium, followed by the indirect test in liquid medium with cultures isolated from smear-negative specimens or in cases of failure of the direct test on agar plates. Total turnaround time of the laboratory reports, including culture isolation and the indirect test is about 3 weeks, but it is highly variable depending on the bacterial contents in the specimens.

The most desirable approach for obtaining maximum information within the shortest turnaround time is to combine molecular and phenotypic methods; these are discussed in Chapters 2 and 9. Therefore, it should be combined with cultivation in both liquid medium and agar plates. Cultures obtained from smear-negative specimens can be subjected to the Hain test for rapid detection of MDR/XDR. The total turnaround time in this case would be less than 3 weeks for most of these smear-negative specimens. Parallel testing by phenotypic methods, in liquid medium and on agar plates, is essential not only for confirmation of the results obtained by the Hain technology but also for obtaining a broader picture of the drug resistance/susceptibility pattern of the isolate. Thus, combined use of molecular and phenotypic methods may provide the most desirable combination of the rapidity and reliability of the results.

7.4 Conclusion

Phenotypic methods of drug susceptibility testing of the *M. tuberculosis* isolates can play a significant role in timely detection of patients with MDR and XDR. An important element of the application of these methods is the direct test for the smear-positive specimens, preferably on agar plates, as a minimal algorithm for countries with limited resources. This option can provide a rapid turnaround time (3 weeks) to report on susceptibility to INH and RIF for 80–85% of specimens. It can be applied to other drugs as well, and it can be complemented with the indirect test for cultures isolated from smear-negative specimens. When resources allow, the addition of the liquid medium system would expedite the results, particularly for smear-negative specimens. Finally, a combination of phenotypic and molecular methods is the best, although the most expensive, option for obtaining the most complete information in the shortest turnaround time

It must be stressed that, regardless of the methods used, any of the procedures for drug susceptibility testing of *M. tuberculosis* require implementation of biosafety standards, usually defined as BSL-3 practices (Richmond *et al.*, 1996; Heifets and Richmond, 2006). There are no phenotypic methods for drug susceptibility testing of *M. tuberculosis* that can be implemented without these standards.

Taking into account the need for costly equipment to comply with biosafety standards, as well as the application of any level of sophistication of the protocol, the most economical approach to drug susceptibility testing, along with bacteriological diagnosis in general, is to have large laboratories with direct centralized services to a country, or to significant parts of that country, and not just reference laboratories that would provide a reference service to the lower level of laboratories.

Direct microscopy smear examination was recommended as the main diagnostic tool when the DOTS strategy was initially introduced. Under the provisions of this approach, the decentralization of laboratory services in developing countries with high tuberculosis prevalence was inevitable, along with the needs of supervision by the reference laboratories of the quality of work at the microscopy stations. Today, the new enhanced DOTS strategy recommends the phased introduction of drug susceptibility testing as a major tool to combat MDR and XDR epidemics (WHO, 2010). Implementation of this approach will require qualified laboratories being able to perform culture isolation and drug susceptibility testing, as well as some molecular testing. The direct delivery of raw specimens to such laboratories will become necessary for the sake of quality of

testing and for shortening the turnaround time of the laboratory reports, as well as for better cost-efficiency of the operation.

References

American Thoracic Society [ATS] (1990) Diagnostic standards and classification of tuberculosis. *American Review of Respiratory Diseases* 142, 3 (Supplement), 725–735.

Bemer, P., Bodmer, T., Munzinger, J., Perrin, M., Vincent, V. and Drugeon, H. (2004) Multicenter evaluation of the MB/BacT system for susceptibility testing of *Mycobacterium tuberculosis*. *Journal of Clinical Microbiology* 42, 1030–1034.

Brossier, F., Veziris, N., Aubry, A., Jarlier, V. and Sougakoff, W. (2010) Detection by GenoType MTBDRsl test of complex mechanism of resistance to second line drugs and ethambutol in multidrug-resistant *Mycobacterium tuberculosis* complex isolates. *Journal of Clinical Microbiology* 48, 1683–1689.

Canetti, G., Froman, S., Grosset, J., Hauduroy P., Langerova, M., Mahler, H.T., *et al.* (1963) Mycobacteria: laboratory methods for testing drug sensitivity and resistance. *Bulletin of The World Health Organization* 29, 565–578.

Canetti, G., Fox, W., Khomenko, A., Mahler, H.T., Menon, M.K., Mitchison, D.A., *et al.* (1969) Advances in techniques of testing mycobacterial drug sensitivity and the use of sensitivity tests in tuberculosis control programs. *Bulletin of The World Health Organization* 41, 21–43.

CDC [Centers for Disease Control and Prevention] (2009) Plan to combat extensively drug-resistant tuberculosis: recommendations of the Federal Tuberculosis Task Force. *Morbidity and Mortality Weekly Report* 58(RR-3), 1–43.

CLSI [Clinical and Laboratory Standard Institute] (2009) *Susceptibility Testing of Mycobacteria, Nocardiae, and Other Aerobic Actinimycetes.* Approved standard – Second Edition. CLSI document M24-A2. Wayne, Pennsylvania.

David, H.L. (1971) *Fundamentals of Drug Susceptibility Testing in Tuberculosis.* CDC/HEW Publication No 00-2165. Atlanta, Georgia.

Farmer, P., Bayona, J., Becerra, M., Furin, J., Henry, C., Hiatt, H., *et al.* (1998) The dilemma of MDR-TB in the global era. *International Journal of Tuberculosis and Lung Disease* 2, 869–876.

Gupta, R., Espinal, M.A. and Raviglione, M.C. (2004) Tuberculosis as a major global health problem in 21st century. In: Heifets, L. (ed.)

Tuberculosis and other mycobacterial infections. *Seminars in Respiratory and Critical Care Medicine* 25(3), 245–253.

Heifets, L.B. (1986) Rapid automated methods (BACTEC System) in clinical mycobacteriology. *Seminars in Respiratory Infections* 1(4), 242–249.

Heifets, L.B. (1988) Qualitative and quantitative drug susceptibility tests in mycobacteriology. *American Review of Respiratory Diseases* 137, 1217–1222.

Heifets, L. (1991) Drug susceptibility tests in the management of chemotherapy of tuberculosis. In: Heifets, L.B. (ed.) *Drug Susceptibility in Chemotherapy of Mycobacterial Infections.* CRC Press, Boca Raton, Florida, pp. 89–121.

Heifets, L. (2000) Conventional methods for antimicrobial susceptibility testing of *M. tuberculosis.* In: Bastian, I. and Portaels, F. (eds) *Multidrug-Resistant Tuberculosis.* Kluwer Academic Publisher, Dordrecht, The Netherlands, pp. 133–143.

Heifets, L. (2002) Susceptibility testing of *M. tuberculosis* to pyrazinamide. *Journal of Medical Microbiology* 51(1), 11–12.

Heifets, L.B. and Gangelosi, G.A. (1999) Drug susceptibility testing of *Mycobacterium tuberculosis*: a neglected problem at the turn of the century. *International Journal for Tuberculosis and Lung Disease* 3(7), 564–581.

Heifets, L. and Gangelosi, G. (2009) Chapter 81: Drug resistant assays for *Mycobacterium tuberculosis.* In: Mayers, D.I. (ed.) *Antimicrobial Drug Resistance.* Humana Press, pp. 1161–1170.

Heifets, L.B. and Richmond, J.Y. (2006) Modern biological safety standards in tuberculosis diagnostic laboratories. In: *Anthology of Biosafety,* IX, Chapter 13, pp. 155–166.

Heifets, L. and Sanchez, T. (2000) New agar medium for testing susceptibility of *Mycobacterium tuberculosis* to pyrazinamide. *Journal of Clinical Microbiology* 38, 1498–14501.

Heifets, L. and Sanchez, T. (2003) and (2005) New agar medium for mycobacteria (HSTB agar). *Patents:* No US 6,579,694 B2, and No US 6,951,733 B2.

Hilleman, D., Rüsch-Gerdes, S. and Richter, E. (2010) Feasibility of the GenoType MTBDR*st* assay for fluoroquinolone, amikacin-capreomycin, and ethambutol resistance testing of *Mycobacterium tuberculosis* strains and clinical specimens. *Journal of Clinical Microbiology* 47, 1767–1772.

Kent, P.T. and Kubica, G.P. (1985) *Public Health Mycobacteriology: A Guide for the Level III Laboratory.* CDC, Atlanta, Georgia.

Krüüner, A., Yates, M.D. and Drobniewski, F.A. (2006) Evaluation of MGIT 960-based antimicrobial testing and determination of critical concentrations of first- and second-line antimicrobial drugs with drug-resistant clinical strains of *M. tuberculosis. Journal of Clinical Microbiology* 44, 811–818.

Lacoma, A., Garcia-Sierra, N., Prat, C., Ruitz-Manzano, J., Haba, L., Rosés, S., *et al.* (2008) Genotype MTBD*plus* assay for molecular detection of rifampin and isoniazid resistance in *Mycobacterium tuberculosis* strains and clinical specimens. *Journal of Clinical Microbiology* 46, 3660–3667.

Madison, B.M., Siddiqi, S.H., Heifets, L., Gross, W., Higgins, M., Warren, N., *et al.* (2004) Identification of a *Mycobacterium tuberculosis* strain with stable, low-level resistance to isoniazid. *Journal of Clinical Microbiology* 42, 1294–1295.

Mitchison, D.A. (1969) What is drug resistance? *Tubercle* 50 (Supplement), 44–47.

Mitchison, D.A. (1998) Standardization of sensitivity tests (letter). *International Journal of Tuberculosis and Lung Disease* 2, 69.

NCCLS [National Committee for Clinical Laboratory Standards] (2003) *Susceptibility Testing of Mycobacteria, Nocardiae, and Other Aerobic Actinomycetes. Approved standard M24-A.* NCCLS, Wayne, Pennsylvania.

Pfyffer, G.E., Bonato, D.A., Ebrahimzade, A., Gross, W, Higgins, M., Warren, N., *et al.* (1999) Multicenter laboratory validation of susceptibility testing of *M. tuberculosis* against second-line and newer antimicrobial drugs by using the radiometric Bactec-460 technique and the proportion method with solid media. *Journal of Clinical Microbiology* 37, 3179–3186.

Piersimoni, C., Olivieri, A., Benacchio, L. and Scarparo, C. (2006) Current perspectives on drug susceptibility testing of *Mycobacterium tuberculosis* complex: the automated non-radiometric systems. *Journal of Clinical Microbiology* 44, 20–28.

Richmond, J.Y., Knudsen, R.C. and Good, R.C. (1996) Bio-safety in the clinical mycobacteriology laboratory. *Clinics in Laboratory Medicine (Clinical Mycobacteriology)* 16, 527–550.

Roberts, G.D., Goodman, N.L., Heifets, L., Larsh, H.W., Lindner, T.H., McClatchy, J.K., *et al.* (1983) Evaluation of the BACTEC radiometric method for recovery mycobacteria and drug susceptibility testing of *M. tuberculosis* acid-fast smear-positive specimens. *Journal of Clinical Microbiology* 18, 689–696.

Siddiqi, S.H., Libonati, J.P. and Middlebrook, G. (1981) Evaluation of a rapid radiometric method for drug susceptibility testing of *M.*

tuberculosis. Journal of Clinical Microbiology 13, 908–912.

Siddiqi, S.H., Hawkins, J.E. and Laszlo, A. (1985) Interlaboratory drug susceptibility testing of *M. tuberculosis* by radiometric and two conventional methods. *Journal of Clinical Microbiology* 22, 919–923.

Tenover, F.C., Crawford, J.T., Heubner, R.E., Geiter, I.J., Horsburg, C.R. and Good, R.C. (1993). The resurgence of tuberculosis: is your laboratory ready? *Journal of Clinical Microbiology* 31, 767–770.

Tortoli, E., Mattei, R., Savarino, A., Bartolini, L. and Beer, J. (2000) Comparison of *M. tuberculosis* susceptibility testing performed with BACTEC 460-TB (Becton Dickinson) and MB/BacT (Organon Teknika) systems. *Diagnostic Microbiology and Infectious Diseases* 38, 83–88.

World Health Organization [WHO] (1997) *TB Treatment Observer*. WHO, Geneva, Switzerland.

WHO (2010) *Multidrug and Extensively Drug-resistant TB (M/XDR-TB): 2010 Global Report on Surveillance and Response*. WHO/HTM/TB 2010.3, Geneva, Switzerland.

8 Genotypic Measures of Antibiotic Susceptibility

Vanessa Mathys,[1] Barun Mathema[2] and Pablo Bifani[3]*

[1]*Tuberculosis and Mycobacteria, Communicable and Infectious Diseases, Scientific Institute of Public Health, Belgium;* [2]*Tuberculosis Center, Public Health Research Institute, University of Medicine and Dentistry, Newark, New Jersey, USA;* [3]*The Novartis Institute for Tropical Diseases, Singapore*

8.1 Introduction: The Challenge of Drug-resistant Tuberculosis

Tuberculosis remains the leading cause of adult mortality attributable to a single infectious disease, despite effective chemotherapy having been available for over 50 years and the development of the tuberculosis control strategy of directly observed therapy, short course (DOTS) (Murray *et al.*, 1991; Bloom and Murray, 1992; Raviglione *et al.*, 1995). Tuberculosis chemotherapy is markedly different from other bacterial pathogens. *Mycobacterium tuberculosis* has an exceptionally long generation time and a capacity for dormancy, when its low metabolic activity renders it a difficult therapeutic target. Moreover, *M. tuberculosis* may reside in pulmonary cavities, solid caseous material or empyema pus where drug penetration is inefficient or the pH sufficiently low to inhibit antibiotic activity (Kaufmann, 2001). Selection for drug-resistant mutants in the patient occurs mainly when patients are treated inappropriately or are exposed to, even transiently, subtherapeutic drug levels; conditions that provide adequate positive selection pressure for emergence and, on occasion, maintenance of drug-resistant organisms *de novo*. The need to maintain high drug levels over many months of treatment, combined with the inherent toxicity of the agents, results in reduced patient compliance and the subsequently higher likelihood of selecting drug-resistant mutants (Davies, 1998). Therefore, in addition to identifying new antituberculosis agents, the means to shorten the length of chemotherapy is paramount, as it would impact clinical management greatly and the emergence of drug resistance.

The emergence of increasingly drug-resistant forms of *M. tuberculosis* represents a growing problem that stands to derail much progress made by global and local tuberculosis control programmes. In recent years, substantial advances have been made in understanding mechanisms of action of antimycobacterial agents and the biochemical basis of drug resistance (reviewed in this chapter) (Ramaswamy and Musser, 1998; Webb and Davies, 1999). In contrast to other pathogenic bacteria, which generally acquire drug-resistance determinants by horizontal transfer, the acquisition of drug resistance in *M. tuberculosis* occurs via *de novo* point mutations, small deletions or insertions in specific chromosomal genes. The genetic basis of drug resistance in *M. tuberculosis* has been defined for many of the commonly used first- and second-line antibiotics (Davies, 1998). Once the bacilli have mutated, selection for drug-resistant mutants occurs in the presence of subtherapeutic drug levels or inappropriate therapy. An alarming trend, and a growing source of public health concern, has been the emergence of multiple drug-resistance tuberculosis (MDR-TB), defined as isolates that are resistant to at least isoniazid (INH) and rifampicin (RIF), the two most potent anti-tubercular drugs (Iseman and Madsen, 1989; Vareldzis et al., 1994). The World Health Organization (WHO) estimates that 50 million individuals worldwide harbour MDR M. tuberculosis (WHO, 1996). MDR-TB is associated with high morbidity and mortality, prolonged treatment to cure and an increased risk of spreading infection with drug-resistant isolates in the community (Iseman and Madsen, 1989; Bifani et al., 1996). A recent global survey of MDR-TB incidence estimated that an average of 3.4% of all new cases (no documented prior history of tuberculosis) had MDR-TB (Dye et al., 2002).

Compounding the tuberculosis crisis, XDR (extensively drug resistant) M. tuberculosis isolates that are defined as resistant to INH, RIF plus a fluoroquinolone and at least one of the injectable drugs (e.g. kanamycin, capreomycin and amikacin) commonly used in second-line treatment for MDR-TB have emerged. The Centers for Disease Control and Prevention (CDC) conducted a global survey of XDR-TB prevalence in 2000–2004 that estimated 9.9% of all MDR-TB isolates were additionally resistant to at least two classes of second-line anti-tuberculosis agents (Shah et al., 2007). This report suggested that XDR-TB might be emerging in many countries with and without an expanding DOTS tuberculosis control programme. While treatment for MDR-TB has improved greatly (mainly in resource-rich settings), outcomes remain far below drug-susceptible counterparts; indices that are worse for XDR-TB (Bifani et al., 1996; Crofton et al., 1997; Iseman, 2000; CDC, 2003; Gandhi et al., 2006). Additionally, using second-line agents, which are often broader-spectrum antibiotics, there is a concern of collateral damage in terms of selection of resistance among other coexisting pathogens. For instance, in South Africa, invasive streptococcal infection that is resistant to levofloxacin has been associated with a history of tuberculosis treatment (Gottberg et al., 2008). Likewise, fluoroquinolones that are widely used to treat community-acquired bacterial infections may also act inadvertently on undiagnosed tuberculosis, in essence by monotherapy and thereby selecting for resistance (Drlica et al., 2008).

In this chapter, we review the genetic basis of drug resistance in M. tuberculosis and correlates to phenotypic antibiotic susceptibility. We focus on anti-tubercular agents and drug resistance-conferring mutations that are most relevant in the clinical and epidemiologic setting.

8.2 Rifampicin

Rifampicin (RIF), a semi-synthetic derivative of rifamycin B, was first introduced as an anti-tubercular in 1966. Together with INH, RIF comprises the cornerstone of present-day anti-tubercular therapy. RIF is the fastest acting, sterilizing anti-tubercular agent, due in part to its ability to kill semi-dormant bacterial subpopulations and hence active against both actively growing and slowly metabolizing M. tuberculosis (Zhang et al., 2005). The loss of RIF as a therapeutic option is associated with higher rates of treatment failure (Espinal et al., 2000). Since the mid-1990s, RIF resistance (RIF[R]) has been used as a surrogate marker for multidrug-resistant M. tuberculosis isolates, given that mono-RIF[R] isolates are rare (Bifani et al., 1996; Ridzon et al., 1998). Various other rifamycin derivatives have been evaluated for activity and reduced cytotoxicity. Of these, rifapentine and rifabutin have been approved by the FDA for the treatment of mycobacterial infections; while others, such as KRM 1648, are under investigation. Rifapentine poses improved pharmacokinetics accumulating in macrophages at concentrations 60 times higher than in the extracellular fluid as well as longer (4–5 times) half-life, allowing for intermittent therapy. Based on clinical trials, rifapentine is now recommended twice a week for the intensive phase of treatment and once a week for continuation therapy. Similarly, rifabutin has a longer half-life than RIF and better *in vitro* activity; however, it has lower *in vivo* activity and increased side effects. Rifabutin is currently used for the prevention of disseminated *M. avium* infection, particularly among HIV/AIDS patients. Both rifapentine and rifabutin share extensive cross-resistance with RIF.

RIF inhibits transcription by binding the DNA-dependent RNA-polymerase (RNAPol) and suppresses the initial chain formation/elongation of the nascent mRNA synthesis. RIF interferes by binding deep in the DNA–RNA channel, both through hydrophobic side-chain interaction and by hydrogen bonding to the key hydroxyl groups of the RIF and the β-subunit of the RNAPol (*rpoβ*). In the process, RIF blocks the elongation selectively at the initiation site, within the addition of the first 2–5 nucleotides (Campbell *et al.*, 2001).

8.2.1 Molecular genetics of rifampicin resistance

The correlation of RIF[R] and mutations in *rpoB* were first described in *E. coli* in 1980 (Ovchinnikov *et al.*, 1981) and in *M. tuberculosis* in 1993 (Honore and Cole, 1993; Telenti *et al.*, 1993). The codon numbering used in *M. tuberculosis* corresponds to the *E. coli* protein, which differs by 81 codons. Numerous studies have shown that >95% of all RIF[R] isolates encode a mutation within the rifampicin resistant-determining region (RRDR), an 81-bp long fragment (codons 507–533). Further, within the RRDR, mutations at His[526] and Ser[531] account for ~80% (~40% each) of all RIF[R] clinical isolates and Asp[516] for a further ~8%. Noteworthy, substitutions at His[526] and Ser[531] correlate to little to no cost in bacterial fitness (Gagneux *et al.*, 2006b). Single nucleotide polymorphisms (SNPs) and in-frame deletions, insertions in other positions of the RRDR and sometimes in the N-terminus of the *rpoB* account for ~4% of the remaining RIF[R] isolates. About ~60 different alterations have been reported, of which ~40 are within the RRDR, and few have yet to be confirmed

to correlate to drug resistance. Often, other mutations within the RRDR are associated with low levels of RIF resistance and low fitness. RIF[R] spontaneous mutants of *M. tuberculosis* and *M. bovis* BCG selected for *in vitro* mirror the clinical distribution of mutations in type and frequency (Morlock *et al.*, 2000; Mathys, unpublished). In some instances, RIF[R] isolates encoding two or more mutations within the RRDR have been reported (Bahrmand *et al.*, 2009). It is possible that these additional mutations are associated with compensatory mechanism(s) or higher levels of resistance; however, adequate experimental work is required before drawing any conclusions. Finally, about 3–5% of all RIF[R] clinical isolates have mechanisms of resistance not encoded by the *rpoB*. Efflux pumps, mechanisms of ADP ribosylation and proteins of unknown functions have been proposed; however, the epidemiological significance of these has yet to be determined (Baysarowich *et al.*, 2008).

8.3 Isoniazid

Isoniazid (INH, isonicotinic acid hydrazide), a structural analogue of nicotinamide, is a synthetic anti-tubercular agent whose activity was first highlighted in 1952 (Bernstein *et al.*, 1952; Fox, 1952) and soon after introduced in clinic. INH was first shown to inhibit the synthesis of cell wall mycolic acids (Winder and Collins, 1970) and later to inhibit the catalysis of the synthesis of mycolic acids leading to the accumulation of long-chain fatty acids in INH-treated samples (Takayama *et al.*, 1972, 1975). Twenty years later, Zhang and colleagues reported that *M. tuberculosis* clinical isolates resistant to INH presented reduced catalase activity, leading to the identification of mutations within the bifunctional catalase-peroxidase enzyme (KatG) (Zhang *et al.*, 1992). Resistance and susceptibility could be reinstated in a wild-type strain through homologous recombination (Zhang *et al.*, 1992, 1993). Subsequent investigations revealed that INH was a prodrug merely activated by KatG, while the target of the active form of INH was the enoyl-ACP reductase (InhA) (Banerjee *et al.*, 1994). InhA encodes a protein implicated in the elongation of the fatty-acid chain in mycolic acid synthesis in the FAS II (fatty acid synthase) system (Banerjee *et al.*, 1994). Recombination of the *inhA* mutant Ser^{94}Ala in a wild-type *M. tuberculosis* is sufficient to confer INH resistance and inhibition of mycolic acid synthesis (Vilcheze *et al.*, 2006), and likewise, overexpression of InhA in a susceptible strain results in INH^R (Larsen *et al.*, 2002). The crystallization of InhA in the presence of INH and NADH made it possible to establish that the activated form of INH did not bind to the InhA directly (Rozwarski *et al.*, 1998). Instead, a covalently bound INH–NAD complex competes for the active site with NADH, the natural substrate, resulting in the inhibition of the synthesis of the mycolic acid α-chain (Argyrou *et al.*, 2006). Consequently, it is hypothesized that INH penetrates the cell by passive diffusion, where it is activated by KatG to form a hypothetical isonicotinoyle radical which binds to NAD, resulting in an INH–NAD complex that would inhibit InhA. These successive steps inhibit mycolic acid synthesis, resulting in the accumulation of long-chain fatty acids and cell death (Timmins and Deretic, 2006; Vilcheze and Jacobs, 2007). In addition to KatG and InhA, several other less frequent targets have been implicated in INH^R isolates. Some of the other targets include an NADH-dehydrogenase (*ndh*II), an arylamine N-acetyltransferase (*nhoA*) and a ferric uptake regulator (*furA*), to mention a few (Ramaswamy *et al.*, 2003). Although in some instances the implication of these alternative targets are supported by extensive experimental data, their prevalence and significance in the clinical setting remain to be explored further. In addition, targets such as the β-ketoacyl-ACP-synthase (KasA) and the dyhydrofolate reductase (DHFR) have been challenged experimentally and clinically (Wang *et al.*, 2010).

8.3.1 Molecular genetics of isoniazid resistance

Review of the literature indicates that approximately 70–80% of all INH^R *M. tuberculosis*

strains encode mutations within the *katG* gene. SNPs account for most of the mutants; however, in- and out-of-frame deletions, insertions and terminations have also been observed (Ramaswamy and Musser, 1998; Slayden and Barry, 2000). SNPs in *katG*-Ser^{315} are by far the most frequently encountered, whereby Ser^{315}Thr alone accounts for ~40–50% of all INH^R strains. Mutations on Ser^{315} have been shown to bypass INH activation while retaining a 50% functional catalase-peroxidase activity (Wengenack *et al.*, 1997), giving a selective advantage to the organism. Mutations in KatG^{315} are associated with resistance to >4 µg/ml in most instances, depending on the substitution. The W-MDR strain from New York City encodes an unusual double nucleotide substitution *katG*-AGC^{315}>ACA^{315} (Bifani *et al.*, 1996). Several other INH^R associated mutations localized within this same locus of *katG*-Ser^{315}. Over 80 different mutations in the *katG* have been reported, of which ~60 are within the 300 aa flanking *katG*-Ser^{315}; thus allowing for ~80% detection of all INH^R strains by only sequencing the direct flanks. Out-of-frame deletions, insertions and terminations lead to a non-functional catalase-peroxidase enzyme associated with low bacterial fitness and very elevated levels of resistance (>256 µg/ml).

Alternatively, mutations in the promoter of the *mabA-inhA* operon occur in 10–25% of clinical isolates resistant to INH (Ramaswamy and Musser, 1998; Slayden and Barry, 2000). Mutations $^{-15}$C>T and $^{-8}$T>C flanking the ribosomal binding site resulting in upregulation of *inhA* and thus increasing the target protein are by far the most common. Intragenic mutations in the InhA remain rare and are usually limited to Ser^{94}Ala and a few others. Overall, mutations in InhA are associated with low levels of INH^R, <1 µg/ml. Although there are numerous studies on the molecular biology of INH^R, there exist some important limitations on the available data. Most laboratories limit their analysis to the 300 aa flanking *katG*^{315} and only examine *mabA-inhA* or the remaining of the *katG* gene in the absence of mutations in *katG*^{315} and seldom explore other genes. An inherent limitation of this approach dictated by cost and complexity is that little is known about the frequency, combinations of and contribution to the resistance of multiple coexisting mutations associated with INH^R. Furthermore, in contrast to observations on RIF^R, the distribution and frequency of INH^R spontaneous mutants does not reflect what is observed in the clinic, hence restricting inferences generated from experimental data (Bergral *et al.*, 2009; Bifani, unpublished).

8.4 Ethionamide

Ethionamide (ETA, 2-ethylthioisonicotinamide), a structural analogue of INH prescribed since 1960, is today an important second-line anti-tubercular agent which is as potent as INH (Rist, 1960). ETA, or its analogue prothionamide (PTH, 2-propyl-thioisonicotinamide), administration is limited for the treatment of MDR-TB, given its significant side effects, including gastrointestinal and hepatic toxicity.

As for INH, ETA is a prodrug requiring activation for inhibitory activity. Recently, a two-gene operon (*ethA-ethR*) implicated in the activation of ETA has been identified (Baulard *et al.*, 2000; DeBarber *et al.*, 2000). The *ethA* gene encodes a monooxygenase (Baeyer–Villiger flavin-containing), which also catalyses the activation of ETA, thiaceta-zone and isoxyl (Fraaije *et al.*, 2004; Dover *et al.*, 2007). The difference in the mechanisms of activation between INH and ETA explains why KatG mutants remain susceptible to ETA but not to INH (Morlock *et al.*, 2003). The expression of EthA is under the control of a repressor EthR (Engohang-Ndong *et al.*, 2004). Overexpression of EthA in *M. smegmatis* induces a hypersusceptibility to ETA, whereas the overexpression of EthR induces a resistance to ETA. EthR controls the expression of EthA, which in turn activates ETA (Baulard *et al.*, 2000). The crystallization of EthR revealed a homodimer of helical structure similar to a transcriptional regulator belonging to the family of TetR/CamR repressors capable of binding DNA and ligands (Aramaki *et al.*, 1995). Interestingly, a fortuitous ligand (hexadecyl octanoate, 1,4-dioxane) was found to fix each EthR monomer during the process of crystallization

(Dover *et al.*, 2004; Frenois *et al.*, 2004). This ligand renders the conformation of EthR incompatible with the function of a repressor, leading to constitutive expression of EthA *in vivo* and hence enhancing the activation of ETA. Consequently, coadministration of such a ligand–ETA complex could reduce the therapeutic dose of ETA required and its accompanying side effect (Frenois *et al.*, 2004, 2006).

8.4.1 Molecular genetics of ethionamide resistance

Analysis of clinical isolates resistant to ETA has only been correlated to mutations in either the *ethA* and/or *inhA* genes. As for other non-essential genes, mutations are scattered throughout the *ethA* and include out-of-frame insertions/deletions, truncations associated with high levels of ETA^R (DeBarber *et al.*, 2000; Morlock *et al.*, 2003; Brossier *et al.*, 2010; Mathys, unpublished). Our own analysis of diverse clinical isolates indicate ~40% bear a mutation within *ethA*, in contrast to others (Brossier *et al.*, 2010; Mathys, unpublished). Cross-resistance with INH has been associated with mutations in *mabA-inhA* promoter (primarily $^{-15}$C>T) and some SNPs within the *inhA* coding region (^{62}I>T, ^{61}A>G, ^{130}C>T, ^{280}T>G) (Lee *et al.*, 2000; Morlock *et al.*, 2003; Guo *et al.*, 2006; Brossier *et al.*, 2010). *MabA-inhA* display both low and high levels of resistance, probably a consequence of concurrent mutations elsewhere (Morlock *et al.*, 2003). Prevalence of InhA-ETA cross-resistance varies depending on the study and, once again, interpretation is limited by the absence of genotyping data. Further, ETA susceptibility testing is performed only on MDR isolates. Cross-resistance associated to the InhA can also stem from increased levels of NADH due to mutations in *ndhII* (NADH-dehydrogenase) (Vilcheze *et al.*, 2005). Other examples of cross-resistance involve EthA, as an activator of thiocarbamide-containing prodrugs including isoxyl and thiacetazone (Dover *et al.*, 2007). Recently, *mshA* has been proposed as a potential additional target for ETA based on extensive genetic evidence (Vilcheze *et al.*, 2008). As for other alternative

GyrA polymorphisms associated with fluoroquinolone resistance

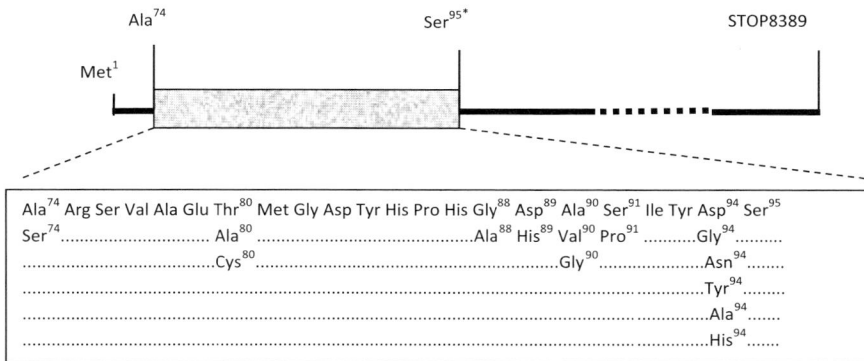

EthA polymorphisms associated with ethionamide resistance

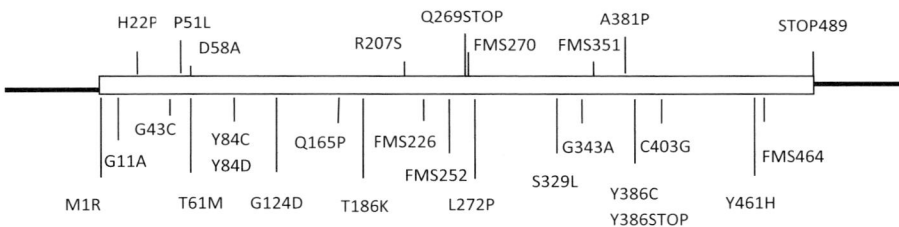

ThyA polymorphisms associated with PAS resistance

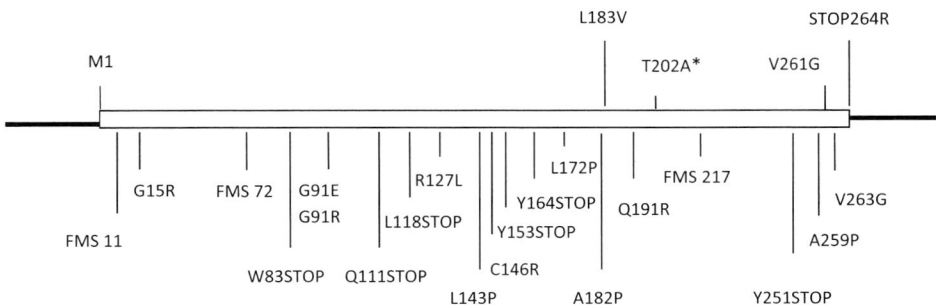

Fig. 8.1. Distribution of polymorphisms associated with fluoroquinolones, ethionamide, *p*-aminosalicylic acid resistance in the GyrA, EthA and ThyA proteins, respectively. Mutations in essential proteins (e.g. GyrA) are restricted to key amino acids and comprise few variations. In contrast, polymorphisms in non-essential proteins are dispersed throughout the corresponding genes (e.g. *ethA* and *thyA*) and include truncations of the proteins. Only selected polymorphisms are shown for EthA and ThyA. FMS = frameshift; A = alanine; C = cysteine; D = aspartic acid; E = glutamic acid; F = phenylalanine; G = glycine; H = histidine; I = isoleucine; K = lysine; L = leucine; M = methionine; N = asparagine; P = proline; Q = glutamine; R = arginine; S = serine; T = threonine; W = tryptophan; V = valine. *GyrA*-Ser^{95} and *thyA*-Thr^{202} are phylogenetic SNPs.

targets, further evaluation of clinical isolates is required, in particular in light of the observation that both the W-Beijing and the Haarlem strain families encode phylogenetic mutations not associated with ETA^R within *mshA* (Mathys, unpublished).

8.5 Pyrazinamide

Pyrazinamide (PZA) is a structural analogue of the nicotinamide, INH and ETA and, likewise, it is a prodrug. None the less, PZA has some distinctive features, including a different mechanism of activation and a unique sterilizing activity on semi-dormant (persistent) tubercular bacilli (McCune *et al.*, 1966; Mitchison, 1985) and is only active in acidified medium (pH 5.5) (McDermott, 1954; Zhang, 1999). Moreover, PZA does not present a bactericidal effect on *M. tuberculosis in vitro*, nor on rapidly growing myco-bacteria. No specific target for pyrazinoic acid (POA) has been discovered; however, a model of activation has been proposed (Zhang and Mitchison, 2003) whereby PZA penetrates the mycobacterial cell wall by passive diffusion and is converted into POA by the pyrazinamidase in the cytoplasm. POA leaves the cell by either passive diffusion or a possible defective efflux mechanism (Konno *et al.*, 1967; Trivedi and Desai, 1987). If the extracellular medium presents an acidic pH, POA is protonated to form HPOA, which is reabsorbed by the cell. As the efflux mechanism of POA is defective, POA accumulates in the cytoplasm of the mycobacterium and causes cellular damage. Moreover, the influx of protons in the cell, via the HPOA, acidifies the cytoplasm and disturbs cellular activity. This model could explain the particular characteristics of the PZA which is only active in an acidic environment.

8.5.1 Molecular genetics of pyrazinamide resistance

Pyrazinamidase is a small protein of 186 aa, encoded by the gene *pncA*. Approximately 70–90% of PZA^R cases are associated with mutations in the *pncA* gene, resulting in the bacilli's inability to activate the prodrug (Butler and Kilburn, 1983). As for EthA, PncA is a non-essential gene allowing for multiple possible mutations dispersed throughout the gene and promoter. No evidence has been found of possible decrease in bacterial fitness associated with PZA resistance, even in the event of a truncation, downregulation or deletion of the gene (Scorpio and Zhang, 1996; Sreevatsan *et al.*, 1997a; Ramaswamy and Musser, 1998). All *M. bovis* isolates are intrinsically resistant to PZA because they encode a phylogenetic mutation C^{169}G which inactivates *pncA* (Singh *et al.*, 2006). Mutations in the *pncA* and promoter present an ideal situation for molecular diagnostics through sequencing, in particular in light of the poor reproducibility of phenotypic assays. Nevertheless, a small number of PZA^R strains are independent of PncA mutations, underlining the need to identify other potential direct or indirect targets.

8.6 Ethambutol

Ethambutol ((S)-2,2'-(ethylenediimino)-di-1-butanol, EMB), as for INH, ETA and PZA, is an antibiotic specifically active on myco-bacteria (Cambau *et al.*, 2003). Side effects comprising retrobulbair neuritis (Melamud *et al.*, 2003) render this drug counter-indicated for treatment in children (Trebucq, 1997). EMB targets an arabinosyl transferase (EmbB) involved in the polymerization of arabinans in the cell wall, though its exact mode of action remains unknown (Mikusova *et al.*, 1995). Inhibition of the enzyme results in the termination of arabinogalactan and lipoarabi-nomannan synthesis, major polysaccharides of the mycobacterial wall (Takayama and Kilburn, 1989; Deng *et al.*, 1995). Accumulation of carbohydrate intermediaries and mycolic acids has been attributed to the loss of anchoring scaffold in the cell wall (Mikusova *et al.*, 1995). *EmbB* is part of the *embA-embB* operon in *M. avium* and *embC-embA-embB* in *M. tuberculosis* and other mycobactera (Alcaide *et al.*, 1997). The EmbB proteins of various mycobacterial species share 65% identity and are all predicted as being integral membrane proteins with 12 transmembrane regions (Telenti *et al.*, 1997; Ramaswamy and Musser, 1998).

8.6.1 Molecular genetics of ethambutol resistance

Resistance to EMB in *M. tuberculosis* correlates primarily to mutations in the *embB* gene (Sreevatsan *et al.*, 1997b; Telenti *et al.*, 1997). *EmbB* are found in ~70% of all the EMB^R clinical strains (Ramaswamy *et al.*, 2000) and are clustered in the ERDR (ethambutol resistance-determining region), likely located in a cytoplasmic loop of the transmembrane protein (Ramaswamy and Musser, 1998). The frequency of SNPs at *embB*-Met^{306} range from 47% to 65%, of which Met^{306}Ile (ATG^{306}>ATA, ATG^{306}>ATC and ATG^{306}>ATT) account for the majority, followed by ATG^{306}>Leu or ATG^{306}>Val (Sreevatsan *et al.*, 1997b; Ramaswamy and Musser, 1998). The implication of mutations at *embB*-Met^{306} on resistance were first demonstrated through homologous recombination in 1997 (Alcaide *et al.*, 1997), but challenged as EMB-susceptible isolates encoding the same mutations were also reported (Mokrousov *et al.*, 2002). Finally, analysis of EMB^R spontaneous mutants and allelic exchange reconfirmed that mutations in *embB*-Met^{306} were sufficient to render 55% of the isolates EMB. Other mutations within *embB* as well as those in the *embCAB*-operon have been linked with EMB^R, albeit at low levels (Safi *et al.*, 2010; Plinke *et al.*, 2010). Further, *rmlD-rmlA2*, involved in the modification of rhamnose and the *iniBAC* promoter may also contribute to EMB^R (Ramaswamy *et al.*, 2000). In spite of these recent discoveries, 30% of the EMB^R strains do not present any polymorphisms within the genes proposed (Ramaswamy *et al.*, 2000; Cambau *et al.*, 2003). SQ109, a homologue of EMB, is presently under evaluation. Interestingly, *embCAB* mutants do not confer cross-resistance.

8.7 Fluoroquinolones

Fluoroquinolones (FQs: ciprofloxacin, gatifloxacin, levofloxacin, moxifloxacin, ofloxacin and sparfloxacin) are potent synthetic antibacterial agents originally derived from nalidixic acid. FQs, currently used as second-line drugs, are under consideration as a potential substitute for INH in the first-line regiment. This will likely reduce the duration of therapy to 4 months (Chang *et al.*, 2010; Nuermberger *et al.*, 2004). Current human trials with moxifloxacin show promising results (Rosenthal *et al.*, 2008); however, a recent report by the WHO describes the presence of XDR-TB (MDR isolates additionally resistant to an FQ and an aminoglycoside or capromycin in 58 countries; WHO, 2009). FQs exert their effects by inhibiting bacterial topoisomerases II and IV (DNA gyrases). Topoisomerase II facilitates DNA unwinding and topoisomerase IV (notably absent in *M. tuberculosis*) activates decatenation (Champoux, 2001; Ginsburg *et al.*, 2003). Consequently, FQs inhibit DNA gyrase, a tetramer constituted of 2 A and B subunits encoded by *gyrA* and *gyrB* (Drlica, 1999). The exact mechanisms of action of FQs remain elusive; however, strand breakage, SOS-mediated autolysis and blockage of replication by the gyrase–FQ complex may enable bacterial inhibition without lethality (Guillemin *et al.*, 1998; Drlica, 1999; Hooper, 2001; Drlica and Malik, 2003; Ginsburg *et al.*, 2003).

8.7.1 Molecular genetics of fluoroquinolone resistance

As for other bacteria, the main mechanism of FQ^R in *M. tuberculosis* results from missense mutations in *gyrA* within the QRDR (quinolone resistance-determining region) and rarely in *gyrB*, corresponding to the DNA–protein complex (Takiff *et al.*, 1994; Alangaden *et al.*, 1995; Sullivan *et al.*, 1995; Kocagoz *et al.*, 1996; Williams *et al.*, 1996; Xu *et al.*, 1996; Perlman *et al.*, 1997). No insertions/deletions, even in-frame, have been reported in *gyrA* or *gyrB*. Instead, 13 possible SNPs in 8 codons within the QRDR account for 42–85% of all FQ^R isolates, of which substitution at D^{94} (D^{94}>A^{94}, D^{94}>N^{94}, D^{94}>G^{94}, D^{94}>Y^{94} and D^{94}>H^{94}) comprise ~60% of all resistant isolates (Sullivan *et al.*, 1995; Yew *et al.*, 1995;

Kocagoz *et al.*, 1996). A correlation between specific mutations in the QRDR and levels of resistance has been described (Kocagoz *et al.*, 1996; Xu *et al.*, 1996; Zhou *et al.*, 2000). Cross-resistance exists only among the FQs in most instances (Alangaden *et al.*, 1995; Yew *et al.*, 1995; Ruiz-Serrano *et al.*, 2000). Mutations outside QRDR, decreased cell wall permeability, active drug efflux pump mechanism, sequestration of drug or drug inactivation are some of the hypotheses proposed for non-QRDR FQ[R] (Jarlier and Nikaido, 1994; Cambau and Jarlier, 1996; Liu *et al.*, 1996; Takiff *et al.*, 1996).

8.8 Para-aminosalic acid

Para-amino-salicylic acid (PAS) was discovered by Lehmann in 1943 (Lehmann, 1946; Youmans *et al.*, 1947). In 1951, INH, PAS and SM constituted the birth of triple therapy (PAS-SM-INH), used until the mid-1960s. Although the efficacy of triple therapy proved positive, PAS was discontinued due to gastrointestinal toxicity, the need for multiple and elevated doses and the advent of more lethal anti-tubercular agents. PAS was only reintroduced in the USA in 1992, following several outbreaks of MDR isolates (CDC, 1992). Currently, a new, less toxic formulation of PAS is used as a second-line antibiotic for the treatment of MDR-TB (WHO, 2000). In spite of this renewed interest, the mechanism of action of PAS remains elusive. Since its discovery, PAS has been assumed to interfere with the folate pathway, given that it presents structural similarities with the sulfonamides, which are analogues of the *p*-aminobenzoic acid, the substrate of the dihydropteroate synthase (FolP1) (Lehninger, 1977). Recent experimental and epidemiological data have not been able to implicate FolP PAS[R] (Nopponpunth *et al.*, 1999; Mathys *et al.*, 2009). Instead, PAS resistance has been shown to be associated in part, downstream of the folate pathway, with the thymidylate synthase (ThyA), but not its analogue ThyX (Rengarajan *et al.*, 2004; Mathys *et al.*, 2009). ThyA and ThyX are responsible for the methylation of uracil.

8.8.1 Molecular genetics of para-aminosalicylic acid resistance

Recently, Rengarajan and colleagues showed by transposon mutagenesis that resistance to PAS was associated with mutations in the *thyA*. Subsequently, it has been shown that approximately 40% of all PAS[R] isolates encode a mutation of the *thyA*, while the mechanism of resistance remains unknown for the remaining ~60% of clinical isolates (Mathys *et al.*, 2009). *thyA* is a non-essential gene in *M. tuberculosis*, given the redundancy of *thyX* (Myllykallio *et al.*, 2002). As such, as for other non-essential drug targets in *M. tuberculosis*, SNPs, deletions and insertions are diverse and scattered throughout the target gene.

8.9 Aminoglycosides and Macrocyclic Polypeptide Antibiotics

Streptomycin (SM) was the first aminoglycoside (AG) discovered and drug approved for the treatment of tuberculosis following human trials in 1947. AGs (SM, amikacin (AK) and kanamycin (KM)) and two macrocyclic polypeptides (viomycin and capreomycin, CAP) share both a common target, the bacterial ribosome, and require intramuscular administration. AG remains an important drug in the tuberculosis therapy arsenal, SM being used regularly in many developing countries, particular for retreatment (WHO Category II) cases, while other AGs and CAPs are used as second line (Peloquin *et al.*, 2004). SM is the least toxic of the three AGs (Peloquin *et al.*, 2004), while AK is the most active in the mouse efficacy model of tuberculosis (Lounis *et al.*, 1997). AG and macrocyclic polypeptides hinder protein synthesis by inhibiting the initiation of translation and the translocation reaction, respectively (Benveniste and Davies, 1973). Extensive molecular data link SM[R] to missense mutations in either the S12 protein (*rpsL*) or 16S RNA (*rrs*) genes, which are components of the 30S subunits of the ribosome. AG tightly binds the 30S ribosomal subunit, while MCP binds the 50S (Benveniste and Davies, 1973; Ho *et al.*, 1997; Chan, 2003).

Table 8.1. Selected characteristics of drug resistance in *M. tuberculosis*.

Anti-tuberculars	Targets, activating enzymes, cross-resistance and comments
Rifamycin – rifampicin (RIF) – rifabutin – rifapentine	Target: RNA polymerase β-subunit: RpoB (*rpoB*) FoR associated with the *rpoB*: >95% within the RRDR, of which His^{526} ~40%, Ser^{531} ~40% and Asp^{516} ~8% FoR associated with other targets or outside the RRDR: <5% Shared cross-resistance within the RRDR for RIF, RFB, RFP and KRM-1648 FoM: 1 × 10^8
Isoniazid (prodrug)	Activating enzyme: bifunctional enzyme catalase-peroxidase: KatG (*katG*) FoR associated with the KatG: ~70–80% Target: enoyl-ACP reductase: InhA (*inhA*) FoR associated with the inhA: 5–25% KatG: no known cross-resistance InhA: cross-resistance with isoniazid and ethionamide Cross-resistance with isoniazid and thiacetazone reported FoM: 1 × 10^6
Ethionamide (prodrug)	Activating enzyme: monooxygenase: EthA-EthR operon (*ethA*) FoR associated with *ethA* mutations: ~40% Cross-resistance (EthA): ETA with isoxyl and thiacetazone (THI) Target: enoyl-ACP reductase InhA (*inhA*) FoR (InhA): 5–25% Cross-resistance (InhA): with isoniazid and ethionamide FoM: 1 × 10^6
Pyrazinamide (prodrug)	Activating enzyme: pyrazinamidase: PncA (*pncA*) FoR associated with the PncA: ~70–90% Active against slow metabolism or dormant bacilli FoM: 1 × 10^5
Ethambutol	Targets: arabinosyl transferase operon *embCAB* FoR (embB): ~70%, of which embB-Met^{306} ~47–65% FoM: 1 × 10^6

Fluoroquinolones
– ciprofloxacin (CIP)
– gatifloxacin (GAT)
– levofloxacin (LEVO)
– moxifloxacin (MOX)
– ofloxacin (OFLOX)
– sparfloxacin (SPA)
	Target: DNA topoisomerase: GyrA and GyrB subunits (*gyrA* and *gyrB*)
	Cross-resistance: GyrA and GyrB: CIP, GAT, LEV, MOX, OFL, SPA
	FoR(GyrA): 80–95% within the QDDR
	FoR(GyrB): 10–15%
	FoM: 1 × 10^7–10^8

p-Aminosalicylic acid (possible prodrug)	Targets: thymidylate synthase: ThyA (*thyA*) Some PAS^R ThyA mutants share cross-resistance with fluorouracil (FU), but FU-resistant mutants are not resistant to PAS High levels PAS^R share cross-resistance with THI; but THI^R mutants are not resistant to PAS FoR(ThyA): ~40% FoM: 1 × 10^5

Aminoglycosides and
macrocyclic
peptides
– streptomycin (SM)
– kanamycin (KM)
– amikacin (AMI)
– capreomycin (CAP)
– viomycin (VIO)
	Targets: SM: S12 ribosomal proteins (*rpsL*); SM, AMI and KAN: 16S rRNA (*rrs*); CAP: methyltransferase (*tlyA*)
	FoR(*rpsL*): ~65%; primarily Lys^{43} and Lys^{88}
	No cross-resistance associated with rpsL-Lys^{43} or Lys^{88}
	FoR (*rrs*): ~10%
	Mutation *rrs*1401 associated with high levels of cross-resistance with AMI, CAP, KM and VIO

Note: FoR = frequency of resistance; FoM: = frequency of mutation.

8.9.1 Molecular genetics of aminoglycosides and macrocyclic resistance

Mutations at either Lys^{43}>Arg(Thr) or Lys^{88}>Arg account for ~65% of all STR^R isolates. While SNPs at positions 43 and 88 are associated with elevated levels of resistance, other *rpsL* mutations are phylogenetic and share no correlation to SM^R (Sreevatsan *et al.*, 1996). In contrast, mutations within the *rrs* have been associated with low levels of SM^R but high levels of resistance to AMI and KM (Alangaden *et al.*, 1998). All together, SNPs in *rpsL* and *rrs* account for only ~75% of all SM^R isolates, and no cross-resistance has been reported with either AK, KM or the macrocyclic polypeptides in mutants with SNPs at position 43 or 88. Cross-resistance with other class members (KM and AK) and the macrocycle polypeptide CAP and viomycin has been correlated to mutation *rrs*1401. Other cross-resistances have not always been complete or reciprocal and depend largely on the mutation (Ho *et al.*, 1997). CAP^R and viomycin^R can result from mutations in the 2'-*O*-methyltransferase (*tlyA*) and the *rrs*; though these do not account for all resistant strains and the full clinical implications have yet to be determined.

8.10 Conclusion

Despite progress made in elucidating the underlying mechanism that confers drug resistance in *M. tuberculosis*, genotypic measures of antibiotic susceptibility remain deceptively simple. This, in part, has to do with a confluence of factors, including the lifestyle of *M. tuberculosis*. That is, the bacilli's long doubling time, subversion of the host immune response, residence in macrophages and in anatomical sites (e.g. cavities) where bacterial populations are dense, thereby rendering drug penetration inefficient and allowing for selection of drug-resistant mutants. In addition to *de novo* acquisition of drug resistance (i.e. acquired resistance), the mainly aerosol transmission route enables rapid dissemination of already resistant organisms (i.e. primary resistance). Compounding

the problem is the long treatment required to cure tuberculosis with inherent drug-associated toxicity hampering therapeutic adherence and thus increasing the likelihood of selecting and maintaining drug-resistant mutants.

Drug resistant-conferring mutations among clinical and laboratory isolates are being used increasingly to study bacterial fitness (Gagneux *et al.*, 2006a,b). These studies have indicated, not surprisingly, a greater diversity of mutations among *in vitro*-generated spontaneous mutants compared to those commonly observed from phenotypically drug-resistant patient isolates. These observations suggest a strong relationship between particular mutants and their inherent fitness, facilitating a progressive *in vivo* infection. Complicating the analysis of bacterial fitness among drug-resistant *M. tuberculosis* is the increasingly immuno-compromised host population (e.g. HIV), where less fit organisms proliferate unchallenged and possibly allow acquiring compensatory alterations to regain fitness (Bifani *et al.*, 2008).

Recently, much progress has been made in rapid diagnostics of drug resistance, particularly first-line agents. Rapid methods typically rely on PCR or other molecular techniques that target hotspot regions. While it is not ideal to study some drug resistance-conferring genomic regions, the majority of mutations in the clinical setting are restricted, facilitating high-throughput rapid analysis. For instance, genotypic (i.e. 81-bp RRDR) correlates for RIF^R are upwards of 95%, making it highly amenable for rapid molecular-based testing (Boehme *et al.*). This is also the case with INH^R, where the majority of mutations are restricted to a few sites in KatG and mabA-inhA (Lacoma *et al.*, 2008). However, interpretation must bear in mind the possibility of heteroresistant subpopulations that collectively may give false positive results.

In this chapter, we have focused on anti-tubercular agents and the corresponding genotypic measures that are of primary clinical and epidemiologic importance. A number of other mutations, some confirmed experimentally, have been described in the literature and have been deposited recently on a website (www.tbdreamdb.com). Of note are mutations in the regions discussed above that have not been confirmed experimentally. Paramount is the experimental confirmation of these genetic alterations, as some are phylogenetic scars or do not confer phenotypic resistance (Motiwala *et al.*, 2010; Feuerriegel *et al.*, 2011).

References

Alangaden, G.J., Manavathu, E.K., Vakulenko, S.B., Zvonok, N.M. and Lerner, S.A. (1995) Characterization of fluoroquinolone-resistant mutant strains of *Mycobacterium tuberculosis* selected in the laboratory and isolated from patients. *Antimicrobial Agents and Chemotherapy* 39, 1700–1703.

Alangaden, G.J., Kreiswirth, B.N., Aouad, A., Khetarpal, M., Igno, F.R., Moghazeh, S.L., *et al.* (1998) Mechanism of resistance to amikacin and kanamycin in *Mycobacterium tuberculosis*. *Antimicrobial Agents and Chemotherapy* 42, 1295–1297.

Alcaide, F., Pfyffer, G.E. and Telenti, A. (1997) Role of *embB* in natural and acquired resistance to ethambutol in mycobacteria. *Antimicrobial Agents and Chemotherapy* 41, 2270–2273.

Aramaki, H., Yagi, N. and Suzuki, M. (1995) Residues important for the function of a multihelical DNA binding domain in the new transcription factor family of Cam and Tet repressors. *Protein Engineering* 8, 1259–1266.

Argyrou, A., Jin, L., Siconilfi-Baez, L., Angeletti, R.H. and Blanchard, J.S. (2006) Proteome-wide profiling of isoniazid targets in *Mycobacterium tuberculosis*. *Biochemistry* 45, 13947–13953.

Bahrmand, A.R., Titov, L.P., Tasbiti, A.H., Yari, S. and Graviss, E.A. (2009) High-level rifampin resistance correlates with multiple mutations in the *rpoB* gene of pulmonary tuberculosis isolates from the Afghanistan border of Iran. *Journal of Clinical Microbiology* 47, 2744–2750.

Banerjee, A., Dubnau, E., Quemard, A., Balasubramanian, V., Um, K.S., Wilson, T., *et al.* (1994) *inhA*, a gene encoding a target for isoniazid and ethionamide in *Mycobacterium tuberculosis*. *Science* 263, 227–230.

Baulard, A.R., Betts, J.C., Engohang-Ndong, J., Quan, S., McAdam, R.A., Brennan, P.J., *et al.* (2000) Activation of the pro-drug ethionamide is regulated in mycobacteria. *Journal of Biological Chemistry* 275, 28326–28331.

Baysarowich, J., Koteva, K., Hughes, D.W., Ejim, L.,

Griffiths, E., Zhang, K., *et al.* (2008) Rifamycin antibiotic resistance by ADP-ribosylation: structure and diversity of Arr. *Proceedings of the National Academy of Sciences* 105, 4886–4891.

Benveniste, R. and Davies, J. (1973) Mechanisms of antibiotic resistance in bacteria. *Annual Review of Biochemistry* 42, 471–506.

Bernstein, J., Lott, W.A., Steinberg, B.A. and Yale, H.L. (1952) Chemotherapy of experimental tuberculosis. V. Isonicotinic acid hydrazide (nydrazid) and related compounds. *American Reviews of Tuberculosis* 65, 357–364.

Bifani, P.J., Plikaytis, B.B., Kapur, V., Stockbauer, K., Pan, X., Lutfey, M.L., *et al.* (1996) Origin and interstate spread of a New York City multidrug-resistant *Mycobacterium tuberculosis* clone family. *Journal of the American Medical Association* 275, 452–457.

Bifani, P., Mathema, B., Kurepina, N., Shashkina, E., Bertout, J., Blanchis, A.S., *et al.* (2008) The evolution of drug resistance in *Mycobacterium tuberculosis*: from a mono-rifampin-resistant cluster into increasingly multidrug-resistant variants in an HIV-seropositive population. *Journal of Infectious Diseases* 198, 90–94.

Bloom, B.R. and Murray, C.J. (1992) Tuberculosis: commentary on a re-emergent killer. *Science* 257, 1055–1064.

Boehme, C.C., Nabeta, P., Hillemann, D., Nicol, M.P., Shenai, S., Krapp, F., *et al.* (2010) Rapid molecular detection of tuberculosis and rifampin resistance. *New England Journal of Medicine* 363, 1005–1015.

Brossier, F., Veziris, N., Truffot-Pernot, C., Jarlier, V. and Sougakoff, W. (2011) Molecular investigation of resistance to the antituberculous drug ethionamide in multidrug-resistant clinical isolates of *Mycobacterium tuberculosis*. *Antimicrobial Agents and Chemotherapy* 55, 355–360.

Butler, W.R. and Kilburn, J.O. (1983) Susceptibility of *Mycobacterium tuberculosis* to pyrazinamide and its relationship to pyrazinamidase activity. *Antimicrobial Agents and Chemotherapy* 24, 600–601.

Cambau, E. and Jarlier, V. (1996) Resistance to quinolones in mycobacteria. *Research in Microbiology* 147, 52–59.

Cambau, E., Lemaitre, N., Sougakoff, W. and Jarlier, V. (2003) Résistance aux antituberculeux. *Antibiotiques* 5, 29–37.

Campbell, E.A., Korzheva, N., Mustaev, A., Murakami, K., Nair, S., Goldfarb, A., *et al.* (2001) Structural mechanism for rifampicin inhibition of bacterial rna polymerase. *Cell* 104, 901–912.

CDC (1992) Update: availability of streptomycin and para-aminosalicylic acid – United States.

Morbidity and Mortality Weekly Report (MMWR) 41, 482.

CDC (2003) Treatment of tuberculosis. *Morbidity and Mortality Weekly Report (MMWR)*. June 20 2003, Vol 52, No RR-11.

Champoux, J.J. (2001) DNA topoisomerases: structure, function, and mechanism. *Annual Review of Biochemistry* 70, 369–413.

Chan, E. (2003) Pyrazinamide, ethambutol, ethionamide, and aminoglycosides. In: Rom, W. and Garay, S. (eds) *Tuberculosis,* 2nd edition. Lippincott Williams and Wilkins, Philadelphia, Pennsylvania.

Chang, K.C., Leung, C.C., Yew, W.W., Lau, T.Y., Leung, W.M., Tam, C.M., *et al.* (2010) Newer fluoroquinolones for treating respiratory infection: do they mask tuberculosis? *European Respiratory Journal* 35, 606–613.

Crofton, J., Chaulet, P., Maher, D., Grosset, J., Harris, W., Horne, N., *et al.* (1997) Guidelines for the management of drug-resistant tuberculosis. *WHO/TB/96.210.*

Davies, J. (1998) Antibiotic resistance in mycobacteria. In: Chadwick, D.J. and Cardew, G. (eds) *Genetics and Tuberculosis.* John Wiley, Chichester, UK.

DeBarber, A.E., Mdluli, K., Bosman, M., Bekker, L.G. and Barry, C.E. 3rd (2000) Ethionamide activation and sensitivity in multidrug-resistant *Mycobacterium tuberculosis. Proceedings of the National Academy of Sciences* 97, 9677–9682.

Deng, L., Mikusova, K., Robuck, K.G., Scherman, M., Brennan, P.J. and McNeil, M.R. (1995) Recognition of multiple effects of ethambutol on metabolism of mycobacterial cell envelope. *Antimicrobial Agents and Chemotherapy* 39, 694–701.

Dover, L.G., Corsino, P.E., Daniels, I.R., Cocklin, S.L., Tatituri, V., Besra, G.S., *et al.* (2004) Crystal structure of the TetR/CamR family repressor *Mycobacterium tuberculosis* EthR implicated in ethionamide resistance. *Journal of Molecular Biology* 340, 1095–1105.

Dover, L.G., Alahari, A., Gratraud, P., Gomes, J.M., Bhowruth, V., Reynolds, R.C., *et al.* (2007) EthA, a common activator of thiocarbamide-containing drugs acting on different mycobacterial targets. *Antimicrobial Agents and Chemotherapy* 51, 1055–1063.

Drlica, K. (1999) Mechanism of fluoroquinolone action. *Current Opinion in Microbiology* 2, 504–508.

Drlica, K. and Malik, M. (2003) Fluoroquinolones: action and resistance. *Current Topics in Medicinal Chemistry* 3, 249–282.

Drlica, K., Zhao, X. and Kreiswirth, B. (2008) Minimising moxifloxacin resistance with tuberculosis. *The Lancet Infectious Diseases* 8, 273–275.

Dye, C., Espinal, M.A., Watt, C.J., Mbiaga, C. and Williams, B.G. (2002) Worldwide incidence of multidrug-resistant tuberculosis. *Journal of Infectious Diseases* 185, 1197–1202.

Engohang-Ndong, J., Baillat, D., Aumercier, M., Bellefontaine, F., Besra, G.S., Locht, C., *et al.* (2004) EthR, a repressor of the TetR/CamR family implicated in ethionamide resistance in mycobacteria, octamerizes cooperatively on its operator. *Molecular Microbiology* 51, 175–188.

Espinal, M.A., Kim, S.J., Suarez, P.G., Kam, K.M., Khomenko, A.G., Migliori, G.B., *et al.* (2000) Standard short-course chemotherapy for drug-resistant tuberculosis: treatment outcomes in 6 countries. *Journal of the American Medical Association* 283, 2537–2545.

Feuerriegel, S., Koser, C., Trube, L., Archer, J., Rusch Gerdes, S., Richter, E., *et al.* (2010) Thr202Ala in thyA is a marker for the Latin American Mediterranean lineage of the *Mycobacterium tuberculosis* complex rather than para-aminosalicylic acid resistance. *Antimicrobial Agents and Chemotherapy* 54, 4794–4798.

Fox, H.H. (1952) The chemical approach to the control of tuberculosis. *Science* 116, 129–134.

Fraaije, M.W., Kamerbeek, N.M., Heidekamp, A.J., Fortin, R. and Janssen, D.B. (2004) The prodrug activator EtaA from *Mycobacterium tuberculosis* is a Baeyer–Villiger monooxygenase. *Journal of Biological Chemistry* 279, 3354–3360.

Frenois, F., Engohang-Ndong, J., Locht, C., Baulard, A.R. and Villeret, V. (2004) Structure of EthR in a ligand bound conformation reveals therapeutic perspectives against tuberculosis. *Molecular Cell* 16, 301–307.

Frenois, F., Baulard, A.R. and Villeret, V. (2006) Insights into mechanisms of induction and ligands recognition in the transcriptional repressor EthR from *Mycobacterium tuberculosis. Tuberculosis (Edinburgh)* 86, 110–1104.

Gagneux, S., Burgos, M.V., Deriemer, K., Encisco, A., Munoz, S., Hopewell, P.C., *et al.* (2006a) Impact of bacterial genetics on the transmission of isoniazid-resistant *Mycobacterium tuberculosis. PLoS Pathogens* 2, e61.

Gagneux, S., Long, C.D., Small, P.M., Van, T., Schoolnik, G.K. and Bohannan, B.J. (2006b) The competitive cost of antibiotic resistance in *Mycobacterium tuberculosis. Science* 312, 1944–1946.

Gandhi, N.R., Moll, A., Sturm, A.W., Pawinski, R.,

Govender, T., Lalloo, U., et al. (2006) Extensively drug-resistant tuberculosis as a cause of death in patients co-infected with tuberculosis and HIV in a rural area of South Africa. The Lancet 368, 1575–1580.

Ginsburg, A.S., Grosset, J.H. and Bishai, W.R. (2003) Fluoroquinolones, tuberculosis, and resistance. The Lancet Infectious Diseases 3, 432–442.

Gottberg, K., Einarsson, U., Ytterberg, C., Fredrikson, S., Von Koch, L. and Holmqvist, L.W. (2008) Use of health care services and satisfaction with care in people with multiple sclerosis in Stockholm county: a population-based study. Multiple Sclerosis 14, 962–971.

Guillemin, I., Jarlier, V. and Cambau, E. (1998) Correlation between quinolone susceptibility patterns and sequences in the A and B subunits of DNA gyrase in mycobacteria. Antimicrobial Agents and Chemotherapy 42, 2084–2088.

Guo, H., Seet, Q., Denkin, S., Parsons, L. and Zhang, Y. (2006) Molecular characterization of isoniazid-resistant clinical isolates of Mycobacterium tuberculosis from the USA. Journal of Medical Microbiology 55, 1527–1531.

Ho, Y.I., Chan, C.Y. and Cheng, A.F. (1997) In-vitro activities of aminoglycoside-aminocyclitols against mycobacteria. Journal of Antimicrobial Chemotherapy 40, 27–32.

Honore, N. and Cole, S.T. (1993) Molecular basis of rifampin resistance in Mycobacterium leprae. Antimicrobial Agents and Chemotherapy 37, 414–418.

Hooper, D.C. (2001) Mechanisms of action of antimicrobials: focus on fluoroquinolones. Clinical Infectious Diseases 32 (Suppl 1), S9–S15.

Iseman, M. (2000) Drug-Resistant Tuberculosis. A Clinican's Guide to Tuberculosis. Lippincott Williams and Wilkins, Philadelphia, Pennsylvania.

Iseman, M.D. and Madsen, L.A. (1989) Drug-resistant tuberculosis. Clinics in Chest Medicine 10, 341–353.

Jarlier, V. and Nikaido, H. (1994) Mycobacterial cell wall: structure and role in natural resistance to antibiotics. FEMS Microbiology Letters 123, 11–18.

Kaufmann, S.H. (2001) How can immunology contribute to the control of tuberculosis? Nature Reviews in Immunology 1, 20–30.

Kocagoz, T., Hackbarth, C.J., Unsal, I., Rosenberg, E.Y., Nikaido, H. and Chambers, H.F. (1996) Gyrase mutations in laboratory-selected, fluoroquinolone-resistant mutants of Mycobacterium tuberculosis H37Ra. Antimicrobial Agents and Chemotherapy 40, 1768–1774.

Konno, K., Feldmann, F.M. and McDermott, W. (1967) Pyrazinamide susceptibility and amidase activity of tubercle bacilli. American Reviews in Respiratory Disease 95, 461–469.

Lacoma, A., Garcia-Sierra, N., Prat, C., Ruiz-Manzano, J., Haba, L., Roses, S., et al. (2008) GenoType MTBDRplus assay for molecular detection of rifampin and isoniazid resistance in Mycobacterium tuberculosis strains and clinical samples. Journal of Clinical Microbiology 46, 3660–3667.

Larsen, M.H., Vilcheze, C., Kremer, L., Besra, G.S., Parsons, L., Salfinger, M., et al. (2002) Over-expression of inhA, but not kasA, confers resistance to isoniazid and ethionamide in Mycobacterium smegmatis, M. bovis BCG and M. tuberculosis. Molecular Microbiology 46, 453–466.

Lee, H., Cho, S.N., Bang, H.E., Lee, J.H., Bai, G.H., Kim, S.J., et al. (2000) Exclusive mutations related to isoniazid and ethionamide resistance among Mycobacterium tuberculosis isolates from Korea. International Journal of Tuberculosis and Lung Disease 4, 441–447.

Lehmann, J. (1946) Para-aminosalicylic acid in the treatment of tuberculosis. The Lancet 247, 15–16.

Lehninger, A.L. (1977) Biochemistry: The Molecular Basis of Cell Structure and Function. Worth Publishers, Inc, New York.

Liu, J., Takiff, H.E. and Nikaido, H. (1996) Active efflux of fluoroquinolones in Mycobacterium smegmatis mediated by LfrA, a multidrug efflux pump. Journal of Bacteriology 178, 3791–3795.

Lounis, N., Ji, B., Truffot-Pernot, C. and Grosset, J. (1997) Comparative activities of amikacin against Mycobacterium avium complex in nude and beige mice. Antimicrobial Agents and Chemotherapy 41, 1168–1169.

McCune, R.M., Feldmann, F.M. and McDermott, W. (1966) Microbial persistence. II. Characteristics of the sterile state of tubercle bacilli. Journal of Experimental Medicine 123, 469–486.

Mathys, V., Wintjens, R., Lefevre, P., Bertout, J., Singhal, A., Kiass, M., et al. (2009) Molecular genetics of para-aminosalicylic acid resistance in clinical isolates and spontaneous mutants of Mycobacterium tuberculosis. Antimicrobial Agents and Chemotherapy 53, 2100–2109.

Melamud, A., Kosmorsky, G.S. and Lee, M.S. (2003) Ocular ethambutol toxicity. Mayo Clinic Proceedings 78, 1409–1411.

Mikusova, K., Slayden, R.A., Besra, G.S. and Brennan, P.J. (1995) Biogenesis of the mycobacterial cell wall and the site of action of ethambutol. Antimicrobial Agents and Chemotherapy 39, 2484–2489.

Mitchison, D.A. (1985) The action of antituberculosis drugs in short-course chemotherapy. *Tubercle* 66, 219–225.

Mokrousov, I., Otten, T., Vyshnevskiy, B. and Narvskaya, O. (2002) Detection of *embB*306 mutations in ethambutol-susceptible clinical isolates of *Mycobacterium tuberculosis* from Northwestern Russia: implications for genotypic resistance testing. *Journal of Clinical Microbiology* 40, 3810–3813.

Morlock, G.P., Plikaytis, B.B. and Crawford, J.T. (2000) Characterization of spontaneous, *in vitro*-selected, rifampin-resistant mutants of *Mycobacterium tuberculosis* strain H37Rv. *Antimicrobial Agents and Chemotherapy* 44, 3298–3301.

Morlock, G.P., Metchock, B., Sikes, D., Crawford, J.T. and Cooksey, R.C. (2003) *ethA*, *inhA*, and *katG* loci of ethionamide-resistant clinical *Mycobacterium tuberculosis* isolates. *Antimicrobial Agents and Chemotherapy* 47, 3799–3805.

Motiwala, A.S., Dai, Y., Jones-Lopez, E.C., Hwang, S.H., Lee, J.S., Cho, S.N., *et al.* (2010) Mutations in extensively drug-resistant *Mycobacterium tuberculosis* that do not code for known drug-resistance mechanisms. *Journal of Infectious Diseases* 201, 881–888.

Murray, C.J., Dejonghe, E., Chum, H.J., Nyangulu, D.S., Salomao, A. and Styblo, K. (1991) Cost effectiveness of chemotherapy for pulmonary tuberculosis in three sub-Saharan African countries. *The Lancet* 338, 1305–1308.

Myllykallio, H., Lipowski, G., Leduc, D., Filee, J., Forterre, P. and Liebl, U. (2002) An alternative flavin-dependent mechanism for thymidylate synthesis. *Science* 297, 105–107.

Nopponpunth, V., Sirawaraporn, W., Greene, P.J. and Santi, D.V. (1999) Cloning and expression of *Mycobacterium tuberculosis* and *Mycobacterium leprae* dihydropteroate synthase in *Escherichia coli*. *Journal of Bacteriology* 181, 6814–6821.

Nuermberger, E.L., Yoshimatsu, T., Tyagi, S., Williams, K., Rosenthal, I., O'Brien, R.J., *et al.* (2004) Moxifloxacin-containing regimens of reduced duration produce a stable cure in murine tuberculosis. *American Journal of Respiratory and Critical Care Medicine* 170, 1131–1134.

Ovchinnikov Yu, A., Monastyrskaya, G.S., Gubanov, V.V., Lipkin, V.M., Sverdlov, E.D., Kiver, I.F., *et al.* (1981) Primary structure of Escherichia coli RNA polymerase nucleotide substitution in the beta subunit gene of the rifampicin resistant rpoB255 mutant. *Molecular and General Genetics* 184, 536–538.

Peloquin, C.A., Berning, S.E., Nitta, A.T., Simone, P.M., Goble, M., Huitt, G.A., *et al.* (2004) Aminoglycoside toxicity: daily versus thrice-weekly dosing for treatment of mycobacterial diseases. *Clinical Infectious Diseases* 38, 1538–1544.

Perlman, D.C., El Sadr, W.M., Heifets, L.B., Nelson, E.T., Matts, J.P., Chirgwin, K., *et al.* (1997) Susceptibility to levofloxacin of *Myocobacterium tuberculosis* isolates from patients with HIV-related tuberculosis and characterization of a strain with levofloxacin monoresistance. Community Programs for Clinical Research on AIDS 019 and the AIDS Clinical Trials Group 222 Protocol Team. *AIDS* 11, 1473–1478.

Plinke, C., Cox, H.S., Zarkua, N., Karimovich, H.A., Braker, K., Diel, R., *et al.* (2010) embCAB sequence variation among ethambutol-resistant *Mycobacterium tuberculosis* isolates without embB306 mutation. *Journal of Antimicrobial Chemotherapy* 65, 1359–1367.

Ramaswamy, S. and Musser, J.M. (1998) Molecular genetic basis of antimicrobial agent resistance in *Mycobacterium tuberculosis*: 1998 update. *Tuberculosis and Lung Disease* 79, 3–29.

Ramaswamy, S.V., Amin, A.G., Goksel, S., Stager, C.E., Dou, S.J., El Sahly, H., *et al.* (2000) Molecular genetic analysis of nucleotide polymorphisms associated with ethambutol resistance in human isolates of *Mycobacterium tuberculosis*. *Antimicrobial Agents and Chemotherapy* 44, 326–336.

Ramaswamy, S.V., Reich, R., Dou, S.J., Jasperse, L., Pan, X., Wanger, A., *et al.* (2003) Single nucleotide polymorphisms in genes associated with isoniazid resistance in *Mycobacterium tuberculosis*. *Antimicrobial Agents and Chemotherapy* 47, 1241–1250.

Raviglione, M.C., Snider, D.E. Jr and Kochi, A. (1995) Global epidemiology of tuberculosis. Morbidity and mortality of a worldwide epidemic. *Journal of the American Medical Association* 273, 220–226.

Rengarajan, J., Sassetti, C.M., Naroditskaya, V., Sloutsky, A., Bloom, B.R. and Rubin, E.J. (2004) The folate pathway is a target for resistance to the drug para-aminosalicylic acid (PAS) in mycobacteria. *Molecular Microbiology* 53, 275–282.

Ridzon, R., Whitney, C.G., McKenna, M.T., Taylor, J.P., Ashkar, S.H., Nitta, A.T., *et al.* (1998) Risk factors for rifampin mono-resistant tuberculosis. *American Journal of Respiratory and Critical Care Medicine* 157, 1881–1884.

Rist, N. (1960) L'activite antituberculeuse de l'ethionamide. *Advances in Tuberculosis Research* 10, 69–126.

Rosenthal, I.M., Zhang, M., Almeida, D., Grosset, J.H. and Nuermberger, E.L. (2008) Isoniazid or moxifloxacin in rifapentine-based regimens for experimental tuberculosis? *American Journal of Respiratory and Critical Care Medicine* 178, 989–993.

Rozwarski, D.A., Grant, G.A., Barton, D.H., Jacobs, W.R. Jr and Sacchettini, J.C. (1998) Modification of the NADH of the isoniazid target (InhA) from *Mycobacterium tuberculosis*. *Science* 279, 98–102.

Ruiz-Serrano, M.J., Alcala, L., Martinez, L., Diaz, M., Marin, M., *et al.* (2000) *In vitro* activities of six fluoroquinolones against 250 clinical isolates of *Mycobacterium tuberculosis* susceptible or resistant to first-line antituberculosis drugs. *Antimicrobial Agents and Chemotherapy* 44, 2567–2568.

Safi, H., Fleischmann, R.D., Peterson, S.N., Jones, M.B., Jarrahi, B. and Alland, D. (2010) Allelic exchange and mutant selection demonstrate that common clinical embCAB gene mutations only modestly increase resistance to ethambutol in *Mycobacterium tuberculosis*. *Antimicrobial Agents and Chemotherapy* 54, 103–108.

Scorpio, A. and Zhang, Y. (1996) Mutations in *pncA*, a gene encoding pyrazinamidase/nicotinamidase, cause resistance to the antituberculous drug pyrazinamide in tubercle bacillus. *Nature Medicine* 2, 662–667.

Shah, N.S., Wright, A., Bai, G.H., Barrera, L., Boulahbal, F., Martin-Casabona, N., *et al.* (2007) Worldwide emergence of extensively drug-resistant tuberculosis. *Emerging Infectious Diseases* 13, 380–387.

Singh, P., Mishra, A.K., Malonia, S.K., Chauhan, D.S., Sharma, V.D., Venkatesan, K., *et al.* (2006) The paradox of pyrazinamide: an update on the molecular mechanisms of pyrazinamide resistance in mycobacteria. *Journal of Communicable Disease* 38, 288–298.

Slayden, R.A. and Barry, C.E. 3rd (2000) The genetics and biochemistry of isoniazid resistance in *Mycobacterium tuberculosis*. *Microbes and Infection* 2, 659–669.

Sreevatsan, S., Pan, X., Stockbauer, K.E., Williams, D.L., Kreiswirth, B.N. and Musser, J.M. (1996) Characterization of rpsL and rrs mutations in streptomycin-resistant *Mycobacterium tuberculosis* isolates from diverse geographic localities. *Antimicrobial Agents and Chemotherapy* 40, 1024–1026.

Sreevatsan, S., Pan, X., Zhang, Y., Kreiswirth, B.N. and Musser, J.M. (1997a) Mutations associated with pyrazinamide resistance in *pncA* of *Mycobacterium tuberculosis* complex organisms. *Antimicrobial Agents and Chemotherapy* 41, 636–640.

Sreevatsan, S., Stockbauer, K.E., Pan, X., Kreiswirth, B.N., Moghazeh, S.L., Jacobs, W.R. Jr., *et al.* (1997b) Ethambutol resistance in *Mycobacterium tuberculosis*: critical role of embB mutations. *Antimicrobial Agents and Chemotherapy* 41, 1677–1681.

Sullivan, E.A., Kreiswirth, B.N., Palumbo, L., Kapur, V., Musser, J.M., Ebrahimzadeh, A., *et al.* (1995) Emergence of fluoroquinolone-resistant tuberculosis in New York City. *The Lancet* 345, 1148–1150.

Takayama, K. and Kilburn, J.O. (1989) Inhibition of synthesis of arabinogalactan by ethambutol in *Mycobacterium smegmatis*. *Antimicrobial Agents and Chemotherapy* 33, 1493–1499.

Takayama, K., Wang, L. and David, H.L. (1972) Effect of isoniazid on the *in vivo* mycolic acid synthesis, cell growth, and viability of *Mycobacterium tuberculosis*. *Antimicrobial Agents and Chemotherapy* 2, 29–35.

Takayama, K., Schnoes, H.K., Armstrong, E.L. and Boyle, R.W. (1975) Site of inhibitory action of isoniazid in the synthesis of mycolic acids in *Mycobacterium tuberculosis*. *Journal of Lipid Research* 16, 308–317.

Takiff, H.E., Salazar, L., Guerrero, C., Philipp, W., Huang, W.M., Kreiswirth, B., *et al.* (1994) Cloning and nucleotide sequence of *Mycobacterium tuberculosis* gyrA and gyrB genes and detection of quinolone resistance mutations. *Antimicrobial Agents and Chemotherapy* 38, 773–780.

Takiff, H.E., Cimino, M., Musso, M.C., Weisbrod, T., Martinez, R., Delgado, M.B., *et al.* (1996) Efflux pump of the proton antiporter family confers low-level fluoroquinolone resistance in *Mycobacterium smegmatis*. *Proceedings of the National Academy of Sciences* 93, 362–366.

Telenti, A., Imboden, P., Marchesi, F., Lowrie, D., Cole, S., Colston, M.J., *et al.* (1993) Detection of rifampicin-resistance mutations in *Mycobacterium tuberculosis*. *The Lancet* 341, 647–650.

Telenti, A., Philipp, W.J., Sreevatsan, S., Bernasconi, C., Stockbauer, K.E., Wieles, B., *et al.* (1997) The *emb* operon, a gene cluster of *Mycobacterium tuberculosis* involved in resistance to ethambutol. *Nature Medicine* 3, 567–570.

Timmins, G.S. and Deretic, V. (2006) Mechanisms of action of isoniazid. *Molecular Microbiology* 62, 1220–1227.

Trebucq, A. (1997) Should ethambutol be recommended for routine treatment of tuberculosis in children? A review of the literature. *International Journal of Tuberculosis and Lung Disease* 1, 12–15.

Trivedi, S.S. and Desai, S.G. (1987) Pyrazinamidase activity of *Mycobacterium tuberculosis* – a test of sensitivity to pyrazinamide. *Tubercle* 68, 221–224.

Vareldzis, B.P., Grosset, J., De Kantor, I., Crofton, J., Laszlo, A., Felten, M., *et al.* (1994) Drug-resistant tuberculosis: laboratory issues. World Health Organization recommendations. *Tuberculosis and Lung Disease* 75, 1–7.

Vilcheze, C. and Jacobs, W.R. Jr (2007) The mechanism of isoniazid killing: clarity through the scope of genetics. *Annual Reviews of Microbiology* 61, 35–50.

Vilcheze, C., Weisbrod, T.R., Chen, B., Kremer, L., Hazbon, M.H., Wang, F., *et al.* (2005) Altered NADH/NAD+ ratio mediates coresistance to isoniazid and ethionamide in mycobacteria. *Antimicrobial Agents and Chemotherapy* 49, 708–720.

Vilcheze, C., Wang, F., Arai, M., Hazbon, M.H., Colangeli, R., Kremer, L., *et al.* (2006) Transfer of a point mutation in *Mycobacterium tuberculosis inhA* resolves the target of isoniazid. *Nature Medicine* 12, 1027–1029.

Vilcheze, C., Av-Gay, Y., Attarian, R., Liu, Z., Hazbon, M.H., Colangeli, R., *et al.* (2008) Mycothiol biosynthesis is essential for ethionamide susceptibility in *Mycobacterium tuberculosis*. *Molecular Microbiology* 69, 1316–1329.

Wang, F., Jain, P., Gulten, G., Liu, Z., Feng, Y., Ganesula, K., *et al.* (2010) *Mycobacterium tuberculosis* dihydrofolate reductase is not a target relevant to the antitubercular activity of isoniazid. *Antimicrobial Agents and Chemotherapy* 54, 3776–3782.

Webb, V. and Davies, J. (1999) Antibiotics and antibiotic resistance in mycobacteria. In: Ratledge, C. and Dale, J. (eds) *Mycobacteria: Molecular Biology and Virulence*. Blackwell Science, Oxford, UK, pp. ??.

Wengenack, N.L., Uhl, J.R., St Amand, A.L., Tomlinson, A.J., Benson, L.M., Naylor, S., *et al.* (1997) Recombinant *Mycobacterium tuberculosis* KatG(S315T) is a competent catalase-peroxidase with reduced activity toward isoniazid. *Journal of Infectious Disease* 176, 722–727.

World Health Organization [WHO] (1996) TB: groups at risk. WHO Report on the Tuberculosis Epidemic. WHO, Geneva, Switzerland.

WHO (2000) Guidelines for establishing DOTS-Plus pilot projects for the management of multidrug-resistant tuberculosis (MDR-TB). *WHO/CDS/TB/2000.279*. WHO, Geneva, Switzerland.

WHO (2009) Global tuberculosis control 2009 – surveillance, planning, financing. WHO Report 2009. WHO/HTM/TB/2009.411. WHO, Geneva, Switzerland.

Williams, K.J., Chan, R. and Piddock, L.J. (1996) gyrA of ofloxacin-resistant clinical isolates of *Mycobacterium tuberculosis* from Hong Kong. *Journal of Antimicrobial Chemotherapy* 37, 1032–1034.

Winder, F.G. and Collins, P.B. (1970) Inhibition by isoniazid of synthesis of mycolic acids in *Mycobacterium tuberculosis*. *Journal of General Microbiology* 63, 41–48.

Xu, C., Kreiswirth, B.N., Sreevatsan, S., Musser, J.M. and Drlica, K. (1996) Fluoroquinolone resistance associated with specific gyrase mutations in clinical isolates of multidrug-resistant *Mycobacterium tuberculosis*. *Journal of Infectious Diseases* 174, 1127–1130.

Yew, W.W., Chau, C.H., Wong, P.C., Lee, J., Wong, C.F., Cheung, S.W., *et al.* (1995) Ciprofloxacin in the management of pulmonary tuberculosis in the face of hepatic dysfunction. *Drugs Under Experimental and Clinical Research* 21, 79–83.

Youmans, G.P., Raleigh, G.W. and Youmans, A.S. (1947) The tuberculostatic action of para-aminosalicylic acid. *Journal of Bacteriology* 54, 409–416.

Zhang, Y. and Mitchison, D. (2003) The curious characteristics of pyrazinamide: a review. *International Journal of Tuberculosis and Lung Disease* 7, 6–21.

Zhang, Y., Heym, B., Allen, B., Young, D. and Cole, S. (1992) The catalase-peroxidase gene and isoniazid resistance of *Mycobacterium tuberculosis*. *Nature* 358, 591–593.

Zhang, Y., Garbe, T. and Young, D. (1993) Transformation with *katG* restores isoniazid-sensitivity in *Mycobacterium tuberculosis* isolates resistant to a range of drug concentrations. *Molecular Microbiology* 8, 521–524.

Zhang, Y., Vilcheze, C. and Jacobs, W.R. (2005) Mechanisms of drug resistance in *Mycobacterium tuberculosis*. In: Cole, S.T., Eisenach, K.D., McMurray, D.N. and Jacobs, W.R. Jr (eds) *Tuberculosis and the Tubercle Bacillus*. ASM Press, Washington, DC.

Zhou, J., Dong, Y., Zhao, X., Lee, S., Amin, A., Ramaswamy, S., *et al.* (2000) Selection of antibiotic-resistant bacterial mutants: allelic diversity among fluoroquinolone-resistant mutations. *Journal of Infectious Diseases* 182, 517–525.

9 Molecular Tools for Fast Identification of Resistance and Characterization of MDR/XDR-TB

Simeon Cadmus[1] and Dick van Soolingen[2]

[1]*Tuberculosis Research Laboratory, Department of Veterinary Public Health and Preventive Medicine, University of Ibadan, Nigeria;* [2]*Mycobacteria Reference Laboratory, National Institute of Public Health and the Environment (RIVM), The Netherlands*

9.1 Introduction

In a bid to provide meaningful solution to the persistent burden of tuberculosis in most developing nations and the world at large, the strategy for the directly observed therapy short course (DOTS) was developed by Dr Karel Styblo in the 1980s. The DOTS strategy (combined five key components: government commitment, diagnosis through microscopy, standardized and supervised treatment, uninterrupted drug supply and regular programme monitoring) contributed immensely to the improvement of global tuberculosis control over a decade. Specifically, it involves the inclusion of the standardized short-course chemotherapy regimens with first-line drugs (isoniazid (INH), rifampicin (RIF), pyrazinamide (PZA) and streptomycin (SM) or ethambutol (EMB), or both) under direct observation, at least in the intensive treatment phase, regardless of patient drug susceptibility pattern (WHO, 1997). In furtherance to this programme, in 2006, the World Health Organization (WHO) launched the Stop TB Strategy to pursue, among other things, DOTS expansion and enhancement and to address TB/HIV, multidrug-resistant tubercu-losis (MDR-TB) and other challenges towards reaching the 2015 Millennium Development Goals (MDGs) (Migliori *et al.*, 2007).

Globally, there were an estimated 8.8 million incident cases of tuberculosis and 650,000 MDR-TB cases in 2010 (WHO, 2012a). However, only about 16% of the estimated MDR-TB patients and 1.4 million tuberculosis patients who suffer from infection with HIV worldwide each year have access to sufficiently sensitive case detection or drug susceptibility testing (WHO, 2012a). Therefore, a major underreporting in the problem of MDR-TB is conceivable. Also, significant diagnostic delay aggravated by the disproportionate frequency of smear-negative disease in HIV-associated tuberculosis is common (Getahun *et al.*, 2007; Perkins and Cunningham, 2007; Uys *et al.*, 2007; Havlir *et al.*, 2008). The failure to recognize and treat MDR-TB patients quickly leads to increased mortality, acquired resistance (including extensively drug-resistant tuberculosis, or XDR-TB) and ongoing transmission (Farmer *et al.*, 1998; Van Rie and Enarson, 2006). There are 27 high-burden MDR-TB countries; the countries that rank first to fifth in terms of total numbers of MDR-TB cases are China

(100,000), India (99,000), the Russian Federation (38,000), Pakistan (15,000) and South Africa (13,000) (WHO, 2010). However, as stated earlier, presumably only the tip of the iceberg of the MDR-TB problem is currently being notified. By the end of 2008, 55 countries and territories had also reported at least one case of XDR-TB (WHO, 2009). However, the problem of XDR-TB most likely has been developing for many years but has not been adequately recognized. In Europe, for instance, in the period from 2003 to 2007, about 10% of the MDR-TB cases in the European Union (EU) were, in fact, already XDR-TB (Devaux *et al.*, 2009). Moreover, on the basis of DNA fingerprint surveillance in the EU, it was shown that about half of the MDR-TB in this region was caused by transmission and not acquired by low-quality treatment (Devaux *et al.*, 2009). In addition, as shown in other geographic regions, the Beijing genotype of *Mycobacterium tuberculosis* was associated with the significant MDR-TB problem in, for example, the Baltic States and the Former Soviet Union States (Devaux *et al.*, 2009) and South Africa (Johnson *et al.*, 2010). Therefore, it is assumed there is also an important bacteriological component in the current emergence of drug resistance globally, although not sufficiently addressed (Parwati *et al.*, 2010). However, in order to meet the global public health challenges related to current tuberculosis control, as described by the WHO, the diagnosis and treatment of MDR-TB and XDR-TB need to be scaled up rapidly.

The treatment of pulmonary tuberculosis involves the prolonged administration of multiple drugs, but is usually highly effective. However, *M. tuberculosis* may be resistant to one or more of the drugs, causing a slow conversion, treatment failures and relapses after curative treatment. The four common first-line drugs used in anti-tuberculosis therapy are INH, RIF, EMB and PZA. When this drug combination fails, MDR-TB (i.e. a tuberculous disease caused by a bacterial strain that is resistant to the two most effective first-line anti-tuberculosis agents, namely INH and RIF, ensues). Further down the spectrum, the previously mentioned problem of XDR-TB is increasingly reported. This form

of tuberculosis with a bad prognosis for the concerned patient is defined as MDR-TB with additional resistance to at least one fluoroquinolone (FQ) and any of the following injectable second-line drugs: kanamycin (KM), amikacin (AK) or capreomycin (CM). Surprisingly, it is estimated that 0–30% of MDR-TB isolates currently tested for second-line drug resistance are, in fact, XDR-TB (WHO, 2008a). It is currently unknown whether XDR-TB is emerging or has been addressed sufficiently in the previous period. Coupled with the emergence of XDR-TB are the technically controversial and recently reported cases of 'totally drug-resistant tuberculosis' (TDR-TB) or 'extremely drug resistant' (XDR-TB), known to be resistant to all first- and second-line anti-tuberculosis drugs that have been found in some patients in Italy, Iran and India (WHO, 2012b). It is currently unknown whether XDR-TB is emerging or has been addressed sufficiently in the previous period. None the less, resistance in general is emerging and is influencing significantly the development of the current worldwide tuberculosis epidemic.

9.2 Principles of Drug Resistance

In *M. tuberculosis* and other members of the *M. tuberculosis* complex, multiple mechanisms can underlie resistance to anti-tuberculosis agents. First, the mycobacterial cell is surrounded by a specific, highly hydrophobic cell wall that has a low permeability to many compounds (Somoskovi *et al.*, 2001). In addition, active drug efflux pumps and degrading or inactivating enzymes, and the genes that are associated with these functions, have been disclosed in *M. tuberculosis* (Ramaswamy and Musser, 1998). The concept of drug resistance in *M. tuberculosis* is believed to be mediated almost exclusively by chromosomal mutations, which affect either the drug target itself or bacterial enzymes that activate prodrugs (Sandgren *et al.*, 2009). The resistance mutations emerge naturally at particular paces (1 in 10^6 for INH and 1 in 10^8 for RIF); however, if combinations of effective drugs are applied, the chance that a resistant mutant is selected for is much lower ($10^6 \times 10^8 = 10^{14}$

in the case of combined use of INH and RIF), because the bacteria resistant to one drug will be killed by the other drug. However, if suboptimal treatment is applied, the bacteria with mutations associated with resistance are selected for and such bacteria will have a relative advantage over the bacteria with the wild-type sequence, and they will form a new bacterial population in the diseased body sites. Since the early 1990s, numerous studies have described the genetic mechanisms of drug resistance in *M. tuberculosis*, and a wealth of data has accumulated on the mutations found in isolates resistant to specific drugs (Ramaswamy and Musser, 1998). An increasing number of studies have identified the genomic mechanisms which confer INH and RIF resistance in the majority of clinical isolates; while for other drugs such as SM and many of the second-line drugs, known resistance mutations occur in only part of the resistant isolates (Ramaswamy and Musser, 1998). Hence, because most mutations associated with INH and RIF are generally only found in restricted genomic sites, molecular tests for these drugs reach a high level of sensitivity and specificity, while for the other drugs mentioned above the positive predictive value can be high, while the sensitivity is low. As documented, RIF resistance is rarely encountered as a monoresistance and therefore usually, in about 95% of cases, this indicates resistance to a number of other anti-tuberculosis drugs (Caws and Drobniewski, 2001; WHO, 2008a). Accordingly, since RIF monoresistance is relatively rare, RIF resistance is a good indicator of MDR-TB. Point mutations in the *rpoB* gene encoding the β-subunit of DNA-dependent RNA polymerase have been shown to account for the majority of RIF resistance worldwide, though with regional variations (Gillespie, 2002). More specifically, 95% of these RIF resistance-causing mutations are located in an 81-bp hotspot region of the *rpoB* gene, spanning codons 507–533, known as the RIF resistance-determining region (RRDR) (Ramaswamy and Musser, 1998). Mutations in codons 516, 526 and 531 of the *rpoB* gene are most commonly associated with high-level RIF resistance (Cavusoglu *et al.*, 2006; Huitric *et al.*, 2006; Rigouts *et al.*,

2007). The mechanism of resistance in the remaining 5% of resistant isolates so far remains undetermined, with the exception of further mutations at codons 381 (Taniguchi *et al.*, 1996), 481 (Nash *et al.*, 1997), 505 (Matsiota-Bernard *et al.*, 1998), 508 (Matsiota-Bernard *et al.*, 1998) and 509 (Nash *et al.*, 1997) of the *rpoB* gene. Molecular assays that have been used to screen the *rpoB* gene for RIF-resistance mutations include DNA sequencing (Kapur *et al.*, 1994), heteroduplex analysis (Williams *et al.*, 1994), PCR single-stranded conformational polymorphism (PCR-SSCP) (Telenti *et al.*, 1993a,b), line probe assay (LPA) (De Beenhouwer *et al.*, 1995; Cooksey *et al.*, 1997; Van Rie *et al.*, 2010), mismatch analysis (Nash *et al.*, 1997) and a recently introduced semi-automated real-time PCR device, the GeneXpert (Boehme *et al.*, 2010).

Although the detection of INH resistance in *M. tuberculosis* is more complex because a number of genes can be implicated, up to 95% of this resistance may be due to mutations in *katG* (Hazbón *et al.*, 2006). If the mutations occurring in the *inhA* gene are also included in the test, a reliable detection of INH resistance can be reached in most areas. The most frequently observed alteration in *katG* is a serine-to-threonine substitution at codon 315 (S315T), located in the active site of the catalase moiety of the *katG* gene. Additionally, mutations in the promoter region of *inhA* account for 8–20% of INH resistance in *M. tuberculosis* (Hazbón *et al.*, 2006). A C-to-T substitution at nucleotide –15 results in the overexpression of *inhA*, an NADH-dependent enoyl-acyl reductase involved in mycolic acid synthesis, and INH resistance arises as a result of drug titration (Hazbón *et al.*, 2006). Although, in general, fitness is reduced by mutations in the *katG* gene, because the bacteria are believed to suffer from a reduced capability to withstand exposure to oxygen radicals in the intracellular environment, this phenomenon varies by mutation (Zhang *et al.*, 1992). Also, the level of resistance is associated with the type of mutation underlying INH resistance. Bacteria with codon 315 mutations have a higher level of resistance than bacteria that utilize other mutations associated with INH resistance (van Doorn *et al.*, 2006). Moreover, while INH resistance in general is a negative risk factor for transmission, codon 315 resistant strains are as transmissible as susceptible ones, while the mutations at this codon are also associated more frequently with multiple resistance (van Doorn *et al.*, 2006).

9.3 Novel and Rapid Molecular Diagnostic Tools

New molecular methods for rapid molecular detection of resistance in *M. tuberculosis* need to be widely deployed and integrated into case-finding strategies to reduce transmission of MDR-TB and to diagnose and treat patients adequately. Recent advances in availability should ensure optimal use of true point-of-care (POC) tests for MDR-TB (Keshavjee and Seung, 2009). With the emergence of resistance to anti-tuberculosis drugs, several high-throughput sequencing methods and genotyping strategies have been developed, and studies to identify the mutations associated with resistance have been undertaken globally in the last few years (Sandgren *et al.*, 2009). The WHO Stop TB Partnership's New Diagnostics Working Group and Foundation for Innovative New Diagnostics (FIND) have classified tools for the diagnosis of active tuberculosis and resistance in three categories, as (i) 'WHO-endorsed' tools (favourably evaluated), (ii) in a 'late-stage development or evaluation' and (iii) tools in 'early-stage development' (Pai *et al.*, 2009). WHO-endorsed tools include molecular LPAs for MDR-TB diagnosis (GenoType® MTBDR*plus*, Hain Lifescience, Nehren, Germany, and INNO-LiPA Rif. TB, Innogenetics, Gent, Belgium) and a rapid-detection and -speciation assay (Capilia TB-Neo, TAUNS, Numazu, Japan). A commercially available tool in late-stage development or evaluation is the GeneXpert MTB/RIF assay (Cepheid, California, USA), a nucleic acid amplification test (NAAT) for *M. tuberculosis* detection and MDR-TB screening. Examples of tools in the early phase of development include the lipoarabinomannan assay, the breathalyser screening test, loop-mediated isothermal amplification technology (TB-LAMP, Eiken Chemical Co Ltd, Tokyo, Japan)

and phage-based tests for rapid diagnosis of MDR-TB (Van Rie *et al.*, 2010).

Though recently introduced, the new Genotype *M. tuberculosis* drug resistance second-line (MTBDR*sl*) assay (Hain Lifescience, Nehren, Germany) is another very promising LPA for the screening of second-line drugs (i.e. FQs, injectable drugs – AK, CM, KM). The implementation of this assay becomes very useful with the emergence of XDR-TB.

9.3.1 Need for molecular assays

M. tuberculosis generally acquires drug resistance via the selection of mutants with *de novo* non-synonymous single nucleotide polymorphisms (nsSNPs), small deletions or insertions in specific chromosomal loci, unlike most other pathogenic bacteria, which often acquire drug resistance via horizontal gene transfer. This feature of *M. tuberculosis* drug resistance, coupled with fast and efficient DNA molecular methods, makes studying drug resistance highly amenable in molecular epidemiology (Mathema *et al.*, 2006).

Calls from the WHO and other international public health authorities translate the demand to expand access rapidly to culture and drug susceptibility tests (DST) in response to the dual threats that HIV and MDR-TB pose as significant challenges to tuberculosis control programmes and tuberculosis laboratory services (WHO, 2007). The costs and complexity of establishing culture and DST capacity to meet the anticipated need, especially in low-income countries where these services are currently scarcely available, present overwhelming challenges (see Chapter 1). Consequently, other diagnostic methods, and in particular fast molecular approaches, are considered as alternatives (Barnard *et al.*, 2008). The fast developments of molecular approaches in tuberculosis diagnosis, especially identification and drug susceptibility, question the necessity to upgrade all tuberculosis laboratories to Biosafety Level 3. It has become likely that within a few years, microscopy and culture can be avoided for the majority of suspects. Only in cases in which resistance is detected may additional culture and extended resistance testing still be required. However, with the current increasing initiatives to apply whole genome sequencing techniques, it is likely that the vast majority of resistance mechanisms can be disclosed within the coming years, facilitating the development of complete full-coverage *Mycobacterium* diagnostic methods.

9.3.2 Advantages in molecular diagnostic tools

One of the main progressions in molecular diagnostic assays is their enhancing sensitivity and the increasing ability to diagnose tuberculosis in clinical material with nearly the same sensitivity as culture (Davies and Pai, 2008). Again, NAAT can be performed on at least one respiratory specimen from each patient with the signs and symptoms of pulmonary tuberculosis, for whom a diagnosis of tuberculosis is being considered but has not yet been established and for whom the test result would alter case management or tuberculosis control activities (CDC, 2009).

In the last decade, molecular tools have been developed based on nucleic acid amplification in conjunction with electrophoresis, sequencing or hybridization. Though most of them are directed at detecting drug resistance in *M. tuberculosis* complex isolates, they are currently also being evaluated for direct detection of DNA of these bacteria and identification of alleles related to drug resistance in clinical specimens (such as sputum). This current trend is aimed at generating laboratory results within the shortest time interval in order to enhance patient care and prevent further spread to the larger population.

One of the methods of detecting mutations is direct sequencing; but although very useful, this approach is still rather expensive and time-consuming. In addition, the technology involved is still limited to few laboratories globally. In most instances, DNA sequencing of the *katG, inhA, inhA* locus, *oxyR-ahpC* and *rpoB* genes is explored. Huang *et al.* (2009) conducted a study involving mutations in *katG, inhA*, the *inhA* locus (*inhA* regulatory

region), the *oxyR-ahpC* intergenic region (*ahpC*) and the *rpoB* gene after PCR amplification and sequencing using specific primers for all resistance genes. Techniques, such as the real-time polymerase chain reaction, that make use of primers complementary to resistance gene sequences to amplify genomic regions where mutations occur and use specific probes (i.e. molecular beacons) to identify mutations, are now available, though still expensive and complicated, even if highly sensitive and specific (Huang *et al.*, 2009). Reverse hybridization-based assays, referred to as LPAs, represent useful tools because of their superior cost-effectiveness and speed. These tests are based on the hybridization of PCR products to specific probes for wild-type and mutated sequences of genes involved in drug resistance, and they show a high specificity and medium/high sensitivity. LPAs, direct DNA sequencing, molecular beacon analysis and biprobe analysis rapidly detect drug resistance accurately against the most important first-line drugs INH and RIF, but these methods are expensive and require extensive training of specialized personnel. The recently introduced reversed line blot method for the detection of resistance against FQs and aminoglycosides is promising (Hillemann *et al.*, 2009) and relatively easy to implement, providing caution is taken regarding analysis of the results, which can be more difficult than assumed.

9.4 Line Probe Assays (LPAs)

Recently, the WHO recommended the use of molecular LPAs for rapid resistance screening in low- and middle-income settings (WHO, 2008b). LPAs use multiple-target PCR amplification and reverse line blot hybridization for the identification of *Mycobacterium* isolates and detection of resistant mutants. There are kits available for the distinction of the *M. tuberculosis* (sub) species and the most frequently encountered non-tuberculous mycobacteria. In addition, there are reliable and favourably evaluated kits for the detection of mutants associated with RIF and INH resistance. Lately, in 2009, an LPA kit was also introduced for the detection of resistance against second-line drugs (Hillemann *et al.*, 2009), as discussed above. LPAs can be performed directly from acid-fast bacilli (AFB) in smear-positive sputum, or from positive cultures, and provide results in 1 day. A recent systematic review concluded that LPAs were highly sensitive and specific for detection of RIF resistance (97% and 99%, respectively) and INH resistance (90% and 99%, respectively) on culture isolates and smear-positive sputum. Overall agreement with conventional DST for detection of MDR-TB was 99% (Ling *et al.*, 2008).

9.4.1 Limitations of the Hain MTBDR*plus* test

Issues to be considered regarding the implementation of LPAs in high tuberculosis burden countries include the supply of consumables and reagents not provided as part of the kit, such as pipette tips and molecular grade water. Furthermore, the necessary infrastructure for performing LPAs should be considered prior to implementation – a minimum of three separate rooms is recommended to minimize the risk of contamination of tests with previously produced amplicons, which induces false positive results. Restricted access to the molecular laboratories and strict adherence to standard operating procedures are essential to reduce the risk of amplicon contamination (Albert *et al.*, 2010).

An additional point of consideration is the interpretation of less obvious test results. For instance, a caveat in the interpretation of the GenoType® MTBDR*plus* assay with respect to RIF resistance detection is that resistance may be suggested by the absence of a wild-type hybridization signal, without confirmation of hybridization on a mutant probe. As a wild-type probe may not hybridize due to a mutation in the RRDR that is not associated with a resistance phenotype (Ma *et al.*, 2006), such RIF-susceptible isolates could be interpreted wrongly as resistant and lead to the unnecessary removal of RIF from treatment regimens. In addition, isolates indicated as resistant due to a mutation at codon 533 may be susceptible (Ma *et al.*, 2006), and

similar caution should be taken. In a study by Huang *et al.* (2009), the performances of the LPA and DNA sequencing in detecting RIF and INH resistance associated mutations in the *rpoB*, *katG*, *inhA* regulatory region and *oxyR-ahpC* genes were compared to that of a conventional agar proportion DST. A total of 242 MDR and 30 pan-susceptible *M. tuberculosis* isolates were evaluated in this study. The sensitivities obtained for RIF resistance detection by the GenoType® MTBDR*plus* test and by resistance gene sequencing were 95.5% and 97.9%, respectively. The sensitivities for INH resistance detection by the GenoType® MTBDR*plus* test and by resistance gene sequencing were 81.8% and 93.4%, respectively. Together, the sensitivity for detection of MDR-TB was 78.5% with the GenoType® MTBDR*plus* test and 91.3% by resistance gene sequencing. The specificity for RIF resistance, INH resistance and MDR-TB detection was 100% by both methods. However, the GenoType® MTBDR*plus* test has the important advantage of a short turnaround time for the diagnosis of drug-resistant *M. tuberculosis* and requires only relative simple equipment. Overall, the two assays performed equally well in detecting RIF resistance ($P\_0.13$), although DNA sequencing demonstrated superior performance in detecting INH resistance ($P < 0.001$) and MDR-TB ($P < 0.001$). The study suggested that additional alleles associated with INH resistance should be evaluated to improve the sensitivity of the GenoType® MTBDR*plus* test, especially in areas with genetically diverse and unknown *M. tuberculosis* strains. The findings of this report are similar to those published by other colleagues. For example, *katG* mutations were found in 97% (77/79) and *inhA* mutations in 24% (19/79) of the INH-resistant isolates from KwaZulu-Natal (Kiepiela *et al.*, 2000), whereas Van Rie and colleagues reported *katG* mutations in 72% of INH-resistant isolates (41/57) and mutation in the *inhA* gene in only 2% (1/57) of the isolates in the Western Cape province of South Africa (Van Rie *et al.*, 2001). Studies from other countries have confirmed this variability in the distribution of mutations associated with INH resistance (Mokrousov *et al.*, 2002; Baker *et al.*, 2005). Mutations in *inhA* were, for instance, also reported as rare in Germany (Hillemann *et al.*, 2007). A high prevalence of *katG* mutations has been reported to account for a high proportion of INH resistance in high tuberculosis prevalence countries and for a much lower proportion in lower tuberculosis prevalence settings, presumably due to ongoing transmission of these strains in high-burden settings (Mokrousov *et al.*, 2002). Furthermore, the GenoType® MTBDR*plus* test may need to include new alleles of RIF- and INH-resistant genes in order to improve sensitivity in the detection of resistance in genetically diverse *M. tuberculosis* strains circulating in various geographic areas.

In conclusion, the results available illustrate that the distribution of mutations resulting in drug resistance in *M. tuberculosis* differs by geographic regions. This may have important implications for the roll-out of rapid genotypic tests for the diagnosis of drug-resistant *M. tuberculosis*, which may impact the progression of *M. tuberculosis* to MDR- and, ultimately, XDR-TB. In particular, a high proportion of what may be genetically related INH- and RIF-monoresistant strains that are not recognized as resistant by the GenoType® MTBDR*plus* assay have already been identified. If rapid genotypic assays for the detection of drug resistance are to be widely used, there is a need to monitor local distribution of drug-resistance mutations continually to ensure that if clonal groups of *M. tuberculosis* with alternative resistance mutations emerge, they are diagnosed properly as drug resistant. In general, potential users of molecular tests should realize that the visualization of mutants associated with resistance in *M. tuberculosis* is an indirect approach; it is likely, but not certain, that these mutations are associated with resistance and it is uncertain whether negative findings exclude all possibilities of resistance problems. In other words, a large part of the mutations that confer resistance are covered by the current molecular tests, but not all. The reliability of molecular tests varies by geographic region. This implies the sensitivity of molecular testing will be lower than 100%. However, this is not a problem if the positive predictive value is sufficiently high. The negative predictive value should not drop below an acceptable level, otherwise such a molecular test becomes useless.

Growth inhibition tests for *M. tuberculosis* isolates therefore remain highly important as a control of the performance of molecular tests. The molecular approach may, in the near future, become nearly perfect when whole genome sequencing will yield more insight into all genomic mechanisms underlying resistance. Translation to simple, cheap and rapid detection of the respective mutations remains a challenge.

Overall, LPAs are accurate and useful for the rapid detection of drug resistance directly in clinical specimens, providing sufficient AFB are present. Currently, if the microscopy is positive, it will generally be possible to amplify the DNA in reversed line blot methods and therefore direct the therapy in an early stage of treatment on the basis of the results. In general, LPAs are expensive and require sophisticated laboratory infrastructure. Their role and utility in low-income, high-burden countries will need to be evaluated further in field studies.

9.4.2 GenoType® MTBDR*sl* assay

Studies have shown that resistance to FQs, AK, CM and EMB in *M. tuberculosis* is most frequently attributed to mutations in the *gyrA*, *rrs* and *embB* genes, respectively (Hillemann *et al.*, 2009). By targeting mutations in codons 90, 91 and 94 in the *gyrA* gene, approximately 70–90% of all FQ-resistant strains can be detected correctly (Antonova *et al.*, 2008; Mokrousov *et al.*, 2008; van Doorn *et al.*, 2008). Previous reports have linked mutations A1401G, C1402T and G1484T in the *rrs* gene to AK, CM and KM resistance (Alangaden *et al.*, 1998; Maus *et al.*, 2005a,b), each of them being responsible for a specific resistance pattern. Mutations G1484T and A1401G were found to cause high-level resistance to all drugs, whereas C1402T caused resistance against CM and KM only. In order to increase the capacity to detect further drug resistance in *M. tuberculosis*, apart from those due to the first-line drugs (particularly INH and RIF, the cause of MDR-TB), the GenoType® *M. tuberculosis* drug-resistance second-line (MTBDR*sl*) assay was developed with a specific focus on the most prevalent *gyrA, rrs* and *embB* gene mutations. Hillemann *et al.* (2009) reported that this assay represented a reliable tool for detection of FQ and AK/CM resistance and it could be applied directly to smear-positive specimens as well as smear-negative specimens known to be culture positive. With a turnaround time of approximately 6 h, the diagnosis of second-line drug resistance can be shortened from weeks (conventional DST) to a single day. The new MTBDR*sl* assay is therefore a major improvement in the routine detection of FQ and AK/CM resistance and, to a lesser extent, to EMB-resistant *M. tuberculosis* strains. Especially in combination with the MTBDR*plus* assay for the detection of MDR *M. tuberculosis*, the detection of XDR *M. tuberculosis* is made possible within 1 or 2 days (Hillemann *et al.*, 2009). Therefore, the introduction of the MTBDR*sl* assay will have a great impact on the diagnosis of drug resistance to strengthen both the management of patient therapy and the prevention of transmission.

The limitations of this assay are that: first, it has to be used in conjunction with other LPAs, hence it cannot be used as a standalone test; and second, its low sensitivity for the detection of EMB resistance: presumably, gene loci other than *embB* codon 306 are also associated with EMB resistance. Therefore, novel mutations with locations besides the probe regions or outside the amplified targets can lead to misinterpretations (Hillemann *et al.*, 2009). Finally, the MTBDR*sl* assay should be evaluated in different settings before routine use, since the prevalence of mutations associated with FQs, AK, CM and EMB resistance varies in different locations (Hillemann *et al.*, 2009).

9.5 The Semi-automated Real-time PCR: The GeneXpert

The GeneXpert is based on the molecular detection of *M. tuberculosis* complex and *rpoB* gene mutations associated with RIF resistance. This is accomplished in the Xpert MTB/RIF test by analysing liquefied sputum samples in less than 2 h. The rapid detection of *M. tuberculosis* and RIF resistance in clinical material allows the physician to make critical patient management decisions regarding therapy during the same medical encounter.

The GeneXpert system integrates and automates sample processing, nucleic acid amplification and detection of the amplified target sequences in simple or complex samples using real-time PCR and reverse transcriptase PCR. The system consists of an instrument, personal computer, barcode scanner and preloaded software for interpretation of the results. The system requires the use of single-use disposable GeneXpert cartridges that hold the PCR reagents and host the PCR process. Because the cartridges are self-contained, the possibility of cross-contamination between samples is eliminated. This is a major step forward.

9.5.1 Strengths and limitations of the GeneXpert

Van Rie *et al.* (2010), in an expert commentary review, concluded that, 'Xpert MTB/RIF is the first novel TB diagnostic that has the potential for use as a true point of care (POC) tool in resource-limited settings. Although the performance characteristics determined by experimental and clinical studies create hope for dramatic improvement in the diagnosis of TB and drug-resistant TB, the current Xpert MTB/RIF assay lacks the robustness (especially with regard to its need for continuous electrical power) and the sensitivity in smear-negative TB to become the "magic bullet" for TB diagnosis in high-TB burden, low-resource settings. In addition it is doubtful whether the sole detection of RIF is sufficient to guide the treatment in areas where poly-resistance is prevalent. The automation and simplicity of the system, however, allow for its use by low-skilled personnel in the absence of biohazard containment infrastructure, and its high specificity for the detection of *M. tuberculosis* and RIF resistance have already caught the interest of clinicians, clinical researchers and funding agencies. The POC diagnosis of RIF resistance, a marker for MDR-TB, and the 72.5% sensitivity of a single Xpert MTB/RIF assay to diagnose smear-negative culture-positive TB cases have created, for the first time, the long-awaited possibility of a POC diagnostic tool to reduce the morbidity and mortality of TB.' Happily, with the endorsement of the WHO in 2010, over 26 of the 145 countries eligible to purchase the Xpert MTB/RIF kits have done so, with greater prospects in the future.

9.6 Conclusions: Future Perspectives of Molecular Diagnosis of MDR-TB/XDR-TB

Owing to the reality of expanding knowledge and advances in molecular and genomic research in the area of drug resistance in tuberculosis, it is envisaged that newer, simpler, more rapid and cheaper molecular inventions and innovations will be brought to bear in unlocking the jigsaw in the diagnosis of MDR-TB and XDR-TB. It is expected that the current developments in whole genome sequencing will enlarge our knowledge on resistance mechanisms in *M. tuberculosis* significantly, and that this will facilitate the development of more sensitive molecular tests. When this is achieved, it is anticipated that the problem of MDR-TB and the emerging pandemic of XDR-TB can be dealt with in a more adequate way. However, solving the problem of tuberculosis is not a matter of waiting for innovative miracles, but working extremely hard in an international but also local multidisciplinary approach.

References

Alangaden, G.J., Kreiswirth, B.N., Aouad, A., Khetarpal, M., Igno, F.R., Moghazeh, S.L., et al. (1998) Mechanism of resistance to amikacin and kanamycin in *Mycobacterium tuberculosis*. *Antimicrobial Agents and Chemotherapy* 42, 1295–1297.

Albert, H., Bwanga, F., Mukkada, S., Nyesiga, B., Ademun, J.P., Lukyamuzi, G., et al. (2010) Rapid screening of MDR-TB using molecular line probe assay is feasible in Uganda. *BMC Infectious Diseases*, 10:41doi:10.1186/1471-2334-10-41.

Antonova, O.V., Gryadunov, D.A., Lapa, S.A.,

Kuz'min, A.V., Larionova, E.E., Smirnova, T.G., et al. (2008) Detection of mutations in *Mycobacterium tuberculosis* genome determining resistance to fluoroquinolones by hybridization on biological microchips. *Bulletin of Experimental Biology and Medicine* 145, 108–113.

Baker, L.V., Brown, T.J., Maxwell, O., Gibson, A.L., Fang, Z., Yates, M.D., et al. (2005) Molecular analysis of isoniazid-resistant *Mycobacterium tuberculosis* isolates from England and Wales reveals the phylogenetic significance of the ahpC-46A polymorphism. *Antimicrobial Agents and Chemotherapy* 49, 1455–1464.

Barnard, M., Albert, H., Coetzee, G., O'Brien, R. and Bosman, M. (2008) Rapid molecular screening for multidrug-resistant tuberculosis in a high-volume public health laboratory in South Africa. *American Journal of Respiratory and Critical Care Medicine* 177, 787–792.

Boehme, C.C., Nabeta, P., Hillermen, D., Nicol, M.P., Shenai, S., Krapp, F., et al. (2010) Rapid molecular detection of tuberculosis and rifampin resistance. *New England Journal of Medicine* 363(11), 1005–1015.

Cavusoglu, C., Turhan, A., Akinci, P. and Soyler, I. (2006) Evaluation of the GenoType MTBDR assay for rapid detection of rifampin and isoniazid resistance in *Mycobacterium tuberculosis* isolates. *Journal of Clinical Microbiology* 44, 2338–2342.

Caws, M. and Drobniewski, F.A. (2001) Molecular techniques in the diagnosis of *Mycobacterium tuberculosis* and the detection of drug resistance. *Annals of the New York Academy of Science* 953, 138–145.

Centers for Disease Control and Prevention [CDC] (2009) Updated guidelines for the use of nucleic acid amplification tests in the diagnosis of tuberculosis. *Morbidity and Mortality Weekly Report* 58, 7–10.

Cooksey, R.C., Morlock, G.P., Glickman, S. and Crawford, J.T. (1997) Evaluation of a line probe assay kit for characterization of *rpoB* mutations in rifampin-resistant *Mycobacterium tuberculosis* isolates from New York City. *Journal of Clinical Microbiology* 35, 1281–1283.

Davies, P.D. and Pai, M. (2008) The diagnosis and misdiagnosis of tuberculosis. *International Journal of Tuberculosis and Lung Disease* 12, 1226–1234.

De Beenhouwer, H., Lhiang, Z., Jannes, G., Mijs, W., Machtelinckx, L., Rossau, R., et al. (1995) Rapid detection of rifampin resistance in sputum and biopsy specimens from tuberculosis patients by PCR and line probe assay. *Tubercle and Lung Disease* 76, 425–430.

Devaux, I., Kremer, K., Heersma, H. and van

Soolingen, D. (2009) Clusters of multidrug-resistant *Mycobacterium tuberculosis* cases, Europe. *Emerging Infectious Diseases* 15, 1052–1060.

Farmer, P., Bayona, J., Becerra, M., Furin, J., Henry, C., Hiatt, H., *et al.* (1998) The dilemma of MDR-TB in the global era. *International Journal of Tuberculosis and Lung Disease* 2, 869–876.

Getahun, H., Harrington, M., O'Brien, R. and Nunn, P. (2007) Diagnosis of smear-negative pulmonary tuberculosis in people with HIV infection or AIDS in resource-constrained settings: informing urgent policy changes. *The Lancet* 369, 2042–2049.

Gillespie, S.H. (2002) Evolution of drug resistance in *Mycobacterium tuberculosis*: clinical and molecular perspective. *Antimicrobial Agents and Chemotherapy* 46, 267–274.

Havlir, D.V., Getahun, H., Sanne, I. and Nunn, P. (2008) Opportunities and challenges for HIV care in overlapping HIV and TB epidemics. *Journal of American Medical Association* 300, 423–430.

Hazbón, M.H., Brimacombe, M., del Valle, M.B., Cavatore, M., Guerrero, M.I., Varma-Basil, M., *et al.* (2006) Population genetics study of isoniazid resistance mutations and evolution of multidrug-resistant *Mycobacterium tuberculosis*. *Antimicrobial Agents and Chemotherapy* 50, 2640–2649.

Hillemann, D., Rusch-Gerdes, S. and Richter, E. (2007) Evaluation of the Genotype MTBDRplus assay for rifampin and isoniazid susceptibility testing of *Mycobacterium tuberculosis* strains and clinical specimens. *Journal of Clinical Microbiology* 45, 2635–2640.

Hillemann, D., Rusch-Gerdes, S. and Richter, E. (2009) Feasibility of the GenoType MTBDRsl/ Assay for fluoroquinolone, amikacin-capreomycin, and ethambutol resistance testing of *Mycobacterium tuberculosis* strains and clinical samples. *Journal of Clinical Microbiology* 47, 1767–1772.

Huang, W., Chen, H., Kuo, Y. and Jou, R. (2009) Performance assessment of the GenoType MTBDR*plus* test and DNA sequencing in detection of multidrug-resistant *Mycobacterium tuberculosis*. *Journal of Clinical Microbiology* 47, 2520–2524.

Huitric, E., Werngren, J., Juréen, P. and Hoffner, S. (2006) Resistance levels and rpoB gene mutations among *in vitro*-selected rifampin-resistant *Mycobacterium tuberculosis* mutants. *Antimicrobial Agents and Chemotherapy* 50, 2860–2862.

Johnson, R., Warren, R.M., van der Spuy, G.D., Gey van Pittius, N.C., Theron, D., Streicher,

E.M., *et al.* (2010) Drug resistant tuberculosis epidemic in the Western Cape driven by a virulent Beijing genotype strain. *International Journal of Tuberculosis and Lung Disease* 14, 119–121.

Kapur, V., Li, L.L., Iordanescu, S., Hamrick, M.R., Wanger, A., Kreiswirth, B.N., *et al.* (1994) Characterization by automated DNA sequencing of mutations in the gene (*rpoB*) encoding the RNA polymerase b subunit in rifampin-resistant *Mycobacterium tuberculosis* strains from New York City and Texas. *Journal of Clinical Microbiology* 32, 1095–1098.

Keshavjee, S. and Seung, K. (2009) Stemming the tide of multidrug-resistant tuberculosis: major barriers to addressing the growing epidemic. In: Giffin, R. and Robinson, S. (eds) Institute of Medicine. *Addressing the Threat of Drug Resistant Tuberculosis: A Realistic Assessment of the Challenge: Workshop Summary*. National Academies Press, Washington, DC, pp. 141–235.

Kiepiela, P., Bishop, K.S., Smith, A.N., Roux, L. and York, D.F. (2000) Genomic mutations in the *katG*, *inhA* and *aphC* genes are useful for the prediction of isoniazid resistance in *Mycobacterium tuberculosis* isolates from Kwa-Zulu Natal, South Africa. *Tubercle and Lung Disease* 80, 47–56.

Ling, D., Zwerling, A. and Pai, M. (2008) GenoType MTBDR assays for the diagnosis of multidrug-resistant tuberculosis: a meta-analysis. *European Respiratory Journal* 32, 1165–1174.

Ma, X., Wang, H., Deng, Y., Liu, Z., Xu, Y., Pan, X., *et al.* (2006) *rpoB* gene mutations and molecular characterization of rifampin-resistant *Mycobacterium tuberculosis* isolates from Shandong Province, China. *Journal of Clinical Microbiology* 44, 3409–3412.

Mathema, B., Kurepina, N.E., Bifani, P.J. and Kreiswirth, B.N. (2006) Molecular epidemiology of tuberculosis: current insights. *Clinical Microbiology Reviews* 19, 658–685.

Matsiota-Bernard, P., Vrioni, G. and Marinis, E. (1998) Characterization of *rpoB* mutations in rifampin-resistant clinical *Mycobacterium tuberculosis* isolates from Greece. *Journal of Clinical Microbiology* 36, 20–23.

Maus, C.E., Plikaytis, B.B. and Shinnick, T.M. (2005a) Molecular analysis of cross resistance to capreomycin, kanamycin, amikacin, and viomycin in *Mycobacterium tuberculosis*. *Antimicrobial Agents and Chemotherapy* 49, 3192–3197.

Maus, C.E., Plikaytis, B.B. and Shinnick, T.M. (2005b) Mutation of *tlyA* confers capreomycin resistance in *Mycobacterium tuberculosis*.

Antimicrobial Agents and Chemotherapy 49, 571–577.

Migliori, G.B., Loddenkemper, R., Blasi, F. and Raviglione, M.C. (2007) 125 years after Robert Koch's discovery of the tubercle bacillus: the new XDR-TB threat. Is 'science' enough to tackle the epidemic? *European Respiratory Journal* 29, 423–427.

Mokrousov, I., Narvskaya, O., Otten, T., Limenschenko, E., Steklova, L. and Vyshnevskiy, B. (2002) High prevalence of *katG* Ser315Thr substitution among isoniazid-resistant *Myco-acterium tuberculosis* clinical isolates from Northwestern Russia, 1996–2001. *Antimicrobial Agents and Chemotherapy* 46, 1417–1424.

Mokrousov, I., Otten, T., Manicheva, O., Potapova, Y., Vishnevsky, B., Narvskaya, O., *et al.* (2008) Molecular characterization of ofloxacin-resistant *Mycobacterium tuberculosis* strains from Russia. *Antimicrobial Agents and Chemotherapy* 52, 2937–2939.

Nash, K.A., Gaytan, A. and Inderlied, C.B. (1997) Detection of rifampin resistance in *Mycobacterium tuberculosis* by means of a rapid, simple, and specific RNA/RNA mismatch assay. *Journal of Infectious Diseases* 176, 533–536.

Pai, M., Minion, J., Sohn, H., Zwerling, A. and Perkins, M.D. (2009) Novel and improved technologies for tuberculosis diagnosis: progress and challenges. *Clinical Chest Medicine* 30, 701–716.

Parwati, I., van Crevel, R. and van Soolingen, D. (2010) Possible underlying mechanisms for successful emergence of the *Mycobacterium tuberculosis* Beijing genotype strains. *The Lancet Infectious Disease* 10, 103–111.

Perkins, M.D. and Cunningham, J. (2007) Facing the crisis: improving the diagnosis of tuberculosis in the HIV era. *Journal of Infectious Disease* 196 (Suppl 1), S15–S27.

Ramaswamy, S. and Musser, J.M. (1998) Molecular genetic basis of antimicrobial agent resistance in *Mycobacterium tuberculosis*: 1998 update. *International Journal of Tuberculosis and Lung Disease* 79, 3–29.

Rigouts, L., Nolasco, O., de Rijk, P., Nduwamahoro, E., Van Deun, A., Arevalo, J., *et al.* (2007) Newly developed primers for comprehensive amplification of the *rpoB* gene and detection of rifampin resistance in *Mycobacterium tuberculosis*. *Journal of Clinical Microbiology* 45, 252–254.

Sandgren, A., Strong, M., Muthukrishnan, P., Weiner, B.K., Church, G.M. and Murray, M.B. (2009) Tuberculosis drug resistance mutation database. *PLoS Medicine* 6(2), e1000002.

Somoskovi, A., Parsons, L.M. and Salfinger, M. (2001) The molecular basis of resistance to isoniazid, rifampicin, and pyrazinamide in *Mycobacterium tuberculosis*. *Respiratory Research* 2, 164–168.

Taniguchi, H., Aramaki, H., Nikaido, Y., Mizuguchi, Y., Nakamura, M., Koga, T., *et al.* (1996) Rifampicin resistance and mutation of the *rpoB* gene in *Mycobacterium tuberculosis*. *FEMS Microbiology Letters* 144, 103–108.

Telenti, A., Imboden, P., Marchesi, F., Lowrie, D., Cole, S., Colston, M.J., *et al.* (1993a) Detection of rifampin resistance mutations in *Mycobacterium tuberculosis*. *The Lancet* 341, 647–650.

Telenti, A., Imboden, P., Marchesi, F., Schmidheini, T. and Bodmer, T. (1993b) Direct, automated detection of rifampin-resistant *Mycobacterium tuberculosis* by polymerase chain reaction and single-strand conformation polymorphism analysis. *Antimicrobial Agents and Chemotherapy* 37, 2054–2058.

Uys, P.W., Warren, R.M. and van Helden, P.D. (2007) A threshold value for the time delay to TB diagnosis. *PLoS ONE* 2, e757.

van Doorn, H.R., de Haas, P.E.W., Kremer, K., Vandenbroucke-Grauls, C.M.J.E., Borgdorff, M.W. and van Soolingen, D. (2006) Public health impact of isoniazid-resistant *Mycobacterium tuberculosis* strains with a mutation at amino-acid position 315 of *katG*: a decade of experience in the Netherlands. *Clinical Microbiology and Infection* 12, 769–775.

van Doorn, H.R., An, D.D., de Jong, M.D., Lan, N.T.N., Hoa, D.V., Quy, H.T., *et al.* (2008) Fluoroquinolone resistance detection in *Mycobacterium tuberculosis* with locked nucleic acid probe real-time PCR. *International Journal of Tuberculosis and Lung Disease* 12, 736–742.

Van Rie, A. and Enarson, D. (2006) XDR tuberculosis: an indicator of public-health negligence. *The Lancet* 368, 1554–1556.

Van Rie, A., Warren, R., Mshanga, I., Jordaan, A.M., van der Spuy, G.D., Richardson, M., *et al.* (2001) Analysis for a limited number of gene codons can predict drug resistance of *Mycobacterium tuberculosis* in a high-incidence community. *Journal of Clinical Microbiology* 39, 636–641.

Van Rie, A., Page-Shipp, L., Scott, L., Sanne, I. and Stevens, W. (2010) Xpert® MTB/RIF for point-of care diagnosis of TB in high-HIV burden, resource-limited countries: hype or hope? *Expert Review of Molecular Diagnostics* 10, 937–946.

Williams, D.L., Waguespack, C., Eisenach, K., Crawford, J.T., Portaels, F. and Salfinger, M. (1994) Characterization of rifampin resistance in pathogenic mycobacteria. *Antimicrobial Agents and Chemotherapy* 38, 2380–2386.

World Health Organization [WHO] (1997) *Global Tuberculosis Programme. Treatment of Tuberculosis: Guidelines for National Programmes*, 2nd edn. Publication WHO/GTB/96.210. World Health Organization, Geneva, Switzerland.

WHO (2007) The global MDR-TB and XDR-TB response plan. WHO/HTM/TB/2007.387. World Health Organization, Geneva, Switzerland.

WHO (2008a) Antituberculosis drug resistance in the world. Fourth global report (http://www.who.int/tb/publications/2008/drs_report4_26feb08.pdf, accessed 5 January 2009).

WHO (2008b) Policy statement. Molecular line probe assays for rapid screening of patients at risk of multidrug resistant tuberculosis (MDR-TB) (http://www.who.int/tb/dots/laboratory/lpa_policy.pdf, accessed 18 November 2009).

WHO (2009) Global tuberculosis control – epidemiology, strategy, financing: WHO report

(WHO/HTM/TB/2009.411). World Health Organization, Geneva, Switzerland.

WHO (2010) Multidrug and extensively drug-resistant TB (M/XDR-TB) 2010. Global Report on Surveillance and Response (http://whqlibdoc.who.int/publications/2010/9787, accessed 18 September 2012).

WHO (2012a) Tuberculosis Global Facts (http://www.who.int/tb/publications/2011/factsheet, accessed 18 September 2012).

WHO (2012b) Totally drug-resistant tuberculosis: a WHO consultation on the diagnostic definition and treatment options (http://www.who.int/tb/challenges/xdr/xdrconsultation/en/, accessed 18 September 2012).

Zhang, Y., Heym, B., Allen, B., Young, D. and Cole, S. (1992) The catalase-peroxidase gene and isoniazid resistance of *Mycobacterium tuberculosis. Nature* 358, 591–593.

Part III

Understanding Treatment

10 Monitoring Therapy by Bacterial Load

Denise M. O'Sullivan

Molecular and Cell Biology Team, Laboratory for the Government Chemist, Teddington, UK

10.1 Introduction

The determination of bacterial load allows the monitoring of antimicrobial therapy; how the patient and bacteria are responding. The monitoring of bacterial load could lead to the challenging of an antibiotic regimen as to whether it is delivering the optimal dose. Bacterial load could identify individuals who could benefit from more aggressive therapy management. In order to evaluate new therapeutics, the monitoring of bacterial load is critical in Phase IIB studies. The measurement of bacterial load could indicate patients who are at increasing risk of treatment failure. In drug-susceptible patients who are receiving the standard regimen recommended by the World Health Organization (WHO) (2-month intensive phase and 4-month continuation phase), the relapse rate is 7% or less and the failure rate is 1–4% (Dye *et al.*, 2005).

10.2 Microscopy

Smear microscopy is the gold standard in the identification of *Mycobacterium tuberculosis* in sputum from patients with pulmonary tuberculosis. It has been reported to have variable sensitivity (30–80%) (Steingart *et al.*, 2006b). Microscopic examination of sputum is useful for monitoring the patient during treatment. Acid-fast microscopy gives a semi-quantitative estimate as to the burden of tuberculosis in the patient. The examination of the smear provides an estimate as to the number of bacilli that are visible per microscopy field. Up to 100 fields are examined to determine smear positivity and then the smear is scored as to the number of acid-fast bacilli. According to WHO guidelines for Ziehl–Neelsen (ZN) staining, >10 bacilli/field is a 3+, 1–10/field is a 2+, 10–99/100 fields is a 1+, 1–9/100 fields is reported as scanty and 0 bacilli/100 fields is reported as smear negative. There are also smear scoring guidelines for fluorochrome microscopy using auramine staining, and there is a separate scoring system provided by the American Thoracic Society which is based on the same principle as the WHO system (2000). In order for a ZN-stained smear to be positive, there must be approximately 10,000 bacilli/ml of sputum. Fluorescence microscopy of auramine-stained smears is approximately 10% more sensitive than light microscopy of ZN-stained smears (Steingart *et al.*, 2006a). Fluorescence microscopy using light-emitting diodes could improve tuberculosis case detection in high tuberculosis burden settings, as they have advantages over conventional fluorescence microscopy. They are cheaper, can be used in resource-poor settings as they do not require a darkroom, require less examination time and they last longer (Albert *et al.*, 2010).

Smears should be prepared when the patient first presents. The preparation of a smear is only possible in the case of pulmonary tuberculosis when the patient is producing sputum, which contains the bacilli (infectious period). Smears should be examined as the patient is progressing through treatment during both the intensive and the continuation phases of treatment. The WHO recommends examination of the smear after the intensive phase of treatment has been completed (WHO, 2009). It is imperative that sputum is examined at the end of treatment, to confirm cure. The term 'conversion rate' is used when monitoring treatment programmes to describe the proportion of patients who have smear-positive disease at the beginning of treatment which becomes smear negative when they are on treatment. Typically, a conversion rate of 2–3 months is an indicator of a good treatment programme (Blumberg *et al.*, 2003; WHO, 2010). The period of sputum smear positivity can typically last 2 months after initiation of treatment (Blumberg *et al.*, 2003), but patients who are responding to treatment can still have positive smears (Telzak *et al.*, 1997; Al-Moamary *et al.*, 1999). Even in drug-susceptible cases where the patient is receiving optimum therapy, 10% remain smear positive after 2 months (Fitzwater *et al.*, 2010). This limits the usefulness of smear microscopy in monitoring bacterial load, as patients can still expectorate bacilli which are dead in their sputum even though they are responding to treatment. If the sputum smear is positive at the end of the intensive phase of treatment, it could, however, indicate that the patient has a drug-resistant strain of *M. tuberculosis*, sub-optimal drug dosing, poor-quality drugs, poor adherence to the regimen or the patient could have extensive disease with cavitation. Smear microscopy is not specific for *M. tuberculosis* and can detect mycobacteria other than tuberculosis (Schluger and Rom, 1994). Approximately 40–60% of patients that have culture-positive tuberculosis are smear nega-tive (Mase *et al.*, 2007) and co-infection with HIV increases the likelihood of smear-negative disease (Getahun *et al.*, 2007).

10.3 Culture

Bacterial load can also be measured by cul-ture, which is more specific and sensitive than smear. However, this is time-consuming, costly and requires appropriate facilities, which are not universally available. It can take up to 12 weeks to get a result by culture, which negates the method's usefulness when it comes to the real-time monitoring of therapy. Culturing of sputum samples requires liquefaction to release the mycobacteria from the cells and mucus in the isolate. Reagents such as *N*-acetyl-L-cysteine (NALC) and sputasol (dithiotheritol) followed by sample vortexing are used to treat the sputum. Culturing also requires decontamination of the sputum sample, which usually involves exposure to strong bases such as sodium hydroxide or acids followed by neutralization (Kubica *et al.*, 1963). This results in removing organic debris and killing the contaminating bacterial and fungal flora, but also a 62–78% reduction in the number of bacilli present (Mitchison *et al.*, 1972; Grandjean *et al.*, 2008). Sodium hydroxide can be used as a mucolytic and decontaminating agent. There are strict incubation periods that must be adhered to, to minimize the reduction in mycobacterial cells while ensuring sufficient killing of the contaminating flora. When smears are prepared from concentrated specimens rather than directly from the sputum, it has been shown to increase the sensitivity of the test (Woods and Witebsky, 1995). Unlike in smear microscopy, where 10^5 bacteria are required to obtain a positive result, culture is much more sensitive, with approximately 10–100 viable bacilli required to obtain a positive result (Rouillon *et al.*, 1976). Sputum sample culture also provides sample for drug susceptibility testing, species identification and determining the strain genotype. Methods which avoid decontamination use selective growth media to inhibit the growth of contaminating flora and directly quantify the bacterial load in the sputum sample. An assay which uses selective media is the sputum serial colony-counting assay. This method is commonly used when evaluating new therapeutics in clinical trials. It deter-mines the number of colony-forming units

(CFU) per ml throughout the treatment at set time points (Mitchison, 2006). The selective growth reagents required for this method are costly and it requires a long incubation time for the results. Early bactericidal studies use serial culture samples collected for up to 5 days after the start of therapy to estimate the potency of different anti-tubercular agents (Jindani *et al.*, 1980; Gillespie *et al.*, 2002).

Sputum culture conversion after 2 months is used to monitor treatment progression and to determine the relapse rate (Mitchison, 1993). Examining changes in CFU from serial sputum samples at weekly or biweekly intervals could also provide a marker for relapse (Brindle *et al.*, 2001). In the work by Brindle *et al.*, the rate of decline in bacterial load was measured as the slope of log CFU counts and it was observed that there was a higher rate of decline in one drug regimen (streptomycin, isoniazid, rifampicin and pyrazinamide) compared to another (streptomycin, isoniazid and thiacetazone). They observed the steepest decline in CFU counts during the initial days of therapy, which was likely to be due to the potent sterilizing activity of isoniazid. Following the first 2 days of therapy, the effect of rifampicin is thought to be involved in the reduction of the bacterial load as well as the bactericidal effect of pyrazinamide. They also observed a difference between HIV-negative and -positive patients, with a greater decline in bacterial load in the initial phases of treatment among HIV-negative patients.

Liquid culture systems such as the BD BACTEC™ Mycobacteria Growth Indicator Tube (MGIT™) mycobacterial detection system and the bioMérieux MB/BacT® and BacT/ALERT® 3D are used in diagnostic clinical laboratories, as they use a culture media which is optimized for the rapid growth of mycobacteria that measure time to positivity (TTP) in days. These automated liquid culture systems can shorten TTP significantly compared to traditional culture, but this can still take 12.6–17.7 days (mean) (Somoskovi *et al.*, 2000). It has been used to monitor tuberculosis patients and has been shown to correlate more closely, when compared to other bacteriological, radiological and clinical evaluations, with the patient response to

treatment (Epstein *et al.*, 1998). The MGIT system detects O_2 consumption by fluorescence and the MB/BacT and BacT/ALERT detection systems monitor the amount of CO_2. When the level of CO_2 reaches a threshold, the machine signals the sample is positive and reports a TTP reading, which can then be correlated to the number of bacteria present (Joloba *et al.*, 2001). The liquid culture systems report a positive sample when there are 10^5–10^6 bacteria present. There is an acceptable range of contamination of 3–5% for liquid culture systems (Della Latta, 2004). If the contamination rate is less than 3%, this would suggest an overly severe decontamination procedure, and a contamination rate of greater than 5% would suggest decontamination was inadequate or sample digestion was incomplete. There is a good correlation between viable counts and TTP, as determined by liquid culture systems (O'Sullivan *et al.*, 2007). The relationship between TTP and CFU in serial samples can be used as a marker of treatment response (the TTP increases as the CFU decreases) (Pheiffer *et al.*, 2008). The relationship between cavitation as observed radiographically, TTP as determined by liquid culture and bacterial load has been investigated (Perrin *et al.*, 2010). It was observed that patients with cavities on their thoracic computed tomography (CT) scan had significantly shorter TTP results and therefore a higher CFU compared to patients with no cavitation. The presence of cavities could therefore require prolonged treatment; however, this is likely to be because of the association between cavitation and high bacterial load. Predicting treatment outcome using culture widely accepts the evaluation of sputum specimens at 2 months (Wallis *et al.*, 2009). However, a systematic review of this subject by Horne *et al.* found this method to have poor sensitivity; 57% for predicting failure and 24% for predicting relapse (Horne *et al.*, 2010). This indicator is still of clinical use, as a positive culture will trigger a follow-up culture at 3 months and it could also provide an early indication of a poor treatment outcome.

It has been shown that a subpopulation of bacterial cells exists *in vitro* which can only be cultured by adding resuscitation-promoting factors (Rpfs), which are mycobacterial proteins that are involved in stimulating growth among non-replicating cells *in vitro* (Mukamolova *et al.*, 2002; Shleeva *et al.*, 2002). As a result, it may be important to add these proteins to the culture to increase the accuracy in measuring the patient's response to chemotherapy, especially as this subpopulation is thought to increase relative to the replicating *M. tuberculosis* cells (Mukamolova *et al.*, 2010).

10.4 Molecular Tools

Methods other than traditional microbiological techniques can be used to monitor bacterial load in clinically useful timescales, which can then predict clinical outcome. These methods described include molecular tests which can use DNA or RNA species. These tests could overcome the low sensitivity and specificity of microscopy and the time-consuming culture methods. The use of PCR in monitoring patients undergoing treatment has been investigated (Kennedy *et al.*, 1994; Levée *et al.*, 1994). Thomsen *et al.* investigated the optical density ratio of PCR for *M. tuberculosis* to an internal inhibition control for 22 patients, compared this to baseline levels which had been previously established and found that the ratio correlated with the extent of the disease (Thomsen *et al.*, 1999). For instance, patients with extensive disease did not reach baseline until at least 1 year after treatment initiation. So, PCR could be used in this setting combined with smear and culture results to indicate suboptimal treatment, non-compliance, resistant *M. tuberculosis* and reduced drug absorption, and could then predict patients who are at risk of relapse. The use of PCR in a semi-quantitative manner as described appears to have more promise compared to using it qualitatively (Chierakul *et al.*, 2001). A negative result from a nucleic acid amplification test could be false, as there may be inhibition of amplification or the limit of detection is too high. These false positives can be controlled for by confirmation by smear microscopy result. The PCR result can continue to remain positive even after patients become culture negative (Yuen *et al.*, 1993). This could be due

to the shedding of dead or non-replicating bacilli from the site of infection, and also DNA which is resistant to degradation. Large-scale studies of the usefulness of PCR in a diagnostic setting have shown it to be less sensitive than culture (Clarridge *et al.*, 1993). The target most often used in PCR is the insertion sequence (IS) element *6110* (Eisenach *et al.*, 1991; Greco *et al.*, 2009). However, careful primer selection is required to increase the specificity of using this target (Kent *et al.*, 1995; Mulcahy *et al.*, 1996). Also, there are strains of *M. tuberculosis* which lack IS*6110* (Das *et al.*, 1995), so it could be useful when combined with another target such as hsp65, *rpoB* or the *M. tuberculosis* complex specific protein MBP-64 (Dinnes *et al.*, 2007). Using a real-time system for PCR product detection removes the need for gel electrophoresis, which makes the PCR process simpler, less cumbersome and there is less risk of cross-contamination. Real-time PCR can use specific fluorescently labelled probes or molecular beacons, which also make the assay more specific.

A new real-time PCR-based system, the Cepheid Xpert MTB/RIF assay, has achieved high sensitivity and specificity in clinical settings (Boehme *et al.*, 2010; Rachow *et al.*, 2011). Although a qualitative test, it has potential to relate Ct (crossing threshold) value generated by target amplification to bacterial load (Rachow *et al.*, 2011). Results are determined by their Ct value, so a low Ct value would relate to a sample with a high concentration of *M. tuberculosis* complex. Rachow *et al.* reported good correlation among the Xpert MTB/RIF assay result, TTP determined by liquid culture and grade of smear positivity. The limit of sensitivity of the Xpert system is 131 CFU/ml (Marlowe *et al.*, 2011).

Messenger RNA (mRNA) methods could overcome the false positivity by only detecting live bacilli compared to dead and live bacilli estimated by DNA methods. Most mRNA species have a short half-life, so they are unstable (Hu and Coates, 1999). Reverse transcriptase PCR targeting the *M. tuberculosis* antigen 85B has been shown to disappear from sputum from patients who are responding to treatment, as indicated by a reduction in viable colony counts (Desjardin *et al.*, 1999). In another study, the levels of antigen 85 in sputum samples were able to predict which patients were 'persisters' (Wallis *et al.*, 1998). Quantitative reverse transcriptase real-time PCR has investigated isocitrate lyase (*icl*) mRNA and found it correlates with *M. tuberculosis* viability as detected by culturing methods (Li *et al.*, 2010). Following 1 month of a standard 4-drug regimen, *icl* mRNA correlated with both liquid and solid culture; however, after 2 months of therapy, it correlated more closely with liquid culture. The use of RNA species is discussed further in Chapter 12.

10.5 Immunological Measures

It is unclear how well the immunological status of a patient correlates with bacterial load. Several immunological assays have attempted to characterize patient improvement during and after treatment. The measuring of cell-mediated immunity has used assays to determine interleukin (IL)-10 and IL-12 levels (Sai Priya *et al.*, 2009). Millington *et al.* found a decline in T-cells secreting interferon-gamma (IFN-γ) and an increase in T-cells secreting IL-2 in relation to antigen load (Millington *et al.*, 2007). Methods have used *ex vivo* enzyme-linked immunospot assay (ELISpot) to quantify the secretion of IFN-γ from Th1-type T-cells (Ewer *et al.*, 2006). It may be possible to estimate bacterial load using ELISpot to quantify the *M. tuberculosis*-specific T-cells (Lalvani, 2004). However, studies have shown conflicting results and have shown that individuals vary in the production of *M. tuberculosis*-specific T-cells in response to bacterial burden (Tibayrenc, 2007). Current immunological assays measuring T-cell response could measure bacterial load in a patient during treatment, although this has also been found to vary over time, but could not be used to measure bacterial load between patients. It is clear that for an immunological test to prove useful in determining mycobacterial load, it will need to include multiple immunological markers. It has been shown that patients who have completed treatment successfully could

still have a strong early secretory antigenic target 6 (ESAT-6) response for up to several years (Wu-Hsieh *et al.*, 2001). ESAT-6, in conjunction with culture filtrate protein 10 (CFP-10), is an *M. tuberculosis* secreted protein which is synthesized and used in IFN-γ release assays such as T-SPOT®.TB and the QuantiFERON®-TB Gold to measure immune response in patients.

10.6 Conclusion

The principal measure of treatment outcome in patients is conversion of positive sputum culture to negative after 2 months. Clinical decisions can be made with respect to the results from culture-based methods. However, these methods are lengthy and require long incubation times. New methods can be used to determine treatment outcome; however, currently, culture remains the standard method. The monitoring of bacterial load is important in anti-tubercular therapy due to lengthy treatment regimens and thus the risk of relapse.

References

Al-Moamary, M.S., Black, W., Bessuille, E., Elwood, R.K. and Vedal, S. (1999) The significance of the persistent presence of acid-fast bacilli in sputum smears in pulmonary tuberculosis. *Chest* 116, 726–731.

Albert, H., Manabe, Y., Lukyamuzi, G., Ademun, P., Mukkada, S., Nyesiga, B., *et al.* (2010) Performance of three LED-based fluorescence microscopy systems for detection of tuberculosis in Uganda. *PLoS ONE* 5, e15206.

American Thoracic Society (2000) Diagnostic Standards and Classification of Tuberculosis in Adults and Children. This official statement of the American Thoracic Society and the Centers for Disease Control and Prevention was adopted by the ATS Board of Directors, July 1999. This statement was endorsed by the Council of the Infectious Disease Society of America, September 1999. *American Journal of Respiratory and Critical Care Medicine* 161, 1376–1395.

Blumberg, H.M., Burman, W.J., Chaisson, R.E., Daley, C.L., Etkind, S.C., Friedman, L.N., *et al.* (2003) American Thoracic Society/Centers for

Disease Control and Prevention/Infectious Diseases Society of America: treatment of tuberculosis. *American Journal of Respiratory and Critical Care Medicine* 167, 603–662.

Boehme, C.C., Nabeta, P., Hillemann, D., Nicol, M.P., Shenai, S., Krapp, F., et al. (2010) Rapid molecular detection of tuberculosis and rifampin resistance. *New England Journal of Medicine* 363, 1005–1015.

Brindle, R., Odhiambo, J. and Mitchison, D. (2001) Serial counts of *Mycobacterium tuberculosis* in sputum as surrogate markers of the sterilising activity of rifampicin and pyrazinamide in treating pulmonary tuberculosis. *BMC Pulmonary Medicine* 1, 2–9.

Chierakul, N., Chaiprasert, A., Tingtoy, N., Arjratanakul, W. and Pattanakitsakul, S.-N. (2001) Can serial qualitative polymerase chain reaction monitoring predict outcome of pulmonary tuberculosis treatment? *Respirology* 6, 305–309.

Clarridge, J.E. 3rd, Shawar, R.M., Shinnick, T.M. and Plikaytis, B.B. (1993) Large-scale use of polymerase chain reaction for detection of *Mycobacterium tuberculosis* in a routine mycobacteriology laboratory. *Journal of Clinical Microbiology* 31, 2049–2056.

Das, S., Paramasivan, C.N., Lowrie, D.B., Prabhakar, R. and Narayanan, P.R. (1995) IS6110 restriction fragment length polymorphism typing of clinical isolates of *Mycobacterium tuberculosis* from patients with pulmonary tuberculosis in Madras, South India. *Tubercle and Lung Disease* 76, 550–554.

Della Latta, P. (2004) Mycobacteriology and antimicrobial susceptibility testing. In: Isenberg, H.D. (ed.) *Clinical Microbiology Procedures Handbook*, Vol 2. ASM Press, Washington DC, pp. 7111–7883.

Desjardin, L.E., Perkins, M.D., Wolski, K., Haun, S., Teixeira, L., Chen, Y., et al. (1999) Measurement of sputum *Mycobacterium tuberculosis* messenger RNA as a surrogate for response to chemotherapy. *American Journal of Respiratory and Critical Care Medicine* 160, 203–210.

Dinnes, J., Deeks, J., Kunst, H., Gibson, A., Cummins, E., Waugh, N., et al. (2007) A systematic review of rapid diagnostic tests for the detection of tuberculosis infection. *Health Technology Assessment* 11, 1–196.

Dye, C., Watt, C.J., Bleed, D.M., Hosseini, S.M. and Raviglione, M.C. (2005) Evolution of tuberculosis control and prospects for reducing tuberculosis incidence, prevalence, and deaths globally. *JAMA: The Journal of the American Medical Association* 293, 2767–2775.

Eisenach, K.D., Sifford, M.D., Cave, M.D., Bates,

J.H. and Crawford, J.T. (1991) Detection of *Mycobacterium tuberculosis* in sputum samples using a polymerase chain reaction. *American Reviews of Respiratory Disease* 144, 1160–1163.

Epstein, M.D., Schluger, N.W., Davidow, A.L., Bonk, S., Rom, W.N. and Hanna, B. (1998) Time to detection of *Mycobacterium tuberculosis* in sputum culture correlates with outcome in patients receiving treatment for pulmonary tuberculosis. *Chest* 113, 379–386.

Ewer, K., Millington, K.A., Deeks, J.J., Alvarez, L., Bryant, G. and Lalvani, A. (2006) Dynamic antigen-specific T-cell responses after point-source exposure to *Mycobacterium tuberculosis*. *American Journal of Respiratory and Critical Care Medicine* 174, 831–839.

Fitzwater, S.P., Caviedes, L., Gilman, R.H., Coronel, J., Lachira, D., Salazar, C., et al. (2010) Prolonged infectiousness of tuberculosis patients in a directly observed therapy short-course program with standardized therapy. *Clinical Infectious Diseases* 51, 371–378.

Getahun, H., Harrington, M., O'Brien, R. and Nunn, P. (2007) Diagnosis of smear-negative pulmonary tuberculosis in people with HIV infection or AIDS in resource-constrained settings: informing urgent policy changes. *The Lancet* 369, 2042–2049.

Gillespie, S.H., Gosling, R.D. and Charalambous, B.M. (2002) A reiterative method for calculating the early bactericidal activity of antituberculosis drugs. *American Journal of Respiratory and Critical Care Medicine* 166, 31–35.

Grandjean, L., Martin, L., Gilman, R.H., Valencia, T., Herrera, B., Quino, W., et al. (2008) Tuberculosis diagnosis and multidrug resistance testing by direct sputum culture in selective broth without decontamination or centrifugation. *Journal of Clinical Microbiology* 46, 2339–2344.

Greco, S., Rulli, M., Girardi, E., Piersimoni, C. and Saltini, C. (2009) Diagnostic accuracy of in-house PCR for pulmonary tuberculosis in smear-positive patients: meta-analysis and metaregression. *Journal of Clinical Microbiology* 47, 569–576.

Horne, D.J., Royce, S.E., Gooze, L., Narita, M., Hopewell, P.C., Nahid, P., et al. (2010) Sputum monitoring during tuberculosis treatment for predicting outcome: systematic review and meta-analysis. *The Lancet Infectious Diseases* 10, 387–394.

Hu, Y. and Coates, A.R.M. (1999) Transcription of the stationary-phase-associated hspX gene of *Mycobacterium tuberculosis* is inversely related to synthesis of the 16-kilodalton protein. *Journal of Bacteriology* 181, 1380–1387.

Jindani, A., Aber, V.R., Edwards, E.A. and Mitchison, D.A. (1980) The early bactericidal activity of drugs in patients with pulmonary tuberculosis. *American Review of Respiratory Disease* 121, 939–949.

Joloba, M.L., Johnson, J.L., Namale, A., Morrissey, A., Assegghai, A.E., Rusch-Gerdes, S., et al. (2001) Quantitative bacillary response to treatment in *Mycobacterium tuberculosis* infected and *M. africanum* infected adults with pulmonary tuberculosis. *International Journal of Tuberculosis and Lung Disease* 5, 579–582.

Kennedy, N., Gillespie, S.H., Saruni, A.O.S., Kisyombe, G., McNerney, R., Ngowi, F.I., et al. (1994) Polymerase chain reaction for assessing treatment response in patients with pulmonary tuberculosis. *Journal of Infectious Diseases* 170, 713–716.

Kent, L., McHugh, T.D., Billington, O., Dale, J.W. and Gillespie, S.H. (1995) Demonstration of homology between IS*6110* of *Mycobacterium tuberculosis* and DNAs of other *Mycobacterium* spp. [published erratum appears in *Journal of Clinical Microbiology* 1995 Nov 33(11), 3082]. *Journal of Clinical Microbiology* 33, 2290–2293.

Kubica, G.P., Dye, W.E., Cohn, M.L. and Middlebrook, G. (1963) Sputum digestion and decontamination with N-acetyl-l-cysteine-sodium hydroxide for culture of mycobacteria. *The American Review of Respiratory Disease* 87, 775–779.

Lalvani, A. (2004) Counting antigen-specific T cells: a new approach for monitoring response to tuberculosis treatment? *Clinical Infectious Diseases* 38, 757–759.

Levée, G., Glaziou, P., Gicquel, B. and Chanteau, S. (1994) Follow-up of tuberculosis patients undergoing standard anti-tuberculosis chemotherapy by using a polymerase chain reaction. *Research in Microbiology* 145, 5–8.

Li, L., Mahan, C.S., Palaci, M., Horter, L., Loeffelholz, L., Johnson, J.L., et al. (2010) Sputum *Mycobacterium tuberculosis* mRNA as a marker of bacteriologic clearance in response to antituberculosis therapy. *Journal of Clinical Microbiology* 48, 46–51.

Marlowe, E.M., Novak Weekley, S.M., Cumpio, J., Sharp, S.E., Momeny, M.A., Babst, A., et al. (2011) Evaluation of the Cepheid Xpert MTB/RIF assay for the direct detection of *Mycobacterium tuberculosis* complex from respiratory specimens. *Journal of Clinical Microbiology* 49, 1621–1623.

Mase, S.R., Ramsay, A., Ng, V., Henry, M., Hopewell, P.C., Cunningham, J., Urbanczik, R., et al. (2007) Yield of serial sputum specimen examinations in the diagnosis of pulmonary tuberculosis: a systematic review [Review Article]. *The International Journal of Tuberculosis and Lung Disease* 11, 485–495.

Millington, K.A., Innes, J.A., Hackforth, S., Hinks, T.S., Deeks, J.J., Dosanjh, D.P., et al. (2007) Dynamic relationship between IFN-gamma and IL-2 profile of *Mycobacterium tuberculosis*-specific T cells and antigen load. *Journal of Immunology* 178, 5217–5126.

Mitchison, D.A. (1993) Assessment of new sterilizing drugs for treating pulmonary tuberculosis by culture at 2 months. *American Review of Respiratory Disease* 147, 1062–1063.

Mitchison, D.A. (2006) Clinical development of antituberculosis drugs. *Journal of Antimicrobial Chemotherapy* 58, 494–495.

Mitchison, D.A., Allen, B.W., Carrol, L., Dickinson, J.M. and Aber, V.R. (1972) A selective oleic acid albumin agar medium for tubercle bacilli. *Journal of Medical Microbiology* 5, 165–175.

Mukamolova, G.V., Turapov, O.A., Young, D.I., Kaprelyants, A.S., Kell, D.B. and Young, M. (2002) A family of autocrine growth factors in *Mycobacterium tuberculosis*. *Molecular Microbiology* 46, 623–635.

Mukamolova, G.V., Turapov, O., Malkin, J., Woltmann, G. and Barer, M.R. (2010) Resuscitation-promoting factors reveal an occult population of tubercle bacilli in sputum. *American Journal of Respiratory and Critical Care Medicine* 181, 174–180.

Mulcahy, G.M., Kaminski, Z.C., Albanese, E.A., Sood, R. and Pierce, M. (1996) IS6110-based PCR methods for detection of *Mycobacterium tuberculosis*. *Journal of Clinical Microbiology* 34, 1348–1349.

O'Sullivan, D.M., Sander, C., Shorten, R.J., Gillespie, S.H., Hill, A.V.S., McHugh, T.D., et al. (2007) Evaluation of liquid culture for quantitation of *Mycobacterium tuberculosis* in murine models. *Vaccine* 25, 8203–8205.

Perrin, F.M., Woodward, N., Phillips, P.P., McHugh, T.D., Nunn, A.J., Lipman, M.C., et al. (2010) Radiological cavitation, sputum mycobacterial load and treatment response in pulmonary tuberculosis. *International Journal of Tuberculosis and Lung Disease* 14, 1596–1602.

Pheiffer, C., Carroll, N.M., Beyers, N., Donald, P., Duncan, K., Uys, P., et al. (2008) Time to detection of *Mycobacterium tuberculosis* in BACTEC systems as a viable alternative to colony counting. *International Journal of Tuberculosis and Lung Disease* 12, 792–798.

Rachow, A., Zumla, A., Heinrich, N., Rojas-Ponce, G., Mtafya, B., Reither, K., et al. (2011) Rapid and accurate detection of *Mycobacterium tuberculosis* in sputum samples by Cepheid

Xpert MTB/RIF assay – a clinical validation study. *PLoS ONE* 6, e20458.

Rouillon, A., Perdrizet, S. and Parrot, R. (1976) Transmission of tubercle bacilli: the effects of chemotherapy. *Tubercle* 57, 275–299.

Sai Priya, V.H., Anuradha, B., Latha Gaddam, S., Hasnain, S.E., Murthy, K.J. and Valluri, V.L. (2009) In vitro levels of interleukin 10 (IL-10) and IL-12 in response to a recombinant 32-kilodalton antigen of *Mycobacterium bovis* BCG after treatment for tuberculosis. *Clinical Vaccine Immunology* 16, 111–115.

Schluger, N.W. and Rom, W.N. (1994) Current approaches to the diagnosis of active pulmonary tuberculosis. *American Journal of Respiratory and Critical Care Medicine* 149, 264–267.

Shleeva, M.O., Bagramyan, K., Telkov, M.V., Mukamolova, G.V., Young, M., Kell, D.B., *et al.* (2002) Formation and resuscitation of 'non-culturable' cells of *Rhodococcus rhodochrous* and *Mycobacterium tuberculosis* in prolonged stationary phase. *Microbiology* 148, 1581–1591.

Somoskovi, A., Kodmon, C., Lantos, A., Bartfai, Z., Tamasi, L., Fuzy, J., *et al.* (2000) Comparison of recoveries of *Mycobacterium tuberculosis* using the automated BACTEC MGIT 960 system, the BACTEC 460 TB system, and Lowenstein–Jensen medium. *Journal of Clinical Microbiology* 38, 2395–2397.

Steingart, K.R., Henry, M., Ng, V., Hopewell, P.C., Ramsay, A., Cunningham, J., *et al.* (2006a) Fluorescence versus conventional sputum smear microscopy for tuberculosis: a systematic review. *The Lancet Infectious Diseases* 6, 570–581.

Steingart, K.R., Ng, V., Henry, M., Hopewell, P.C., Ramsay, A., Cunningham, J., *et al.* (2006b) Sputum processing methods to improve the sensitivity of smear microscopy for tuberculosis: a systematic review. *The Lancet Infectious Diseases* 6, 664–674.

Telzak, E.E., Fazal, B.A., Pollard, C.L., Turett, G.S., Justman, J.E. and Blum, S. (1997) Factors influencing time to sputum conversion among patients with smear-positive pulmonary tuberculosis. *Clinical Infectious Diseases* 25, 666–670.

Thomsen, V.O., Kok-Jensen, A., Buser, M., Philippi-Schulz, S. and Burkardt, H.J. (1999) Monitoring treatment of patients with pulmonary tuberculosis: can PCR be applied? *Journal of Clinical Microbiology* 37, 3601–3607.

Tibayrenc, M. (2007) *Encyclopedia of Infectious Diseases: Modern Methologies.* Wiley and Sons, Inc, Hoboken, New Jersey.

Wallis, R.S., Perkins, M., Phillips, M., Joloba, M., Demchuk, B., Namale, A., *et al.* (1998) Induction of the antigen 85 complex of *Mycobacterium tuberculosis* in sputum: a determinant of outcome in pulmonary tuberculosis treatment. *Journal of Infectious Diseases* 178, 1115–1121.

Wallis, R.S., Doherty, T.M., Onyebujoh, P., Vahedi, M., Laang, H., Olesen, O., *et al.* (2009) Biomarkers for tuberculosis disease activity, cure, and relapse. *The Lancet Infectious Diseases* 9, 162–172.

Woods, G.L. and Witebsky, F.G. (1995) Mycobacterial testing in clinical laboratories that participate in the College of American Pathologists' Mycobacteriology E survey: results of a 1993 questionnaire. *Journal of Clinical Microbiology* 33, 407–412.

World Health Organization [WHO] (2009) *Treatment of Tuberculosis: Guidelines,* 4th edn. World Health Organization, Geneva, Switzerland.

WHO (2010) Monitor TB Case Detection and Treatment. *Management of Tuberculosis: Training for Health Facility Staff,* 2nd edn. World Health Organization, Geneva, Switzerland.

Wu-Hsieh, B.A., Chen, C.-K., Chang, J.-H., Lai, S.-Y., Wu, C.H.H., Cheng, W.-C., *et al.* (2001) Long-lived immune response to early secretory antigenic target 6 in individuals who had recovered from tuberculosis. *Clinical Infectious Diseases* 33, 1336–1340.

Yuen, K.Y., Chan, K.S., Chan, C.M., Ho, B.S., Dai, L.K., Chau, P.Y., *et al.* (1993) Use of PCR in routine diagnosis of treated and untreated pulmonary tuberculosis. *Journal of Clinical Pathology* 46, 318–322.

11 Modelling Responses to Tuberculosis Treatment

G.R. Davies

Institute of Translational Medicine, University of Liverpool, UK

11.1 Introduction

Renewed interest in drug development for improved treatment of tuberculosis has recently led to a re-evaluation of existing measures of treatment response. While it is widely accepted that the definitive outcome for tuberculosis trials is the absence of bacteriological relapse up to 2 years after the cessation of treatment, a key debate in the field centres on the extent to which intermediate surrogates can capture treatment effects on this reference end point and which statistical representation offers optimal power for their use in clinical trials. This chapter gives an overview of the challenges this problem poses for the development of new drugs, summarizes the state of current efforts to overcome them and gives some insight into future developments.

11.2 Conceptualizing Treatment Response

Response to treatment for tuberculosis can be conceptualized as a dependent chain of possible composite clinical and laboratory events (Lienhardt and Davies, 2010) (Fig. 11.1). The most appropriate end points for quantifying the success or failure of a particular regimen can therefore depend on its overall potency,

and this hierarchy of end points relates directly to the historical development of tuberculosis treatment (Fox *et al.*, 1999).

The earliest trials of monotherapy with streptomycin (SM), para-amino-salicylic acid (PAS) and isoniazid (INH) provided dramatic evidence that such agents could prevent early death from the disease (MRC, 1948, 1952). Typically, the case fatality rate in the comparator arm of these studies was 30% during the first few months of the trial. These desperate circumstances provided investigators with an unequivocal and statistically powerful end point on which to establish the efficacy of such drugs even prior to completion of treatment by the majority of participants in the trial. The same clinical situation has recently returned with the advent of extensively drug-resistant tuberculosis (XDR-TB), which may carry an even higher case-fatality rate (Gandhi *et al.*, 2010).

Even when such unambiguous results could be obtained quickly, however, the effects of treatment were noticed to be time dependent. Though SM, for instance, provided durable benefits, after 5 years of follow-up these were marginal by comparison with the early results in these trials (Fox *et al.*, 1954). Detailed microbiological study of the evolution of *Mycobacterium tuberculosis* strains during these trials revealed the rapid emergence of resistance in a significant proportion

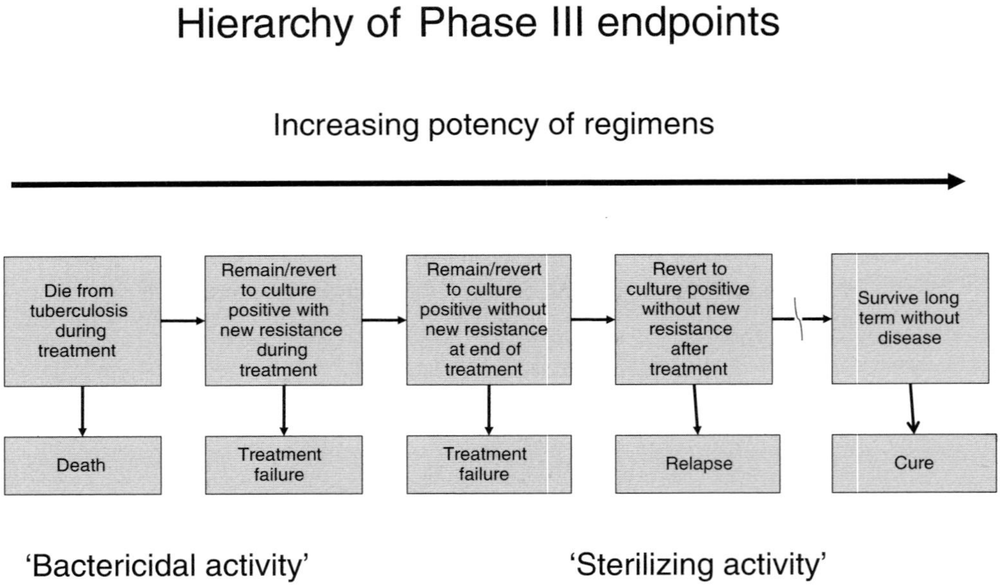

Hierarchy of Phase III endpoints

Increasing potency of regimens

Fig. 11.1. Chain of outcomes in Phase III trials of anti-tuberculosis treatment.

of patients, with subsequent failure of therapy (Mitchison, 1950). It was soon widely acknowledged that monotherapy could not be relied on to achieve a permanent cure and interest began to focus on the capacity of multiple drugs to prevent the emergence of resistance during therapy (MRC, 1950, 1953). While drug combinations with even modest potency could achieve this, they still required prolonged therapy of up to 24 months to ensure stable cure (MRC, 1973).

Once more potent agents became available, offering the possibility of shortening the duration of therapy, a new problem was identified. Though drugs such as rifampicin (RIF) and pyrazinamide (PZA) halved the duration of treatment at a stroke, if the duration of the regimen was too short, apparent cure was soon followed by an unacceptably high rate of relapse (EAMRC, 1974, 1981). Characteristically, however, the organisms responsible were not drug resistant, giving rise to the concept of subpopulations of organisms capable of persisting during therapy in the absence of genotypic resistance (Mitchison, 1979).

Hence, the distinct ways in which tuberculosis treatment can fail offer some empirical insight into the pharmacodynamic mechanisms underlying successful therapy. In particular, a combination of drugs must be collectively potent enough to result in a significant net decrease in bacillary load in order to prevent death of the host and reduce the probability that resistance mutation events will occur. Both these goals are dependent to some extent on the speed with which particular drugs can achieve this. Historically, this property of a regimen has often been referred to as 'bactericidal activity' (Mitchison, 1992). It is also clear, however, that bactericidal activity alone may not suffice for a stable cure. The ability of a combination regimen to reduce bacillary numbers in itself may effectively prevent the emergence of resistance, but if it cannot ultimately eliminate them (or at least reduce them below some threshold at which the host's immune system can complete the task) then relapse will occur. This capability has typically been referred to as 'sterilizing activity' and understanding and quantifying this phase of the pharmacodynamics of anti-tuberculosis drugs has attracted much research interest in recent years (Davies, 2010). From a practical perspective, it must currently be equated with relapse rates post-treatment and the extent to which earlier measures reflect this remains uncertain. Whether bactericidal and sterilizing activities should be conceived of as simply ends of a spectrum created by increasing drug potency or as qualitatively distinct, arising from the nature of the targets of the different drug classes, has also remained an open question.

11.3 The Problem of Surrogate End Points

Early prediction of efficacy or toxicity in Phase I/II trials is a generic problem in most areas of clinical trial activity. The challenge is to select surrogate end points correctly from among candidate biomarkers which can reliably capture changes in a given clinical or reference end point appropriate for Phase III trials (Burzykowski *et al.*, 2005). Typically, such reference end points occur infrequently enough that a very large sample size would be required to achieve adequately powerful comparisons between treatments, and they may require prolonged follow-up to obtain. Hence, they are usually not appropriate for the purposes of proof-of-concept, dose finding and defining optimum combinations of drugs in early development. A practically useful surrogate end point can be characterized by the following (De Gruttola *et al.*, 2001):

- a biologically plausible relationship with the reference end point, preferably mechanism based
- useful statistical properties
- successful evaluation against the reference end point.

Recently, a general statistical framework has been proposed for understanding and evaluating the relationship between proposed surrogate and reference end points (Buyse *et al.*, 2000). In particular, two key concepts have been clarified by these advances. Firstly,

surrogacy is clearly a matter of degree, with the dual consequence that evaluation is a cumulative process across many trials and ultimately unlikely to provide theoretically 'perfect' surrogate end points capable of completely substituting for any reference end point (Prentice, 1989). Secondly, a critical distinction has to be made between surrogacy at the level of individual participants and that of trial cohorts. While the former may provide a useful clinical predictor of response, it is usually the latter which is of interest in drug development. These aspects of a surrogate end point are not always closely linked in practice and are, in fact, logically and statistically independent (Baker and Kramer, 2003), which again suggests that evaluation across many trials should be preferred to large cohorts of individuals within a single trial. Another important consideration is that even biomarkers which initially show some empirical statistical association will be unlikely to be taken up if they lack a plausible causal explanation for the relationship. Increasingly, this must be framed in terms of specific biological mechanisms of action and pharmacodynamic considerations for the class of drugs concerned.

11.3.1 Bacteriological versus non-bacteriological biomarkers

Bacteriological data have always formed part of the definition of composite 'clinical' end points since the earliest trials. Since the pharmacodynamic target of current anti-tuberculosis drugs is to kill viable *M. tuberculosis* organisms, measures of bacillary elimination based on laboratory culture would be expected *a priori* to have some usefulness as surrogate end points. As the potency of regimens has improved, these have received more emphasis and priority over other aspects of response. In general, because development of anti-tuberculosis drugs has focused on pulmonary disease, where repeated clinical samples are readily accessible, data on this approach come almost exclusively from studies of sputum.

That bacteriological end points at an

early stage of treatment could be used to
predict the ultimate outcome was proposed
initially on the basis of the aggregated data
from the extensive series of short-course
chemotherapy trials conducted by the British
Medical Research Council (Aber and Nunn,
1978; Mitchison, 1996). Data from these trials
(12 trials comprising 6974 patients in 49
treatment arms) were recently retrieved and
re-analysed at the trial level and this analysis
confirmed that, particularly for RIF-based
regimens, there was a moderately strong
relation between 2- and 3-month culture
results and poor treatment outcome (R^2 was
0.67 and 0.46, respectively) (Phillips and
Fielding, 2007, 2008). However, the relationship appeared less strong over all the regimens included in the analysis and there must
therefore remain some caution over the
generalizability of this observation to future
combination regimens containing drugs with
new mechanisms of action.

Given the imperfections of historical
bacteriological data, several other techniques
and biomarkers have been developed and
proposed as a means of supplementing or
supplanting them for use as surrogate end
points. Those most advanced have been
reviewed recently (Perrin *et al.*, 2007; Wallis *et
al.*, 2009) and can be considered broadly as
organism or host based. Organism-based
biomarkers include new methods of
automated broth-based culture and nucleic
acid-based techniques (discussed further
below), while relevant host-based biomarkers
include serial peripheral blood IFN-γ release
assays and transcriptomic approaches. To
date, very few of these alternative biomarkers
have undergone any large-scale evaluation
against the current standard bacteriological
approach. Whether the majority of these
novel techniques will find any secure place as
surrogate end points in the development
process remains to be seen. While it seems
currently unlikely that any single one will
replace sputum bacteriology in the near
future, it may be that some could be useful
adjuncts as covariates to such data, perhaps
providing better insight into additional
bacillary or host determinants of response
that influence sterilizing activity.

11.3.2 Empirical versus model-based approaches

Traditionally, bacteriological response has
been represented as culture positivity at fixed
time-points as treatment progresses (Fox *et
al.*, 1999). The structure of short-course chemotherapy regimens with an initial intensive and
simplified continuation phase tended to focus
the attention of trialists and, later, tuberculosis
programme managers on results at 2 and
subsequently 5 and 6 months. The choice of
these occasions was based arbitrarily on con-
venience and clinical considerations. Though
simple to interpret, when expressed as a
simple proportion, this approach is statistically inefficient (Fedorov *et al.*, 2009; Yoo,
2009). An additional problem is that as the
potency of regimens improves and the rate of
culture conversion at 2 months in the comparator arm increases, statistical power to
detect treatment differences diminishes. Such
an empirical approach employs no specific
model of the pharmacodynamics of treatment.
Hence, it is insensitive both quantitatively in
the sense that it will only reliably detect large
treatment effects and qualitatively in that
differences in the pattern of bacillary
elimination due to different classes of drugs
cannot be detected using only a single or very
sparse measurements.

Typically, however, samples for culture
have often been obtained on at least a monthly
basis in Phase III trials and on a weekly basis
throughout the intensive phase in Phase II
trials. The analysis of such repeated measurements has frequently been expressed as a
series of univariate analyses with or without
correction for multiplicity and usually
prioritizing the 2-month result as primary.
This is clearly not faithful to the correlated
nature of these data in time, and in recent
years it has become more common to make
use of more modern survival techniques
(Holtz *et al.*, 2006; Conde *et al.*, 2009). By
representing bacillary elimination as a hazard
of culture conversion over time, this approach
implicitly adopts a non-parametric model of
pharmacodynamics which makes use of all
the available data and hence has greater
power to detect treatment effects. Within a

regression framework, it also becomes simpler to adjust the model for important covariates, and logistic regression models are also increasingly used for this purpose, using the 2-month culture conversion end point alone (Burman *et al.*, 2006).

Within the context of modern drug development, the continued use of these empirical approaches in tuberculosis appears anomalous. In the early stages of clinical development, it is critical to refine and expand information about drug response and this is often achieved more effectively using continuous, time-dependent measures and modelling and simulation methodology (Zhang *et al.*, 2006). This 'learning' approach is to be contrasted with the shift in focus in Phase III to a 'confirming' paradigm under which unambiguous and simple response measures are collected when or after treatment is completed (Sheiner, 1997). A strictly empirical approach to response in Phase II trials is a significant obstacle to implementing the learning paradigm in tuberculosis, making the achievement of the goals of early development difficult or impossible at reasonable sample sizes.

11.4 Early Bactericidal Activity

An alternative method of assessing drug activity in tuberculosis is based on explicitly quantitative bacteriological methods. By standardizing sputum preparation and using solid media highly selective for mycobacteria, a reproducible count of viable colonies in sputum specimens can be obtained and followed over time (Mitchison, 1950; Mitchison *et al.*, 1971). The first study to use this serial sputum colony-counting approach followed patients on individual and pairs of drugs over the first 14 days of therapy (Jindani *et al.*, 1980). Using an analysis of variance approach based on the linear slopes of the decline in colony counts summarized over different time periods for individual patients, clear differences in the potency of the drugs studied could be demonstrated. Such measurements have since become known as 'early bactericidal activity' (EBA) and studies mak-

ing use of it have become the standard design for Phase IIa studies for all new agents (Donald *et al.*, 2003).

EBA studies have provided useful insights into the pharmacology of many classes of drugs. Since they can be conducted with as few as 10–20 patients per arm, they are well suited to initial proof-of-concept and dose-finding studies. For INH, which exhibits the highest EBA (approximately –0.5 $\log_{10}$ colony-forming units (CFU)/ml/day), a complete dose–response curve can be obtained which clearly identifies the minimum and maximum effective doses, and activity can be related to pharmacokinetic exposure and acetylator status (Donald *et al.*, 1997, 2004). For rifamycins, EBA studies have drawn attention to incomplete dose-finding data (Diacon *et al.*, 2007) and differences in activity across members of the class according to differences in the free drug concentration (Sirgel *et al.*, 2005). The technique has also been used to compare the relative potencies of antimycobacterial fluoroquinolones and identify equivalent dose regimens (Johnson *et al.*, 2006). However, the activity of INH is clearly time dependent, waning after only 2–5 days of treatment, while some classes of drugs such as PZA, aminoglycosides and nitroimidazopyrans have delayed or very weak EBA (Jindani *et al.*, 1980; Donald *et al.*, 2001, 2002; Diacon *et al.*, 2010), suggesting that EBA may represent imperfectly the capability of drugs to achieve long-term cure. Since no ethics committee has agreed to longer than 14 days of monotherapy with anti-tuberculosis drugs, for reasons of patient safety and the possible emergence of resistance, this is a major limitation of the approach.

The EBA methodology is highly dependent on the variance of the measurements on which it is based. Since this ranges more than twofold over different centres that have attempted such studies (Sirgel *et al.*, 2000), the sample sizes typically proposed can sometimes be unduly optimistic. Both laboratory experience with the technique and careful patient selection are important, since efforts to correct for sputum quality have not been successful (Sirgel *et al.*, 2001). Furthermore, variance of the measurements increases with time, which diminishes the efficiency of the technique to detect delayed treatment effects. The traditional statistical approach to analysis of EBA data is based on computation of a summary statistic for each patient based on their measurements in a series of arbitrary time intervals (e.g. days 0–2, 2–7, 7–14, etc.), followed by analysis of the variance of these statistics across treatment groups. This is a simple and effective way to circumvent the problem of correlation between repeated measurements in study subjects (Matthews *et al.*, 1990). However, it embodies strong assumptions of piecewise linearity within the selected time intervals and begs the question of the pharmacodynamic significance of those intervals. A particular problem is that the summary statistics absorb the inter-individual variability in colony counts as well as the intra-individual variability, which compromises significantly their power to detect treatment effects. This is exacerbated when combination regimens are evaluated, because they inevitably incorporate INH, which has the highest variance in its EBA among all drugs studied to date. Since the correlation between early EBA measures (such as EBA_{0-2} $_{0-5}$) and the baseline measurement is fairly high (usually ~0.5–0.7), one way to improve this situation would be use the baseline measurement as a covariate in the analysis in order to account for inter-individual variability in the counts (analysis of covariance, or ANCOVA). Interestingly, many study protocols incorporate 1 or 2 pre-treatment samples, but these measurements are never used in the analysis. A number of linear summary statistics based on the ANCOVA approach have been proposed (Frison and Pocock, 1992, 1997), which could be used to take advantage of this additional data.

11.5 Mixed Models

An alternative approach to representing multiple hierarchical levels of variability in statistical modelling is that of mixed effects modelling (Davidian and Giltinan, 1995). Though relatively novel in medical statistics (Diggle *et al.*, 2002), this idea has been used extensively in the fields of education (Gold-

stein *et al.*, 2002) and pharmacokinetics for many years (Sheiner *et al.*, 1977). The basic principle is that instead of computing summary estimates of the parameters of interest for each individual, the mixed effects approach focuses on obtaining estimates of these parameters for the population as a whole (the 'fixed' effects), while representing the variability of those parameters with a probability distribution whose parameters in turn are to be estimated (the 'random' effects). Thus, estimates of a particular individual's parameters are not obtained directly using this method (but can be obtained indirectly as model predictions) and if, as is usually the case in clinical trials, these individual values are not the primary focus of the analysis, the mixed effects representation of the data is both parsimonious and efficient. The total variance is partitioned in the model between inter and intra-individual components and it is the explicit modelling of inter-individual variability that lends the technique its power when applied to repeated measures data. The methodology can be applied to any type of outcome measure, though in pharmacokinetic–pharmacodynamic analyses it is typically applied in a continuous context. To date, no published examples of applying this approach to EBA data have appeared.

11.5.1 Extended serial sputum colony-counting studies

The phenomenon of delayed or unexpectedly weak EBA, specifically the anomalous case of PZA and recent discrepant results in the development programme of TMC207 (bedaquiline), in the context of other evidence of possibly strong sterilizing activity, has raised concerns about the interpretation of such studies (Rustomjee *et al.*, 2008a; Diacon *et al.*, 2009). Since there is no possibility of extending EBA studies of monotherapy beyond 14 days, one proposal has been to study instead combination regimens over a longer period in an attempt to define more clearly the pattern of response and give better assurance that this corresponds to long-term outcome.

The first such study compared two distinct combination regimens in a cohort of 100 patients in Nairobi, Kenya, over the first month of therapy, sampling their sputum at days 0, 2, 7, 14 and 28 (Brindle *et al.*, 1993). Approximately half were receiving streptomycin-isoniazid-thiacetazone (SHT), a 'standard' regimen, and half streptomycin-isoniazid-rifampicin-pyrazinamide (SHRZ), a 'short-course' regimen. The initial analysis of these data concluded that response to treatment was similar in both groups and did not differ by HIV status (Brindle *et al.*, 2001). A recent review and re-analysis of these data applied instead a mixed effects modelling approach, with different results (Davies *et al.*, 2006a). Firstly, the profile of response was noticed to be unequivocally non-linear, with an early phase of rapid elimination of bacilli lasting up to 7 days succeeded by a later phase where elimination proceeded at less than 20% of the initial rate, continuing until the end of the study period (Fig. 11.2). Secondly, using a biphasic model with two distinct phases of exponential decay, it was

possible to show that, though the two regimens in the study did not differ in terms of the rate of early phase elimination, the SHRZ regimen accelerated late-phase activity significantly. Given the size of the treatment groups and the already established superior efficacy of the SHRZ regimen in prior clinical trials, this result was of great interest. Lastly, though HIV-positive subjects in this study had lower baseline bacillary loads, their status did not affect the rate of bacillary elimination from their sputum. A great deal of the variability in the model was accounted for by random effects in the intercepts rather than the rates of the two phases of decay.

The biphasic nature of elimination in this model raises interesting questions of interpretation. The same profile of response could, in principle, be due to two different scenarios: simultaneous elimination of distinct and heterogeneous subpopulations of organisms present prior to the commencement of therapy or rapid adaptation to drug action and

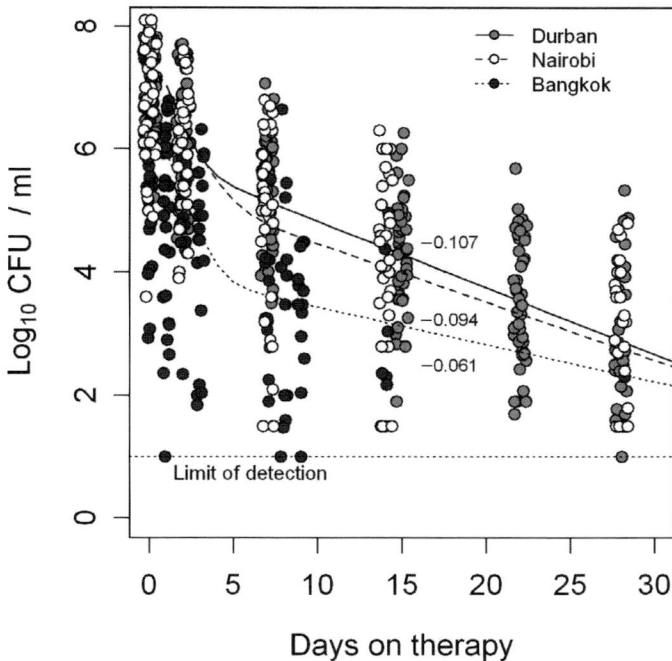

Fig. 11.2. Serial sputum colony-counting data and fitted model predictions from three studies using similar short-course regimens. The figures refer to the estimated rates of late-phase elimination of organisms (log CFU/mL/day).

selection from a single more homogeneous initial population. These two scenarios are not identifiable in this basic model due to the lack of information with which to classify organisms into the two putative subpopulations and hence estimate any rate of transition between them. In addition, extrapolation and simulation of the model predictions suggested that even organisms undergoing slow elimination were not likely to comprise the subpopulation of organisms capable of causing relapse after treatment was stopped.

Given the findings of this analysis, further evaluation of the biphasic model for response to tuberculosis treatment was carried out. Conditional on the estimates of the model parameters estimated in the original study, features of the study design were optimized using an analysis of the Fisher's information matrix of the model and an approximate linearization method for computation of sample size (Davies *et al.*, 2006b). This suggested that greatly improved precision of studies based on such a model could be achieved at sample sizes as low as 40–60/ arm, provided that the total number of sampling points be doubled to 10 and the duration of sampling be increased to include the entire intensive phase of 56 days.

Subsequently, a study employing a similar design was conducted in South Africa (Rustomjee *et al.*, 2008b). This study evaluated substitution of three different fluoroquinolones (ofloxacin, moxifloxacin and gatifloxacin) for ethambutol in the first-line regimen. The design thus comprised four arms of 50 patients each and obtained sputum samples at 0, 2 days and then weekly until day 56. Analysis of the colony-counting data using the biphasic mixed effects model separated the four arms into two groups on the basis of late-phase elimination, with the control and ofloxacin arms distinct from the moxi-/gatifloxacin arms. The estimated parameters for the control regimen (HRZE) were similar to those observed in the previous analysis. In the moxi-/gatifloxacin arms, the elimination rate was approximately 24% faster than the former, a highly statistically significant result compatible with the rank order of activity obtained in an *in vitro* model of stationary phase *M. tuberculosis* (Para-

masivan *et al.*, 2005). Once again, HIV did not affect the rate of elimination materially, but a simple measure of radiological extent of disease was associated with lower activity. The results of this study are in agreement with those obtained under a similarly intensive sampling scheme in another study of substitution of moxifloxacin for ethambutol in Brazil (Conde *et al.*, 2009). This slightly larger study relied on a survival analysis of the rate of culture conversion, which suggested significantly faster conversion in the moxifloxacin arm. Another multicentre study of the same regimens used 2-month culture conversion as its primary end point and concluded that there was no difference between the regimens, despite suggestions of more rapid culture conversion in the moxifloxacin arm at earlier time points (Burman *et al.*, 2006).

A third observational pharmacokinetic–pharmacodynamic study based on a colony-counting design of two balanced blocks of five sampling points each was completed recently in Thailand (Davies *et al.*, 2008). Though baseline bacillary load was lower than in the two African studies, the rate parameters of the model estimated from this data set were similar. Again, HIV status did not appear to influence the rate of bacillary elimination. In this study, INH exposure was related significantly to early-phase elimination in the presence of the other companion drugs, but there was no apparent relationship between RIF or PZA exposure and late-phase elimination.

Given a particular study design, the relative performance of the possible analytical approaches has also been evaluated using trial simulation techniques (Davies, 2009). Assuming that the biphasic model of elimination is a reasonable description of the data, the late phase of the model can be approximated by a linear mixed effects model from day 7 onwards. This approach has been used to simulate large numbers of trial scenarios under the alternative hypothesis of a real treatment effect and the resulting data sets analysed using the different possible statistical methods to compute the power of each approach. The results of this study appear to bear out the limited experience to date. An analysis of covariance approach based on the quantitative information in the colony counts appeared to be uniformly the most powerful method under all scenarios. However, non- and semi-parametric survival methods based on culture conversion also performed quite well and were reasonably robust to interval censoring caused by sparse sampling schemes. Not unexpectedly, restricting the analysis to proportions positive at 2 months alone reduced the expected power of these designs severely, generally doubling the sample size required to detect a given treatment effect size (Fig. 11.3).

Taken together, these early data on colony-counting techniques support its fur- ther evaluation and raise the possibility of efficient, possibly factorial Phase II designs which may be capable of sequential or fully adaptive dose and companion drug opti- mization in humans.

11.5.2 Liquid culture

In the most recent clinical trials, automated liquid culture techniques have increasingly been used alongside more traditional solid media (see Chapter 3). The technique may have a lower limit of detection with respect to bacillary load and may, in addition, enable the resuscitation of organisms in altered growth states that lack the capacity to grow on solid media, particularly later in treatment. Another attractive feature is that, *in vitro* at least, time to positivity (TTP) in the liquid culture system is proportional to the load of organisms inoculated. This inherently quan- titative aspect of liquid culture data raises the possibility of another measure of bacillary load that is not as labour-intensive to obtain as colony counts. Unfortunately, a number of alternative culture systems exist with dif- ferent detection systems and protocols for

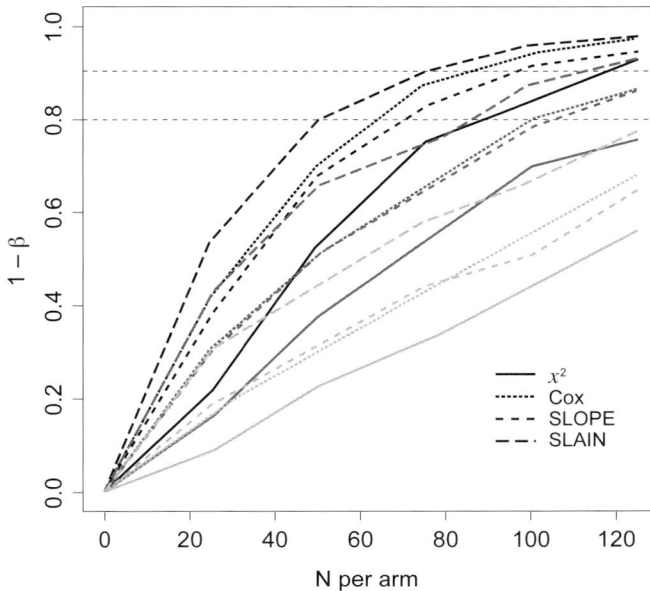

Fig. 11.3. Simulated power curves for four different analytical approaches over three different treatment effect sizes: a χ^2 test of culture conversion at 2 months, Cox proportional hazards modelling, the SLOPE summary statistic based on ANOVA and the SLAIN summary statistic based on ANCOVA. Within each panel colour refers to the effect size used in the simulations: mid-grey = 0.015; light grey = 0.020; black = 0.025. The dotted horizontal lines correspond to 80% and 90% power.

processing of the samples, which can make interpretation of existing data problematic.

When used simply as an alternative to solid media for the purposes of evaluating culture conversion at specific time points, liquid culture tends to result in higher culture positivity rates overall, which persist later in the course of treatment. Paradoxically, this can, in fact, result in a loss of sensitivity of a simple analysis of proportions due to a reduction in the culture conversion rate in the comparator arm, which is a critical determinant of its power. However, the prolonged period over which culture positivity persists in liquid media is generally an advantage for survival approaches, provided that sampling persists long enough to capture a large enough number of culture conversion events.

The only published analyses of liquid culture data have focused mostly on its use for prediction of solid culture results. In a recent example, it was demonstrated that very short baseline TTP was associated with delayed culture conversion at 2 months and with subsequent relapse of disease (Hesseling *et al.*, 2010). The radiological extent of disease was also an important covariate in this analysis. A previous analysis by the same investigators proposed a response ratio based on TTP measurements obtained during the first 2 weeks as an alternative means of predicting poor treatment outcome (Pheiffer *et al.*, 2008). However, in this study, the positive predictive value of this ratio was only 14% and the results appeared to depend on the timing of sampling during treatment.

More extensive data on changes in TTP during treatment are available from recent clinical trials, but much remains unpublished to date. In a recently completed clinical trial of adjuvant vitamin D treatment, extensive liquid culture data were collected over the first 2 months of therapy. Over time, these data appeared to follow a linear decline in TTP and were adequately modelled using a linear mixed effects approach (Martineau *et al.*, 2011).

11.5.3 Molecular markers

Given the potentially altered growth characteristics of bacilli *in vivo*, considerable interest

has centred on the application of molecular methods to try to overcome this limitation, since this technology offers potentially greater scope for improved sensitivity. Extensive studies under *in vitro* conditions have identified a tractable number of genes implicated in responses to hypoxia, nutrient limitation and drug pressure (Butcher, 2004; see Chapter 12). Several of these have also been identified as undergoing upregulation in sputum during treatment in humans (Garton *et al.*, 2008; see Chapter 13). Such genes could conceptually be used either as an alternative quantitative measure of total bacillary load or as a means of monitoring the changing metabolic state of the whole population of organisms over time. Most studies of this approach have addressed the former application. For this purpose, DNA hybridization has not proved to be a useful measure, since it persists long after the destruction of viable organisms. mRNA reflects ongoing transcription better and is believed to continue constitutively at low but measurable levels even in stationary phase bacilli.

Several studies have reported results with mRNA amplification from sputum during treatment. One recent study compared PCR of the DNA IS*6110* element with RT-PCR of mRNA for antigen 85B against culture conversion (Mdivani *et al.*, 2009). The former remained persistently positive late into treatment, suggesting that it would be unlikely to be a useful predictor of treatment failure. Antigen 85B mRNA, however, declined in tandem with culture results, becoming undetectable at a similar rate (see Chapter 12).

Another study evaluated RT-PCR of multiple targets (fbpB, hspX, icl1 and rrnA-P1) in the context of response to different single and combination drug regimens (Li *et al.*, 2010). Expression of hspX and icl1, both relating to proteins well-known to be upregulated in the stationary phase, correlated well with decline in bacillary load, though the contrasting sensitivity of the amplification of the different targets appeared to be responsible for variable calibration against rates of culture conversion. The analysis of all of these studies relied on empirical statistical techniques such as correlation and repeated measures analysis of variance and did not employ a modelling approach. None of these studies clearly expressed the relative variability of the mRNA measurements against culture results and it is difficult to comment on their suitability for use in clinical trials without this information. However, the ability to examine qualitatively different aspects of *M. tuberculosis* physiology simultaneously is an attractive aspect of this approach and could give some insight into differing patterns of pharmacodynamics induced by various classes of drugs.

11.6 Adjuncts to Modelling Responses and Joint Modelling

Several studies have now observed that the performance of quantitative models of treatment response is frequently enhanced by the addition of other important covariates which capture some additional aspect of pharmacodynamics, whether this reflects factors related to the host or the organism. Clearly, correctly identifying and incorporating this information into such models is critical to their success.

Radiological measures of severity of disease at baseline have often been identified as independent predictors of disease outcome since the earliest clinical trials (MRC, 1948). However, precisely which features are important has not been clearly established and various approaches have been developed to give an overall measure of severity. The proportion of lung involvement, especially when expressed as bilateral or unilateral disease, has been a consistent predictor of poor response (Davies *et al.*, 2006a; Rustomjee *et al.*, 2008b). The only qualitative feature with similar predictive power appears to be the presence or absence of cavitation (Burman *et al.*, 2006; Dorman *et al.*, 2009). Both these features are usually correlated with high sputum bacillary load and hence help to explain the variability of this measure.

Where pharmacokinetic information is available, it may be expected that measurements of drug exposure could also explain

some of the inter-individual variability in treatment response. Recent advances in animal and *in vitro* models of tuberculosis therapy have established concentration response relationships successfully and the nature of the relevant pharmacokinetic–pharmacodynamic index using dose fractionation methods (Jayaram *et al.*, 2003, 2004; Gumbo *et al.*, 2004, 2007). So far, in clinical studies this has only been clearly demonstrated for INH, a drug with a strong pharmacokinetic–pharmacodynamic relationship in EBA studies and highly polymorphic pharmacogenetic determinants of metabolism, resulting in a wide range of exposures. To date, this goal has not been reproduced convincingly for any other TB drug, particularly not those with known or putative sterilizing activity (Davies and Nuermberger, 2008). Several possible reasons for this have been advanced: lack of concomitant information about the susceptibility of individual organisms in terms of their minimum inhibitory concentration (MIC), assay and sampling variability in the pharmacokinetic assays, narrow dose range and limited sample size of the relevant studies.

The extent of variability in the characteristics of *M. tuberculosis* in individual patients remains uncertain. Though animal models support the use of area under the curve (AUC)/MIC as a general index of treatment success for many tuberculosis drugs, usually only a limited number of strains are evaluated. There is currently no convincing evidence that the different natural lineages of *M. tuberculosis* have any impact on treatment success (Nahid *et al.*, 2010). In the absence of genotypic high-level resistance, the variance in the *in vitro* distribution of MIC_{90}s for INH and RIF is less than tenfold (Schön *et al.*, 2009), but since no human studies have yet evaluated it extensively as a covariate, no data exist as to its predictive value. Another approach has been to attempt to quantify phenotypic drug tolerance by studying the time-kill properties of patient strains on re-exposure to drug pressure in liquid culture systems. One small study claimed to show that this could be related to rapidity of treatment response (Wallis *et al.*, 1999). Observations that stationary phase bacilli exhibiting phenotypic drug tolerance frequently accumulate droplets of triacylglycerol during changes of intermediary metabolism *in vitro* (Garton *et al.*, 2002) have prompted investigations of whether staining with neutral lipid dyes could be used to discriminate and perhaps quantify different subpopulations of bacilli *in vivo* (Garton *et al.*, 2008). Independent information of this kind could be used to improve selection among the models referred to above, which cannot currently discriminate between the simultaneous and evolutionary models of bacillary heterogeneity.

In addition to the identification of covariates for the models of response, another statistical approach gaining increasing currency is that of the joint modelling of more than one response (Diggle *et al.*, 2008). Conceptually, this involves simultaneous modelling of the joint distribution of two distinct outcome variables, and in practical terms has usually involved combining clinical data expressed as survival times and repeated measurements of some continuous biomarker which is related to survival. Provided that the biomarker does explain an important proportion of the variability in the other outcome, this can lead to more precise inferences. For example, joint modelling of the profiles of culture conversion could be considered alongside some other meaningful measure of host response; for example, T cell ELISpot measurements or measurements of mRNA transcripts for specific bacillary genes.

11.6.1 Mechanistic modelling approaches

There have been attempts by theoretical biologists to construct systems models representing assumptions about how tuberculosis therapy works and drawing indirectly from the results of animal and clinical data (Lipsitch and Levin, 1998). Usually, they have only been capable of a sensitivity analysis approach to their assumptions, particularly regarding such phenomena as post-antibiotic effect and bacillary heterogeneity, and have not incorporated explicit modelling of drug effects.

However, the rapid growth in information about all aspects of the biology of *M. tuberculosis* has resulted recently in the capability to study the total transcriptome and proteome dynamically under different conditions *in vitro*, and even in limited numbers of clinical samples. These advances have enabled the construction of a complete metabolic map of *M. tuberculosis* (http://tbcyc. tbdb.org/MTH37RVV) and the development of related dynamic systems models of these processes (Jamshidi and Palsson, 2007; Fang *et al.*, 2009), which have enabled global identification of critical metabolic subsystems which could be targeted by new drugs. Impressive as this is, the local mechanisms of action of many classes of drugs have already been clearly defined and the critical components of the implicated pathways can sometimes be quantified as biomarkers (Raman *et al.*, 2005, 2009; Wang and Marcotte, 2008). These new techniques could be exploited to provide considerable supplementary information about drug response. How best to incorporate such information into pharmacokinetic–pharmacodynamic models has attracted recent attention under the rubric of 'disease modelling' and overlaps with similar developments in systems biology where the idea of 'multi-scale modelling' has facilitated a flexible approach to incorporating molecular mechanisms into the lowest level of hierarchical representations of biological structures (Young *et al.*, 2008). This kind of approach will certainly help to integrate current scientific knowledge derived from related disciplines and, by making use of a simulation strategy, help to generate and refine new research questions. Relatively simple disease models supported by additional biomarker data may even be capable of being fitted to data from clinical studies.

11.7 Conclusion

Treatment response in tuberculosis is best thought of as a process rather than a single event, different aspects of which are appropriate to different treatment situations and phases of clinical drug development. Among currently proposed biomarkers, only bacterio-logical responses have so far received significant, albeit imperfect, support as surrogate end points. However, the laboratory methods used and the way in which the data are handled are crucial to getting the best performance out of these measures. Statistical modelling approaches based on capturing treatment effects over the entire period of therapy should be preferred over simpler and less efficient end points, especially in the early phases of development, when learning about pharmacokinetics and pharmacodynamics is prioritized over definitive confirmation of efficacy. New biomarkers currently in development are unlikely to replace bacteriological end points, but may have a significant role to play in improving their performance. How this new information can be combined with current approaches remains to be seen, but a number of different novel modelling approaches capable of incorporating it have been developed recently and promise to reduce the uncertainty that currently plagues early phase clinical development of new anti-tuberculosis drugs.

References

Aber, V. and Nunn, A. (1978) Factors affecting relapse following short-course chemotherapy. *Bulletin of the International Union Against Tuberculosis* 53(4), 260–264.

Baker, S.G. and Kramer, B.S. (2003) A perfect correlate does not a surrogate make. *BMC Medical Research Methodology* 3, 16.

Brindle, R.J., Nunn, P.P., Githui, W., Allen, B.W., Gathua, S. and Waiyaki, P. (1993) Quantitative bacillary response to treatment in HIV-associated pulmonary tuberculosis. *American Review of Respiratory Diseases* 147, 958–961.

Brindle, R., Odhiambo, J. and Mitchison, D. (2001) Serial counts of *Mycobacterium tuberculosis* in sputum as surrogate markers of the sterilizing activity of rifampicin and pyrazinamide in treating pulmonary tuberculosis. *BMC Pulmonary Medicine* 1, 2.

Burman, W.J., Goldberg, S., Johnson, J.L., Muzanye, G., Engle, M., Mosher, A.W., *et al.* (2006) Moxifloxacin versus ethambutol in the first 2 months of treatment for pulmonary tuberculosis. *American Journal of Respiratory*

and *Critical Care Medicine* 174(3), 331–338.

Burzykowski, T., Molenberghs, G. and Buyse, M. (2005) *The Evaluation of Surrogate Endpoints.* Springer, New York.

Butcher, P. (2004) Microarrays for *Mycobacterium tuberculosis. Tuberculosis* 84, 131–137.

Buyse, M., Molenberghs, G., Burzykowski, T., Renard, D. and Geys, H. (2000) The validation of surrogate endpoints in meta-analyses of randomized experiments. *Biostatistics (Oxford, England)* 1(1), 49–67.

Conde, M.B., Efron, A., Loredo, C., De Souza, G.R., Graça, N.P., Cezar, M.C., *et al.* (2009) Moxifloxacin versus ethambutol in the initial treatment of tuberculosis: a double-blind, randomised, controlled phase II trial. *The Lancet* 373(9670), 1183–1189.

Davidian, M. and Giltinan, D. (1995) *Nonlinear Models for Repeated Measurement Data.* Chapman and Hall, London.

Davies, G. (2009) Effect of analytical approach, sampling scheme and laboratory method on power of surrogate endpoints in tuberculosis Phase II trials: a simulation study. In: *Gordon Conference on Tuberculosis Drug Development.* Oxford.

Davies, G.R. (2010) Early clinical development of anti-tuberculosis drugs: science, statistics and sterilizing activity. *Tuberculosis (Edinburgh)* 90(3), 171–176.

Davies, G.R. and Nuermberger, E.L. (2008) Pharmacokinetics and pharmacodynamics in the development of anti-tuberculosis drugs. *Tuberculosis (Edinburgh)* 88 (Suppl 1), S65–74.

Davies, G.R., Brindle, R., Khoo, S.H. and Aarons, L.J. (2006a) Use of nonlinear mixed-effects analysis for improved precision of early pharmacodynamic measures in tuberculosis treatment. *Antimicrobial Agents and Chemotherapy* 50(9), 3154–3156.

Davies, G., Khoo, S. and Aarons, L. (2006b) Optimal sampling strategies for early pharmacodynamic measures in tuberculosis. *Journal of Antimicrobial Chemotherapy* 58, 594–600.

Davies, G., Cheirakul, N., Saguenwong, N., Chaiprasert, A., Chuchuttaworn, C., Eompo-kalap, B., *et al.* (2008) A factorial study of the effect of HIV, tuberculosis and pharmacogenetics on the pharmacokinetics and pharmacodynamics of anti-tuberculosis drugs. In: *Conference on Retroviruses and Opportunistic Infections.* Boston, USA.

De Gruttola, V.G., Clax, P., DeMets, D.L., Downing, G.J., Ellenberg, S.S., Friedman, L., *et al.* (2001) Considerations in the evaluation of surrogate endpoints in clinical trials. summary of a

National Institutes of Health workshop. *Controlled Clinical Trials* 22(5), 485–502.

Diacon, A., Patientia, R.F., Venter, A., van Helden, P.D., Smith, P.J., McIlleron, H., *et al.* (2007) Early bactericidal activity of high-dose rifampin in patients with pulmonary tuberculosis evidenced by positive sputum smears. *Antimicrobial Agents and Chemotherapy* 51(8), 2994–2996.

Diacon, A.H., Pym, A., Grobusch, M., Patientia, R., Rustomjee, R., Page-Shipp, L., *et al.* (2009) The diarylquinoline TMC207 for multidrug-resistant tuberculosis. *The New England Journal of Medicine* 360(23), 2397–2405.

Diacon, A.H., Dawson, R., Hanekom, M., Narunsky, K., Maritz, S.J., Venter, A., *et al.* (2010) Early bactericidal activity and pharmacokinetics of PA-824 in smear-positive tuberculosis patients. *Antimicrobial Agents and Chemotherapy* 54(8), 3402–3407.

Diggle, P., Heagerty, P., Liang, K.Y. and Zeger, S. (2002) *Analysis of Longitudinal Data.* Oxford University Press, Oxford.

Diggle, P.J., Sousa, I. and Chetwynd, A.G. (2008) Joint modelling of repeated measurements and time-to-event outcomes: the fourth Armitage lecture. *Statistics in Medicine* 27(16), 2981–2998.

Donald, P., Sirgel, F.A., Botha, F.J., Seifart, H.I., Parkin, D.P., Vandenplas, M.L., *et al.* (1997) The early bactericidal activity of isoniazid related to it's dose size in pulmonary tuberculosis. *American Journal of Respiratory and Critical Care Medicine* 156, 895–900.

Donald, P., Sirgel, F.A., Venter, A., Smit, E., Parkin, D.P., Van de Wal, B.W., *et al.* (2001) The early bactericidal activity of amikacin in pulmonary tuberculosis. *International Journal of Tuberculosis and Lung Disease* 5(6), 533–538.

Donald, P., Sirgel, F.A., Venter, A., Smit, E., Parkin, D.P., Van de Wal, B.W., *et al.* (2002) The early bactericidal activity of streptomycin. *International Journal of Tuberculosis and Lung Disease* 6(8), 693–698.

Donald, P., Sirgel, F.A., Venter, A., Parkin, D.P., Seifart, H.I., van de Wal, B.W., *et al.* (2003) Early bactericidal activity of antituberculosis agents. *Expert Reviews in Anti-Infective Therapy* 1(1), 141–155.

Donald, P., Sirgel, F.A., Venter, A., Parkin, D.P., Seifart, H.I., Van de Wal, B.W., *et al.* (2004) The influence of human N-acetyltransferase genotype on the early bactericidal activity of isoniazid. *Clinical Infectious Diseases* 39, 1425–1430.

Dorman, S.E., Johnson, J.L., Goldberg, S., Muzanye, G., Padayatchi, N., Bozeman, L.,

et al. (2009) Substitution of moxifloxacin for isoniazid during intensive phase treatment of pulmonary tuberculosis. *American Journal of Respiratory and Critical Care Medicine* 180(3), 273–280.

EAMR Council (1974) Controlled clinical trial of four short-course (6-month) regimens of chemotherapy for treatment of pulmonary tuberculosis. Third report. *The Lancet* 2, 237–240.

EAMR Council (1981) Controlled clinical trial of five short-course (4 month) chemotherapy regimens in pulmonary tuberculosis. Second report of the fourth study. *American Review of Respiratory Disease* 123, 165–170.

Fang, X., Wallqvist, A. and Reifman, J. (2009) A systems biology framework for modeling metabolic enzyme inhibition of *Mycobacterium tuberculosis*. *BMC Systems Biology* 3, 92.

Fedorov, V., Mannino, F. and Zhang, R. (2009) Consequences of dichotomization. *Pharmaceutical Statistics* 8(1), 50–61.

Fox, W., Sutherland, I. and Daniels, M. (1954) A five year assessment of patients in a controlled trial of streptomycin in pulmonary tuberculosis. *Quarterly Journal of Medicine* 23, 347–366.

Fox, W., Ellard, G.A. and Mitchison, D.A. (1999) Studies on the treatment of tuberculosis undertaken by the British Medical Research Council Tuberculosis Units 1946–1986, with subsequent relevant publications. *International Journal of Tuberculosis and Lung Disease* 3(10), S231–S279.

Frison, L. and Pocock, S.J. (1992) Repeated measures in clinical trials: analysis using mean summary statistics and its implications for design. *Statistics in Medicine* 11(13), 1685–1704.

Frison, L.J. and Pocock, S.J. (1997) Linearly divergent treatment effects in clinical trials with repeated measures: efficient analysis using summary statistics. *Statistics in Medicine* 16(24), 2855–2872.

Gandhi, N.R., Shah, N.S., Andrews, J.R., Vella, V., Moll, A.P., Scott, M., *et al.* (2010) HIV coinfection in multidrug- and extensively drug-resistant tuberculosis results in high early mortality. *American Journal of Respiratory and Critical Care Medicine* 181(1), 80–86.

Garton, N.J., Christensen, H., Minnikin, D.E., Adegbola, R.A. and Barer, M.R. (2002) Intracellular lipophilic inclusions of mycobacteria *in vitro* and in sputum. *Microbiology (Reading, England)* 148(Pt 10), 2951–2958.

Garton, N.J., Waddell, S.J., Sherratt, A.L., Lee, S.M., Smith, R.J., Senner, C., *et al.* (2008) Cytological and transcript analyses reveal fat and lazy persister-like bacilli in tuberculous sputum. *PLoS Medicine* 5(4), e75.

Goldstein, H., Browne, W. and Rasbash, J. (2002) Multilevel modelling of medical data. *Statistics in Medicine* 21, 3291–3315.

Gumbo, T., Louie, A., Deziel, M.R., Parsons, L.M., Salfinger, M. and Drusano, G.L. (2004) Selection of a moxifloxacin dose that supresses drug resistance in *Mycobacterium tuberculosis* by use of an *in vitro* pharmacodynamic infection model and mathematical modelling. *Journal of Infectious Diseases* 190, 1642–1651.

Gumbo, T., Louie, A., Deziel, M.R., Liu, W., Parsons, L.M., Salfinger, M., *et al.* (2007) Concentration-dependent *Mycobacterium tuberculosis* killing and prevention of resistance by rifampin. *Antimicrobial Agents and Chemotherapy* 51(11), 3781–3788.

Hesseling, A.C., Walzl, G., Enarson, D.A., Carroll, N.M., Duncan, K., Lukey, P.T., *et al.* (2010) Baseline sputum time to detection predicts month two culture conversion and relapse in non-HIV-infected patients. *The International Journal of Tuberculosis and Lung Disease* 14(5), 560–570.

Holtz, T.H., Sternberg, M., Kammerer, S., Laserson, K.F., Riekstina, V., Zarovska, E., *et al.* (2006) Time to sputum culture conversion in multidrug-resistant tuberculosis: predictors and relationship to treatment outcome. *Annals of Internal Medicine* 144(9), 650–659.

Jamshidi, N. and Palsson, B. (2007) Investigating the metabolic capabilities of *Mycobacterium tuberculosis* H37Rv using the *in silico* strain iNJ661 and proposing alternative drug targets. *BMC Systems Biology* 1(1), 26.

Jayaram, R., Gaonkar, S., Kaur, P., Suresh, B.L., Mahesh, B.N., Jayashree, R., *et al.* (2003) Pharmacokinetics–pharmacodynamics of rifampin in an aerosol infection model of tuberculosis. *Antimicrobial Agents and Chemotherapy* 47(7), 2118–2124.

Jayaram, R., Shandil, R.K., Gaonkar, S., Kaur, P., Suresh, B.L., Mahesh, B.N., *et al.* (2004) Isoniazid pharmacokinetics–pharmacodynamics in an aerosol infection model of tuberculosis. *Antimicrobial Agents and Chemotherapy* 48(8), 2951–2957.

Jindani, A., Aber, V.R., Edwards, E.A. and Mitchison, D.A. (1980) The early bactericidal activity of drugs in patients with pulmonary tuberculosis. *American Review of Respiratory Diseases* 121, 939–949.

Johnson, J., Hadad, D.J., Boom, W.H., Daley, C.L., Peloquin, C.A., Eisenach, K.D., *et al.* (2006) Early and extended early bactericidal activity of levofloxacin, gatifloxacin and moxifloxacin in

pulmonary tuberculosis. *International Journal of Tuberculosis and Lung Disease* 10, 605–612.

Li, L., Mahan, C.S., Palaci, M., Horter, L., Loeffelholz, L., Johnson, J.L., *et al.* (2010) Sputum *Mycobacterium tuberculosis* mRNA as a marker of bacteriologic clearance in response to antituberculosis therapy. *Journal of Clinical Microbiology* 48(1), 46–51.

Lienhardt, C. and Davies, G. (2010) Methodological issues in the design of clinical trials for the treatment of multidrug-resistant tuberculosis: challenges and opportunities. *The International Journal of Tuberculosis and Lung Disease* 14(5), 528–537.

Lipsitch, M. and Levin, B.R. (1998) Population dynamics of tuberculosis treatment: mathematical models of the roles of non-compliance and bacterial heterogeneity in the evolution of drug resistance. *The International Journal of Tuberculosis and Lung Disease* 2(3), 187–199.

Martineau, A.R., Timms, P.M., Bothamley, G.R., Hanita, Y., Islam, K., Claxton, A.P., *et al.* (2011) High dose vitamin D_3 during intensive-phase antimicrobial treatment of pulmonary tuberculosis: a double-blind randomised controlled trial. *The Lancet* 377, 242–250.

Matthews, J.N., Altman, D.G., Campbell, M.J. and Royston, P. (1990) Analysis of serial measurements in medical research. *BMJ (Clinical Research Ed.)* 300(6719), 230–235.

Mdivani, N., Li, H., Akhalaia, M., Gegia, M., Goginashvili, L., Kernodle, D.S., *et al.* (2009) Monitoring therapeutic efficacy by real-time detection of *Mycobacterium tuberculosis* mRNA in sputum. *Clinical Chemistry* 55(9), 1694–1700.

Mitchison, D. (1950) Development of streptomycin resistant strains of tubercle bacilli in pulmonary tuberculosis. Results of simultaneous sensitivity tests in liquid and on solid media. *Thorax* 5, 144–161.

Mitchison, D. (1979) Basic mechanisms of chemotherapy. *Chest* 76(6 Suppl), 771–781.

Mitchison, D. (1992) The Garrod Lecture. Understanding the chemotherapy of tuberculosis-current problems. *Journal of Antimicrobial Chemotherapy* 29, 477–493.

Mitchison, D. (1996) Modern methods for assessing the drugs used in the chemotherapy of mycobacterial disease. *Journal of Applied Bacteriology* 81, 72S–80S.

Mitchison, D., Allen, B.W., Carrol, L., Dickinson, J.M. and Aber, V.R. (1971) A selective oleic acid albumin agar medium for tubercle bacilli. *Journal of Medical Microbiology* 5(2), 165–175.

MRC (1948) Streptomycin treatment of pulmonary tuberculosis. *British Medical Journal* 2, 769–782.

MRC (1950) Treatment of pulmonary tuberculosis with streptomycin and para-aminosalicylic acid. *British Medical Journal* 2, 1073–1085.

MRC (1952) The treatment of pulmonary tuberculosis with isoniazid. *British Medical Journal* 2, 735–746.

MRC (1953) Isoniazid in combination with strepto-mycin or with PAS in the treatment of pulmonary tuberculosis. *British Medical Journal* 2, 1005–1014.

MRC (1973) Co-operative controlled trial of a standard regimen of streptomycin, PAS and isoniazid and three alternative regimens of chemotherapy in Britain. *Tubercle* 54, 99–129.

Nahid, P., Bliven, E.E., Kim, E.Y., MacKenzie, W.R., Stout, J.E., Diem, L., et al. (2010) Influence of *M. tuberculosis* lineage variability within a clinical trial for pulmonary tuberculosis. *PloS One* 5(5), e10753.

Paramasivan, C., Sulochana, S., Kubendiran, G., Venkatesan, P. and Mitchison, D.A. (2005) Bactericidal action of gatifloxacin, rifampin, and isoniazid on logarithmic- and stationary-phase cultures of *Mycobacterium tuberculosis*. *Antimicrobial Agents and Chemotherapy* 49, 627–631.

Perrin, F., Lipman, M.C., McHugh, T.D. and Gillespie, S.H. (2007) Biomarkers of treatment response in clinical trials of novel antituberculosis agents. *The Lancet Infectious Diseases* 7(7), 481–490.

Pheiffer, C., Carroll, N.M., Beyers, N., Donald, P., Duncan, K., Uys, P., et al. (2008) Time to detection of *Mycobacterium tuberculosis* in BACTEC systems as a viable alternative to colony counting. *The International Journal of Tuberculosis and Lung Disease* 12(7), 792–798.

Phillips, P. and Fielding, K. (2007) The evaluation of culture conversion during treatment for tubercu-losis as a surrogate marker for relapse. In: *Conference of the International Union Against Tuberculosis and Lung Disease*, 2007, Cape Town.

Phillips, P.P.J. and Fielding, K. (2008) Surrogate markers for poor outcome to treatment for tuberculosis: results from extensive multi-trial analysis. In: *Conference of the International Union against Tuberculosis and Lung Disease*, 2008, Cape Town.

Prentice, R.L. (1989) Surrogate endpoints in clinical trials: definition and operational criteria. *Statistics in Medicine* 8(4), 431–440.

Raman, K., Rajagopalan, P. and Chandra, N. (2005) Flux balance analysis of mycolic acid pathway: targets for anti-tubercular drugs. *PLoS Com-putational Biology* 1(5), e46.

Raman, K., Vashisht, R. and Chandra, N. (2009) Strategies for efficient disruption of metabolism in *Mycobacterium tuberculosis* from network analysis. *Molecular bioSystems* 5(12), 1740–1751.

Rustomjee, R., Diacon, A.H., Allen, J., Venter, A., Reddy, C., Patientia, R.F., et al. (2008a) Early bactericidal activity and pharmacokinetics of the diarylquinoline TMC207 in treatment of pulmonary tuberculosis. *Antimicrobial Agents and Chemotherapy* 52(8), 2831–2835.

Rustomjee, R., Lienhardt, C., Kanyok, T., Davies, G.R., Levin, J., Mthiyane, T., et al. (2008b) A Phase II study of the sterilising activities of ofloxacin, gatifloxacin and moxifloxacin in pulmonary tuberculosis. *The International Journal of Tuberculosis and Lung Disease* 12(2), 128–138.

Schön, T., Juréen, P., Giske, C.G., Chryssanthou, E., Sturegård, E., Werngren, J., et al. (2009) Evaluation of wild-type MIC distributions as a tool for determination of clinical breakpoints for *Mycobacterium tuberculosis*. *The Journal of Antimicrobial Chemotherapy* 64(4), 786–793.

Sheiner, L.B. (1997) Learning versus confirming in clinical drug development. *Clinical Pharma-cology and Therapeutics* 61(3), 275–291.

Sheiner, L.B., Rosenberg, B. and Marathe, V.V. (1977) Estimation of population characteristics of pharmacokinetic parameters from routine clinical data. *Journal of Pharmacokinetics and Biopharmaceutics* 5(5), 445–479.

Sirgel, F., Donald, P.R., Odhiambo, J., Githui, W., Umapathy, K.C., Paramasivan, C.N., et al. (2000) A multicentre study of the early bactericidal activity of anti-tuberculosis drugs. *Journal of Antimicrobial Chemotherapy* 45, 859–870.

Sirgel, F., Venter, A. and Mitchison, D. (2001) Sources of variation in studies of the early bactericidal activity of antituberculosis drugs. *Journal of Antimicrobial Chemotherapy* 47, 177–182.

Sirgel, F., Fourie, P.B., Donald, P.R., Padayatchi, N., Rustomjee, R., Levin, J., et al. (2005) The early bactericidal activities of rifampin and rifapentine in pulmonary tuberculosis. *American Journal of Respiratory and Critical Care Medicine* 171, 1–8.

Wallis, R., Patil, S., Cheon, S.H., Edmonds, K., Phillips, M., Perkins, M.D., et al. (1999) Drug tolerance in mycobacterium tuberculosis. *Antimicrobial Agents and Chemotherapy* 43(11), 2600–2606.

Wallis, R.S., Doherty, T.M., Onyebujoh, P., Vahedi, M., Laang, H., Olesen, O., et al. (2009) Biomarkers for tuberculosis disease activity, cure, and relapse. *The Lancet Infectious Diseases* 9(3), 162–172.

Wang, R. and Marcotte, E.M. (2008) The proteomic response of *Mycobacterium smegmatis* to anti-tuberculosis drugs suggests targeted pathways. *Journal of Proteome Research* 7(3), 855–865.

Yoo, B. (2009) The impact of dichotomization in longitudinal data analysis: a simulation study. *Pharmaceutical Statistics* 9(4), 298–312.

Young, D., Stark, J. and Kirschner, D. (2008) Systems biology of persistent infection: tuberculosis as a case study. *Nature Reviews. Microbiology* 6(7), 520–528.

Zhang, L., Sinha, V., Forgue, S.T., Callies, S., Ni, L., Peck, R., *et al.* (2006) Model-based drug development: the road to quantitative pharmacology. *Journal of Pharmacokinetics and Pharmacodynamics* 33(3), 369–393.

12 Measuring Gene Expression by Quantitative PCR (qPCR)

Isobella Honeyborne

Centre for Clinical Microbiology, Department of Infection, University College London, UK

12.1 Introduction

Quantification of gene expression requires isolation and detection of RNA. There are two main ways in which extracted RNA can be used to study *Mycobacterium tuberculosis*. The first is to compare changes in the transcriptome (mRNA expression level) during phases of growth or with different stress factors; for example, drug treatment, hypoxia and starvation.

The ability to elucidate how the bacteria respond under different circumstances will inform our understanding of the basic biology of the organism and help to identify novel drugs which can subvert these survival mechanisms. Like many bacteria, *M. tuberculosis* is remarkably adaptable. *M. tuberculosis* is able to tolerate reduced oxygen tension in the granuloma, host adaptive immune responses and subvert post-phagocytic destruction within the macrophage to use this cell as a living space. These different conditions are likely to induce changes in genes important in adapting to a generic stress response. Additionally, particular gene pathways may respond by increased or decreased expression in order to cope with a specific set of conditions. Detecting tran-

scriptome changes is therefore important in understanding how the bacteria are adapting and surviving in the host. To obtain a broad picture of the changes in gene pathways, microarray technology is generally used. Microarrays can screen a large number of genes simultaneously. Reverse transcription quantitative PCR (RT-qPCR) is then used to confirm the findings for changes in the expression of specifically identified genes.

The second use for measuring gene expression by qPCR reflects quantification of cell numbers. It is theoretically possible to determine the number of *M. tuberculosis* bacteria in a clinical sample by detecting the amount of a particular high abundance, constitutively expressed gene. Sputum is a useful sample for this purpose, since it can be collected non-invasively and is usually readily available from individuals with pulmonary tuberculosis. Use of a standard curve with qPCR cycle threshold values for sputum samples with a known bacterial load should then allow the unknown sputum bacterial load to be determined. The remainder of this chapter will focus on using qPCR of such constitutively expressed genes to determine the bacterial number.

12.2 The Need for Molecular-based Quantification of Bacterial Load

To date, although there are several commercially available molecular-based kits for the detection and diagnosis of tuberculosis, there are none available that offer quantification. This is surprising since real-time PCR technology has been available for upwards of a decade. The reasons why a commercial assay is not already available will be explored later in this section.

Assessment of bacterial load in sputum is generally used as a research tool or to ascertain the efficacy of novel drugs. For clinical diagnosis of tuberculosis, the bacterial burden of the sample is only assessed at the level of the sputum smear. Although it is of limited use in clinical decision making, a smear can be graded according to how many bacilli are seen per microscope field of view. This can then be used to approximate the bacterial load of the sample. Notably, this does not differentiate between live and dead bacilli and the detection of tuberculosis by sputum smear requires approximately 10^4 bacilli/ml sputum. There are a large number of tuberculosis-positive individuals who are smear negative, and of this group, paediatric tuberculosis is particularly difficult to diagnose by this method.

The use of culture in many laboratories increases the detection rate of tuberculosis. Inoculation of decontaminated sputum sediment on to solid culture, such as Löwenstein–Jensen slopes, can be used to semi-quantify the bacterial load by counting the number of colonies that grow. Liquid culture can be used similarly by assessing how long the culture takes to be become positive. These methods, however, are confounded by several effects, with the major drawback being the slow replication rate of tuberculosis. In solid culture, bacterial colonies are unlikely to be seen for at least 2–3 weeks, and for liquid culture the speed of detection is dependent on the number of bacteria present in the starting inoculum. Those samples most likely to be missed by smear, due to a low bacilli load, will also likely take the longest to flag positive in the automated liquid culture

system. Despite the decontamination process, a proportion of samples will be overgrown and therefore invalidated by growth of other microorganisms. Additionally, there may be *M. tuberculosis* bacteria present that are refractive to the particular culture media but which are not dead. Recent studies have suggested that these may represent an important population (Shleeva *et al.*, 2002; Davies *et al.*, 2008; Mukamolova *et al.*, 2010).

If decontamination is not used, then the solid culture media can be made selective for tuberculosis by the addition of antimicrobials, and can be used to quantitate bacilli load directly in sputum samples. In some cases, the results are still invalidated by the growth of other microorganisms. The sputum serial colony-counting (SSCC) assay uses such selective media to determine the number of *M. tuberculosis* colony-forming units (CFU) in sputum at multiple time points during treatment (see Chapter 11).

The drawbacks of the currently available culture-based methods for detecting bacterial load highlight how useful a molecular-based assay would be for quantification. There are two main advantages of using molecular quantitation over culture. The first would be the use of primer and probe sets specific for *M. tuberculosis* complex bacteria to circumvent the problems with invalidation by growth from other organisms. The second that samples could be enumerated rapidly, regardless of the number of bacteria present.

Although bacterial load is not commonly used during routine clinical management of tuberculosis disease, culture-based methods are used to determine the efficacy of novel tuberculosis drugs by measuring the decline in bacterial numbers during early therapy (Donald *et al.*, 2000; Brindle *et al.*, 2001). Previous studies have identified culture positivity after 2 months of therapy as a risk factor (Aber and Nunn, 1978; Mitchison, 1993) associated with later relapse. Recently, high presenting bacterial load has been highlighted as a hazard factor for risk of later relapse (Hesseling *et al.*, 2010). It is important to detect all bacteria with the potential to cause disease, regardless of the life cycle they are in. As discussed in Chapter 11, mathematical modelling of SSCC measurement during the first 2 months of treatment has found the data are best fitted to a biexponential decay curve. This has been suggested as being reflective of two principle subpopulations of bacteria which respond to treatment differently.

A recent study shortened treatment from 6 to 4 months for those with sputum culture negative for tuberculosis at 2 months of treatment (Johnson *et al.*, 2009). A higher proportion of this group went on to relapse with the identical strain to the first episode during the 2-year follow-up period. This suggests that either there were bacteria present in the sputum that were refractive to culture or that the bacteria were archived in the lung in a place inaccessible to expectorated sputum.

In summary, it is clear that bacterial load ascertained from culture-based methods is a useful method for determining bacterial load but is likely not to give an accurate reflection of the true viable bacteria in the sample.

12.3 Why There Is Not Currently a Molecular Assay for Enumeration of *M. tuberculosis* in Sputum

Ideally, molecular techniques would identify the number of bacteria present in a sample that were at any stage of the bacterial life cycle and capable of causing disease. The perfect molecule for measuring this would be both abundant, and therefore readily detectable, but would also decay rapidly following cell death, so that only live cells would be quantified.

DNA has been shown to be detected following culture negativity in a controlled murine model, which is suggestive that this molecule is unreflective of live cell status (de Wit *et al.*, 1995). This observation has also been confirmed in several studies using longitudinal data from tuberculosis-infected individuals during chemotherapy in Tanzania (Kennedy *et al.*, 1994), and DNA was detected in 25% of specimens collected in tuberculosis-positive patients administered with at least 180 days of treatment (Hellyer *et al.*, 1996). At

this time point, all patients were found simultaneously to be negative for *M. tuberculosis* by culture, as would be expected, since after 6 months of treatment the vast majority of individuals have been cured of active disease.

It is widely accepted that RNA is a shorter-lived species than DNA and therefore its degradation might be expected to match disappearance in bacteria as they are killed. Either ribosomal (rRNA) or messenger (mRNA) can be followed. mRNA is a useful molecule, since it has been shown to decay rapidly after cell death (Hellyer *et al.*, 1999a); however, it is not very abundant. There are an estimated 0.1 copies of the highly expressed antigen 85B mRNA per CFU (Desjardin *et al.*, 1999). Previous studies and our data suggest that you cannot detect abundant mRNA species in samples containing $<10^4$ bacilli/ml (Desjardin *et al.*, 1999). Additionally, some *in vitro* data found 85B mRNA disappearance to be pre-emptive of the decline in bacterial numbers (Hellyer *et al.*, 1999a). rRNA is much more available for detection, with an estimated 800 molecules/CFU (Desjardin *et al.*, 1999). It would be expected, therefore, that it would be detected more readily than even non-repetitive DNA sequences in samples containing few bacteria. The literature, however, has reported that the 16S rRNA molecule does not decay rapidly enough to be useful as a marker of cell viability (Desjardin *et al.*, 1999; Hellyer *et al.*, 1999a). However, the *in vitro* study did find changes in the 16S rRNA level after 72 h of isoniazid treatment (Hellyer *et al.*, 1999a).

Other studies of mycobacteria also support the rapid decline of 16S rRNA following bacterial cell death. One such study found that *M. aurum* ingestion by peritoneal macrophages resulted in ribosome destruction being an early event, occurring after 4 days (Silva *et al.*, 1987). Macrophages form a major part of the granuloma, although they are not present in the acellular necrotic centre. It is hypothesized that dead bacteria will be expelled from the sputum and those remaining destroyed by macrophages present in the periphery of the granuloma structure. Further work needs to be done, however, to ascertain the extent to which rRNA is detectable following ingestion of tuberculosis by alveolar macrophages following bacterial cell death. In *ex vivo* samples, detection of rRNA beyond culture negativity could represent a population of live bacteria refractive to culture (Moore *et al.*, 1996). In a recent study of 111 patients with severe tuberculosis disease, we measured tuberculosis-specific 16S rRNA longitudinally during treatment. We found a rapid decline of 16S rRNA after 72 h of therapy (0.99 $\log_{10}$). In the same study, we found that only 1 of 43 patients was positive for tuberculosis using the 16S assay after 168 days of treatment (unpublished observation).

12.3.1 Sensitivity of nucleic acid-based detection

mRNA has been demonstrated to decay rapidly following *in vitro* drug treatment of *M. tuberculosis* (Hellyer *et al.*, 1999a) and in sputum (Desjardin *et al.*, 1999; Hellyer *et al.*, 1999b; Li *et al.*, 2010). Genes that have previously been measured include *fbpB* (encodes 85B protein), *hspX* (encodes alpha-crystalline homologue protein), *rrnA-P1* (a non-encoding region for the ribosomal promoter) and *icl* (encodes isocitrate lyase). *icl* expression appears to be the highest of the genes tested to date; however, it does not appear to correlate with decline of CFU between days 0 and 2 (Li *et al.*, 2010). *icl* and *rrnA-P1* showed some correlation with CFU between days 2 and 7. In the same study, after 2 months of therapy, 66% (25 of 38) of individuals tested were still culture positive; detection of *icl*, however, was found in only 28% of the same samples (7 of 25). Detection of these genes may have some use during very early therapy and, potentially, combinations of genes could prove useful. However, sensitivity of mRNA detection still remains an issue. Due to the greater abundance of rRNA compared to mRNA, we have developed an assay based on detection of 16S rRNA. Using a serial dilution from a known number of bacteria and spiking *M. tuberculosis* into negative sputum samples, we have

detected and enumerated accurately between 10^7 and 10^2/ml sputum using this method (Honeyborne *et al.*, 2011).

12.3.2 Problems and preservation of sputum RNA

Rapid decay of RNA is a useful attribute for measuring live cells; however, the friability of this molecule means that preserving it so that it is available must be addressed. It is important for transcriptome studies that RNA transcripts are preserved immediately following expectoration, otherwise bacteria present in sputum may change their expression in response to altered environmental conditions not relevant to the experiment. Treating bacteria with solutions containing guanidine thiocyanate (GTC) has been found to preserve the RNA effectively (Monahan *et al.*, 2001).

GTC penetrates host cells and the myco-bacterial cell wall protects the tuberculosis bacteria, preserving the intracellular components including RNA. In the method used in our laboratory, based on the method of Monahan *et al.* (2001), successful amplification of RNA has been performed from sputum samples frozen in GTC. This is somewhat surprising since it would be expected that the bacterial cell wall would lose its integrity on thawing. However, we have extracted RNA repeatedly and successfully from sputum frozen at –80°C in GTC-containing solutions, even with repeat freeze–thaw cycles of the sputum in GTC. We have extracted *M. tuberculosis* RNA successfully and amplified it in RT-qPCR reactions after the sputum has been frozen at –80°C for up to 10 years.

Following the treatment of sputum with GTC, the solution is centrifuged at 2000 g to pellet the bacteria out of the sample. Nucleic acid in aqueous solutions will not pellet at this centrifugal force. Some nucleic acid released from cells is, however, recovered during this process. We have shown this by spiking a naked *in vitro* transcribed mRNA 1957-bp fragment into sputum in GTC and find that it is possible to detect the gene by RT-qPCR following extraction. Approximately

500-fold of the mRNA is lost during this process, however.

12.3.3 Extraction of RNA and inhibitors

There are inhibitors present in sputum samples and if these are not accounted for, then a count based on direct correlation between cycle threshold as measured by RT-qPCR will not be accurate.

The loss of RNA and inhibitors present in a sample are proportional for the synthetic spiked mRNA and bacterial genes *sigA* and 16S rRNA tested (Fig. 12.1). This was determined when 51 tuberculosis-negative sputum samples were spiked with the same number of *M. tuberculosis* bacteria and internal control and RNA extracted from each sample. When *sigA* mRNA, 16S rRNA and the internal control gene were measured, there was a large range of cycle threshold values obtained for each measured gene. As would be expected, comparison of the detection of two bacterial genes (16S rRNA and *sigA*) found there was a correlation between their recovery ($R^2 = 0.87$). When detection of the internal control was similarly compared to that of the 16S rRNA and *sigA*, a similar correlation was found between the internal control and 16S rRNA and between the internal control and *sigA* of $R^2 = 0.84$ and 0.81, respectively. The range in cycle threshold values was caused by RNA loss and inhibitors, transferred with the RNA that affected the reverse transcriptase and Taq polymerase. However, these effects were the same for the internal control and the bacterial genes measured. This therefore allows the internal control to be used to normalize cycle threshold values obtained for bacterial genes in unknown samples.

In summary, the low abundance of mRNA, the questionability of whether rRNA is a short-lived molecule, preservation of RNA in sputum and inhibitors are likely to be the main reasons why a commercially available molecular-based assay of quantification has not been readily available to date.

If RNA is extracted carefully without the introduction of RNases, it does not degrade rapidly at 4°C. We measured samples stored at 4°C 3 months later and identical cycle threshold values were obtained. In all likelihood, multiple freeze–thaw cycles degrade RNA more rapidly and should be avoided.

The use of 16S rRNA and an internal control has allowed us to develop a molecular assay to quantify tuberculosis bacteria in sputum samples.

If a serial dilution of tuberculosis is made and spiked into tuberculosis-negative sputum, RNA can be extracted and detected. If inhibition is taken into account by normalizing against the internal control, then a reproducible method of quantification is available between 10^7 and 10^2 bacilli/ml sputum (Fig. 12.2). Samples tested were between 10^7 and 10^2 bacilli/ml sputum were shown to be enumerated within $0.5 \log_{10}$ in 98% (n = 86) of cases.

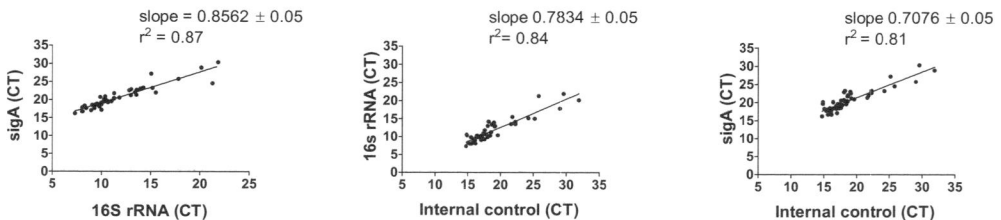

Fig. 12.1. Detection of tuberculosis mRNA (*sigA*), 16S rRNA and artificially spiked internal control. Each point is a sample with 10^7 bacilli and 50 ng internal control. (Adapted from Copyright © American Society for Microbiology, *Journal of Clinical Microbiology*, Vol 49, 2011, pp. 3905–3911, DOI 10.1128/JCM.00547-11.)

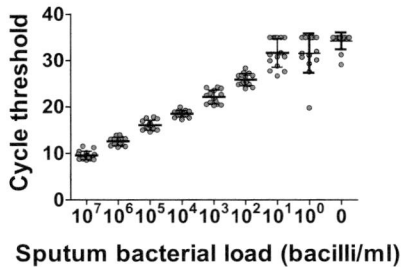

Fig. 12.2. Serial dilutions of H37Rv and 50 ng internal control were spiked into tuberculosis-negative sputum samples. RNA was extracted and the cycle threshold measured for 16S rRNA and the internal control. The recovery of the internal control was used to normalize the detection of the 16S rRNA and the cycle threshold (CT) value for each dilution plotted (the mean ± standard deviations are defined by the lines at each bacterial concentration). (Adapted from Copyright © American Society for Microbiology, *Journal of Clinical Microbiology*, Vol 49, 2011, pp. 3905–3911, DOI 10.1128/JCM.00547-11.)

12.4 Measurement of 16S rRNA in Patient Sputum Samples

16S rRNA normalized against our novel internal control has been used successfully to screen patient sputum samples over time (Honeyborne, 2011). Modelling of bacterial decay in response to chemotherapy has previously been performed using solid agar counting on media selective for tuberculosis by the addition of antimicrobials, as described. These studies typically found biphasic decay in bacterial load when measured over time. Modelling of bacterial load using 43 patients and measuring the bacterial load using the 16S rRNA assay found similar biphasic decay. Comparison of the decay of 16S rRNA determined bacterial load in our study compared to bacterial load ascertained by SSCC in other studies. The biexponential mixed effects model with parameters differing by relapse status resulted in the best fit (model 4) (Fig. 12.3). A and B represent the intercepts on the $\log_{10}$ scale of the first and second phases of elimination, and α and β represent the corresponding gradients of the decline of counts during that phase. There was a significant difference in the fitted lines between relapsed and cured patients ($P = 0.0031$), with the difference coming in the A and B parameters, reflecting the bacterial load at presentation (Fig. 12.3). There was no significant difference in the gradient α in the first ($P = 0.122$) or second phase. Comparison between the 16S rRNA measured bacterial load and other studies measuring bacterial decline using solid agar counts found the transition times were longer using 16S rRNA assay than solid culture, occurring at 8.15 days and 9.36 days for cured and relapsed, respectively, compared to other studies of cured patients, which found the transition time to be around 2.62 and 2.12 days (Fig. 12.3). These differences may be due to a plethora of reasons, including 16S rRNA not decaying immediately following bacterial cell death or measurement of bacteria that are refractive to culture.

At day 56, we compared liquid culture positivity to samples positive by the 16S rRNA assay. However, a culture result was not available as 14% of samples (15 of 110) were found to have contaminated cultures. This was in comparison to 0.9% (1 of 110) where the internal control had failed and a 16S rRNA assay result was not available; 64% (60 of 94) had a culture and 16S rRNA result that matched. There were an additional 24 samples that were found to be positive by culture but negative by 16S rRNA, and 10 that contained $\geq 10^2$ bacilli/ml sputum by 16S rRNA but were negative by culture (Table 12.1).

Ninety-six per cent (25 of 26) of sputum samples that were found to contain $\geq 10^3$ bacilli/ml sputum as measured by the abundance of 16S rRNA were also found to be culture negative.

12.5 Conclusion

In summary, future studies measuring bacterial numbers in sputum samples might find it worthwhile to have data for both the 16S rRNA assay and culture. Those that are negative by both assays at day 56 might be better candidates for treatment shortening.

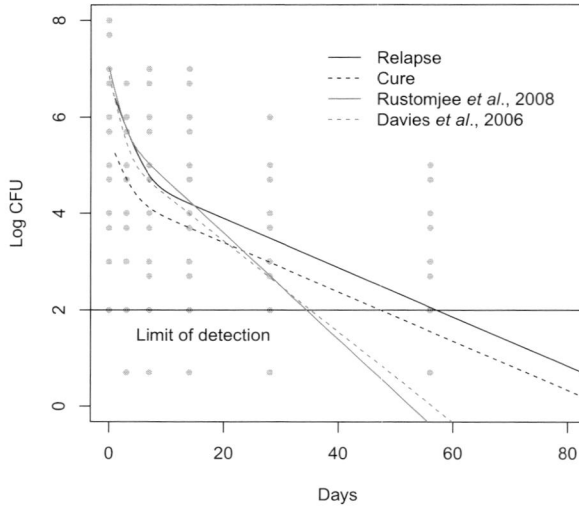

	Parameter estimates with 95% confidence intervals					
Model	A	α	B	β	AIC[a]	Results of likelihood ratio test
1. Mono-exponential	5.29 (5.07, 5.51)	0.07 (0.06, 0.08)			801.8	
2. Bi-exponential	5.95 (5.57, 6.34)	0.38 (0.19, 0.75)	4.78 (4.43, 5.14)	0.05 (0.05, 0.07)	783.1	p<.0001[†]
3. Bi-exponential mixed effects (pooled)	5.82 (5.47, 6.17)	0.22 (0.18, 0.27)	4.24 (3.79, 4.68)	0.04 (0.04, 0.05)	702.7	p<.0001[‡]
4. Bi-exponential mixed effects Cure	5.46 (5.07, 5.86)	0.19 (0.15, 0.25)	4.06 (3.58, 4.55)	0.04 (0.04, 0.05)	694.9	p=0.0031[§]
Relapse	6.68 (5.69, 7.66)	0.28 (0.15, 0.54)	4.72 (3.68, 5.77)	0.04 (0.04, 0.05)		
Test[II]	p=0.0013	p=0.112	p=0.082			

Notes: Lower panel: [a]AIC = Akaike Information Criterion – a lower number indicates a model that fits the data better; [b]comparing models 1 and 2; [c]comparing models 2 and 3; [d]comparing models 3 and 4; [e]Wald test comparing parameter estimates between models for cured and relapse patients.

Fig. 12.3. Mathematical modelling of longitudinal data of bacterial decline for 43 patients using data from day 0 to day 56. Upper panel: the best fit, mixed effect biphasic decay model for patients who went on to cure and those who relapsed, showing the OLFLOTUB (Rustomjee *et al.*, 2008) and Davies streptomycin and isoniazid or rifampin and pyrazinamide (SHRZ) (Davies *et al.*, 2006) studies where bacterial decline was measured using solid agar colony and also found the best fit was a biphasic decay. Lower panel: fit of nested sums of various exponential models. Parameters A and B are the intercepts for the various phases of killing ($\log_{10}$ bacterial load/ml sputum), α and β are the corresponding rates of decrease in bacterial load ($\log_{10}$ bacterial load/ml sputum), as derived from the model. (Adapted from Copyright © American Society for Microbiology, *Journal of Clinical Microbiology*, Vol 49, 2011, pp. 3905–3911, DOI 10.1128/JCM.00547-11.)

Table 12.1. Liquid culture and 16S rRNA sputum tuberculosis detection after 8 weeks of therapy for 110 individuals. Upper panel: total sputum samples positive and negative for each assay. Lower panel: distribution of positive and negative culture at each bacterial load measured using 16S rRNA. (Adapted from Copyright © American Society for Microbiology, *Journal of Clinical Microbiology*, Vol 49, 2011, pp. 3905–3911, DOI 10.1128/JCM.00547-11.)

16S rRNA	Liquid culture	
+	+	37
–	–	23
+	–	10
–	+	24
Result	Contaminated	15
Failed	Result	1

16S rRNA measured bacterial load/ml sputum	Liquid culture	
	+	–
$1–5 \times 10^2$	12	9
$1–5 \times 10^3$	22	1
$1–5 \times 10^4$	2	0
$1–5 \times 10^5$	1	0

References

Aber, V.R. and Nunn, A.J. (1978) Short-term chemotherapy of tuberculosis. Factors affecting relapse following short term chemotherapy. *Bulletin of the International Union against Tuberculosis and Lung Disease* 53(4), 276–280.

Brindle, R., Odhiambo, J. and Mitchison, D. (2001) Serial counts of *Mycobacterium tuberculosis* in sputum as surrogate markers of the sterilising activity of rifampicin and pyrazinamide in treating pulmonary tuberculosis. *BMC Pulmonary Medicine* 1, 2.

Davies, A.P., Dhillon, A.P., Young, M., Henderson, B., McHugh, T.D. and Gillespie, S.H. (2008) Resuscitation-promoting factors are expressed in *Mycobacterium tuberculosis*-infected human tissue. *Tuberculosis (Edinburgh)* 88(5), 462–468.

Davies, G.R., Brindle, R., Khoo, S.H. and Aarons, L.J. (2006) Use of nonlinear mixed-effects analysis for improved precision of early pharmacodynamic measures in tuberculosis treatment. *Antimicrobial Agents and Chemotherapy* 50(9), 3154–3156.

de Wit, D., Wootton, M., Dhillon, J. and Mitchison, D.A. (1995) The bacterial DNA content of mouse organs in the Cornell model of dormant tuberculosis. *Tuberculosis and Lung Disease* 76(6), 555–562.

Desjardin, L.E., Perkins, M.D., Wolski, K., Haun, S., Teixeira, L., Chen, Y., *et al.* (1999) Measurement of sputum *Mycobacterium tuberculosis* messenger RNA as a surrogate for response to chemotherapy. *Amercian Journal of Respiratory and Critical Care Medicine* 160(1), 203–210.

Donald, P.R., Sirgel, F.A., Kanyok, T.P., Danziger, H., Venter, A., Botha, F.J., *et al.* (2000) Early bactericidal activity of paromomycin (aminosidine) in patients with smear-positive pulmonary tuberculosis. *Antimicrobial Agents and Chemotherapy* 44(12), 3285–3287.

Hellyer, T.J., Fletcher, T.W., Bates, J.H., Stead, W.W., Templeton, G.L., Cave, M.D., *et al.* (1996) Strand displacement amplification and the polymerase chain reaction for monitoring response to treatment in patients with pulmonary tuberculosis. *Journal of Infectious Diseases* 173(4), 934–941.

Hellyer, T.J., DesJardin, L.E., Hehman, G.L., Cave, D. and Eisenach, K.D. (1999a) Quantitative analysis of mRNA as a marker for viability of *Mycobacterium tuberculosis*. *Journal of Clinical Microbiology* 37(2), 290–295.

Hellyer, T.J., DesJardin, L.E., Teixeira, L., Perkins, M.D., Cave, M.D. and Eisenach, K.D. (1999b) Detection of viable *Mycobacterium tuberculosis* by reverse transcriptase-strand displacement amplification of mRNA. *Journal of Clinical Microbiology* 37(3), 518–523.

Hesseling, A.C., Walzl, G., Enarson, D.A., Carroll, N.M., Duncan, K., Lukey, P.Y., *et al.* (2010) Baseline sputum time to detection predicts month two culture conversion and relapse in non-HIV-infected patients. *The International Journal of Tuberculosis and Lung Disease* 14(5), 560–570.

Honeyborne, I., McHugh, T.D., Phillips, P.P., Bannoo, S., Bateson, A., Carroll, N., *et al.* (2011) Molecular bacterial load assay, a culture-free biomarker for rapid and accurate quantification of sputum *Mycobacterium tuberculosis* bacillary load during treatment. *Journal of Clinical Microbiology* 49(11), 3905–3911.

Johnson, J.L., Hadad, D.J., Dietze, R., Maciel, E.L., Sewali, B., Gitta, P., *et al.* (2009) Shortening treatment in adults with noncavitary tuberculosis and 2-month culture conversion. *American Journal of Respiratory and Critical Care Medicine* 180(6), 558–563.

Kennedy, N., Gillespie, S.H., Saruni, A.O., Kisyombe, G., McNerney, R., Ngowi, F.I., *et al.* (1994) Polymerase chain reaction for assessing treatment response in patients with pulmonary tuberculosis. *Journal of Infectious Diseases* 170(3), 713–716.

Li, L., Mahan, C.S., Palaci, M., Horter, L., Loeffelholz, L., Johnson, J.L., *et al.* (2010) Sputum *Mycobacterium tuberculosis* mRNA as a marker of bacteriologic clearance in response to antituberculosis therapy. *Journal of Clinical Microbiology* 48(1), 46–51.

Mitchison, D.A. (1993) Assessment of new sterilizing drugs for treating pulmonary tuberculosis by culture at 2 months. *American Review Respiratory Disease* 147(4), 1062–1063.

Moore, D.F., Curry, J.I., Knott, C.A. and Jonas, V. (1996) Amplification of rRNA for assessment of treatment response of pulmonary tuberculosis patients during antimicrobial therapy. *Journal of Clinical Microbiology* 34(7), 1745–1749.

Monahan, I.M., Mangan, J.A. and Butcher, P.D. (2001) Extraction of RNA from intracellular *Mycobacterium tuberculosis*: methods, considerations, and applications. In: Parish, T. and Stoker, N.G. (eds) Mycobacterium tuberculosis *Protocols: Methods in Molecular Medicine*. Humana Press, Totowa, New Jersey.

Mukamolova, G.V., Turapov, O., Malkin, J., Woltmann, G. and Barer, M.R. (2010) Resuscitation-promoting factors reveal an occult population of tubercle bacilli in sputum. *American Journal of Respiratory and Critical Care Medicine* 181(2), 174–180.

Rustomjee, R., Lienhardt, C., Kanyok, T., Davies, G.R., Levin, J., Mthivane, T., *et al.* (2008) A Phase II study of the sterilising activities of ofloxacin, gatifloxacin and moxifloxacin in pulmonary tuberculosis. *International Journal of Tuberculosis and Lung Disease* 12(2), 128–138.

Shleeva, M.O., Bagramyan, K., Telkov, M.V., Mukamolova, G.V., Young, M., Kell, D.B., *et al.* (2002) Formation and resuscitation of 'non-culturable' cells of *Rhodococcus rhodochrous* and *Mycobacterium tuberculosis* in prolonged stationary phase. *Microbiology* 148(Pt 5), 1581–1591.

Silva, M.T., Appelberg, R., Silva, M.N. and Macedo, P.M. (1987) *In vivo* killing and degradation of *Mycobacterium aurum* within mouse peritoneal macrophages. *Infection and Immunity* 55(9), 2006–2016.

13 Transcriptomic Approaches to Mapping Responses to Drug Therapy for Tuberculosis

Simon J. Waddell[1] and Philip D. Butcher[2]

[1]*Brighton and Sussex Medical School, University of Sussex, Brighton, UK;*
[2]*Centre for Infection and Immunity, Division of Clinical Sciences,*
St George's University of London, UK

13.1 Introduction

Understanding how anti-tuberculosis drugs work is fundamental to developing novel chemotherapy strategies; transcriptional profiling of the response of *Mycobacterium tuberculosis* bacilli to drug exposure offers important clues to the mode of action of both new and existing compounds (Sacchettini *et al.*, 2008; Barry and Blanchard, 2010). Global gene expression profiling by microarray was first applied to *M. tuberculosis* in 1999, when Wilson and colleagues explored the action of isoniazid (INH) and ethionamide (ETA) on log-phase bacilli (Wilson *et al.*, 1999). Since then, contrasting and dissecting the transcriptional responses of *M. tuberculosis* bacilli to antimycobacterial agents has become an integral element of the drug discovery toolbox. Global mRNA profiling is particularly suited to tackling three key scenarios in the drug development pipeline. First, to identify targets for rational drug design by defining pathways used by bacilli in axenic, intracellular or *in vivo* models of *M. tuberculosis* infection. Second, in a hypothesis-generating capacity, to characterize the mode of action of compounds isolated from whole cell screens or mechanisms of resistance in drug-resistant strains. Third, as an unsupervised global approach, to confirm compound-target selectivity and detect mutagenic signatures during hit-to-lead medicinal chemistry. As such, while the experimental set-up is involved and the results often difficult to interpret, transcriptional profiling contributes considerably to multiple stages of early antibacterial drug discovery; as summarized in Fig. 13.1. This chapter focuses on the applications of gene expression profiling, derived predominantly from microarray analyses, towards the development of novel compounds and a greater understanding of drug action in *M. tuberculosis*.

13.2 Identifying Compound Class and Mechanism of Action

The genome-wide measurement of transcript abundance offers a molecular landscape of pathways used by *M. tuberculosis* bacilli in the particular microenvironment modelled. Thus, the comparison of mRNA profiles in the presence or absence of a compound that inhibits a key target captures the effects that

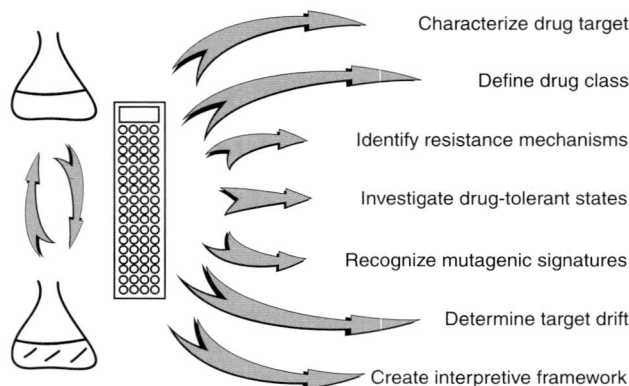

Fig. 13.1. The applications of *M. tuberculosis* transcriptional profiling through the drug development process, from the comparison of drug-treated with drug-free mRNA signatures derived from log-phase bacilli.

abrogation of this enzyme might have on every cellular process. This global approach has therefore been employed to reveal, at the transcriptional level, which pathways are influenced by the actions of antimycobacterial compounds. The first proof-of-principle study, by Wilson *et al.* (1999), demonstrated that the mechanism of action of a known drug, INH, could be inferred from the genes expressed divergently after INH treatment. Genes associated with the FAS-II cycle (*fabD*, *acpM*, *kasA*, *kasB*, *accD6*), involved in the elongation of mycolic acids, were induced after INH (or ETA) exposure. Thus, although the enoyl-ACP reductase InhA (encoded by *inhA*), the target of INH, was not itself upregulated in the presence of INH, genes in the FAS-II pathway were significantly differentially expressed. This approach was expanded by the studies of Betts *et al.* (2003) and Waddell *et al.* (2004), where common and drug-specific signatures were defined for a range of antimycobacterial compounds. The former investigation employed a stepwise linear-discriminant analysis that was able to predict the antibiotic applied (from three compounds all targeting fatty acid biosynthesis) based on the expression pattern of 21 genes. The seminal work of Boshoff and colleagues categorized the responses of *M. tuberculosis* bacilli to 75 different drugs or drug combinations and demonstrated that compounds with similar modes of action

generated analogous transcriptional signatures (Boshoff *et al.*, 2004), therefore confirming that the class of an antibiotic could be defined by the bacterial transcriptional response to drug exposure.

Contrasting these drug class-specific gene expression signatures may also reveal novel modes of action for existing (and newly discovered) compounds. For example, the profile derived after exposure to triclosan, an inhibitor of mycolic acid synthesis (InhA), did not cluster with known cell wall-targeting drugs but rather with a group of compounds that acted by inhibiting mycobacterial respiration. This led the authors to propose an alternative mechanism for triclosan-mediated killing (Boshoff *et al.*, 2004). Likewise, the transcriptional response of *M. tuberculosis* to the nitroimidazole PA-824 revealed signatures representative of both cell wall inhibition and respiratory poisoning. This multifactorial profile highlighted to the authors that PA-824 might have dual mechanisms of action; targeting cell wall biosynthesis in log-phase growth and mediating killing via nitric oxide in hypoxic non-replicating bacilli (Manjunatha *et al.*, 2009). The use of such an interpretive framework of drug-induced transcriptional patterns to classify novel compounds has been highlighted recently (Makarov *et al.*, 2009). The mycobacterial response to benzothiazinones (BTZs) was highly similar to the signature derived after exposure of *M. tuberculosis* bacilli to ethambutol (EMB). Subsequent investigations demonstrated that this new class of anti-mycobacterial compound prevented the generation of arabinogalactan precursors, specifically decaprenylphosphoryl arabinose mediated by Rv3790, a decaprenylphosphoryl-beta-d-ribose 2'-epimerase (Makarov *et al.*, 2009; Trefzer *et al.*, 2010). Furthermore, the BTZ-target epimerase Rv3790 acts in the same pathway two enzymatic steps upstream of the arabinosyl-transferases (encoded by *embC/A/B*) that are inhibited by EMB (Belanger *et al.*, 1996). Thus, BTZ and EMB, both targeting the mycobacterial cell wall by preventing formation of arabinogalactan-mycolyl structures, exert similar stresses on multiple processes within the cell. Correspondingly, the transcriptional profiles derived from these two compounds overlap considerably (Makarov *et al.*, 2009). In such a way, a drug-induced transcriptional signature alongside profiles of target knockdown or conditional overexpression linked to changes in minimum inhibitory concentration (MIC) becomes an effective method of target validation for drug discovery programmes.

A useful feature of these analyses is the ability to scrutinize crude extracts demonstrating antimycobacterial activity. This is particularly relevant to natural product screens, where, for example, the RNA signature derived after exposure of *M. tuberculosis* to an unrefined sample of the marine tunicate *Eudistoma amplum* is analogous to that of the purified active compound, ascididemin (Boshoff *et al.*, 2004).

13.3 The Multifactorial Nature of INH Exposure as a Paradigm of Complex *M. tuberculosis* Responses

The effects of drug-mediated enzyme inhibition may influence multiple metabolic processes in the mycobacterial cell, all of which may be reflected in the changing *M. tuberculosis* transcriptome. Here, we describe briefly the mechanism of INH killing to exemplify the complexity of drug-induced stresses and how this may contribute to the INH-induced transcriptional signature. These consider-ations are also summarized in Fig. 13.2; for a detailed review of INH activity, see Vilcheze and Jacobs (2007). INH enters the bacterium by passive diffusion, where the prodrug is converted to an active INH–NAD adduct by a catalase-peroxidase-peroxynitritase (encoded by *katG*). The transformation of INH into the INH–NAD adduct requires NAD+ and KatG catalase activity, which might usually perform antioxidative/nitrosative functions. This process may also generate nitric oxide radicals, with toxic consequences (Timmins and Deretic, 2006). Thus, conversion of INH to the active INH–NAD adduct may influence the mycobacterial NAD+/NADP+ pool and the ability of bacilli to respond to reactive oxygen and nitrogen intermediates. Efflux pumps (such as IniB/A/C) may remove both INH and INH–NAD moieties from the cell. The INH–NAD adduct acts primarily to inhibit elongation of mycolic acids (targeting the enoyl-ACP reductase, encoded by *inhA*), although additional targets (products of *kasA*, *fabG1/mabA* and *dfrA*) have been proposed (Argyrou *et al.*, 2006; Timmins and Deretic, 2006; Vilcheze and Jacobs, 2007; Wang *et al.*, 2010). Abrogation of enoyl-ACP reductase activity as part of fatty acid synthesis (FAS-II) results in defective mycolic acid biosynthesis. This results in the build-up of precursors from FAS-I and intermediate saturated fatty acids that feed into FAS-II, and perhaps also an excess of cofactors that normally form complex structures with full-length mycolic acids. Finally, the inability to generate mature full-length mycolic acids presumably leads to a breakdown in the structure of the mycobacterial cell wall and cell death as membrane integrity is impaired. It is a combination of these effects that are captured in the INH-transcriptional signature, reflecting changes in the flux of fatty acid intermediates (*fadB*, *acpM*, *kasA*, *kasB*, *accD6*, *fbpC*), removal or impact of toxic intermediates (*aphC*, *efpA*, *iniB/A/C*) and maintenance of membrane potential and the cell wall structure.

Thus, besides identifying drug mode of action, mapping the transcriptional responses to antimicrobial compounds acts as a tool for exploring complex patterns of differential gene regulation in response to multiple

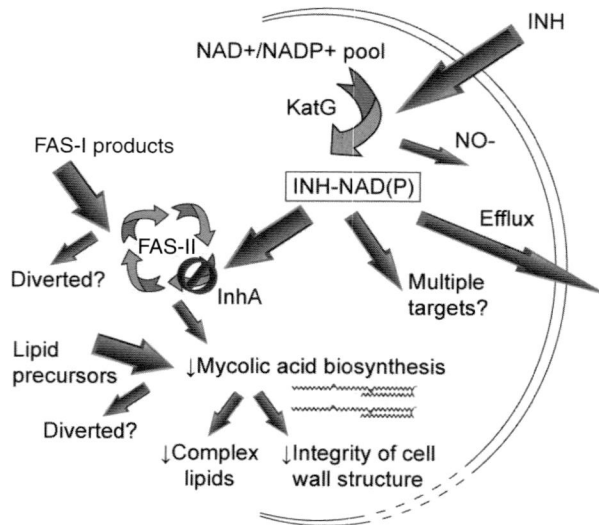

Fig. 13.2. The multifactorial impact of INH exposure on *M. tuberculosis* bacilli, highlighting the multiple stimuli that likely contribute to the complex drug-induced transcriptional signature.

stimuli. For example, in addition to identifying molecular markers for cell cycle arrest, chemical inhibition of FtsZ and FtsI highlighted regulatory networks associated with the cessation of septum formation and mycobacterial replication (Slayden *et al.*, 2006; Slayden and Belisle, 2009).

13.4 Temporal and Concentration-dependent Signatures

A number of additional parameters, other than mechanism of action, influence the bacterial response to drug exposure, including secondary effects that result from bacterial killing. Modification of experimental conditions may be used to define drug action further and the regulation of gene expression in *M. tuberculosis*. For example, the *kas* operon (*Rv2243–Rv2247*) was induced maximally after 2 h exposure to ×1 MIC thiolactomycin (which targets the β-ketoacyl-ACP synthases encoded by *kasA* and *kasB*), while the highest induction of the *kas* operon by INH (which inhibits the enoyl-ACP reductase coded by

inhA also in the FAS-II cycle) was after 6 h treatment with ×5 MIC INH. Thus, the contrasting kinetics of these responses highlights the different primary targets of these FAS-II inhibitory drugs (Betts *et al.*, 2003). The length of antimycobacterial drug treatment clearly impacts on the transcriptional response observed, in most cases with a greater number of genes (with increasing magnitude) differentially expressed with time compared to drug-free control cultures. Commonly selected time points range from 2 to 6 h post-exposure to define the initial drug-induced modifications. This relatively discrete primary response is likely to be most useful for recognizing the key pathways targeted. Later time intervals of 12–48 h, incorporating the secondary effects of drug exposure as bacilli are killed, may be more applicable to distinguishing between compound classes. The concentration of compound administered may also influence differential expression patterns, with an increase in dose often correlating with greater transcriptional regulation (both magnitude of expression and number of genes). MICs from ×1 to ×50 are routinely used, with ×10 MIC a common starting point (Boshoff *et al.*, 2004; Waddell *et al.*, 2004). Subinhibitory concentrations usually accompanied by longer time intervals have also been assessed; such as 0.5× MIC mefloquine for 24 h (Danelishvili *et al.*, 2005), or 0.5× MIC and 0.25× MIC ciprofloxacin for 24 h (O'Sullivan *et al.*, 2008). Both temporal and dose-dependent signatures are contingent on the dynamics of mycobacterial killing that will vary for each compound profiled. The metabolic state of bacilli will also mediate the efficacy and transcriptional adaptations to drug exposure. This will be discussed further in the following sections; suffice to say that most studies describe signatures derived from log-phase bacilli, as this is the setting where maximal antimicrobial activity is usually achieved.

Technical parameters such as the choice of assay (quantitative RT-PCR, microarray platform, RNAseq) also contribute to variation between studies and must be considered. However, a high degree of correlation between gene expression patterns determined by qRT-PCR and microarray methodologies and the identification of core sets of genes induced by the same drug in multiple reports, for example INH (Wilson *et al.*, 1999; Betts *et al.*, 2003; Boshoff *et al.*, 2004; Waddell *et al.*, 2004; Fu, 2006), demonstrate that the technical variation between methodologies can be minimized. Other experimental details such as the stabilization of RNA during extraction may contribute significantly to variation in signatures (Waddell and Butcher, 2010). Gene expression analyses are, in most cases, comparative; therefore, the choice of comparator condition also impacts on the divergent transcriptional patterns generated. Studies usually contrast drug-exposed to drug-free or, more usefully, carrier-control cultures, where the same volume of solvent used to re-suspend the antimicrobial compounds (usually sterilized water, ethanol or DMSO) acts as the control. Finally, the gene expression signature will be biased fundamentally towards the pathways that are regulated at the transcriptional level. The accumulation of precursors or the deprivation of intermediates resulting from drug action will only be reflected through transcriptionally regulated

feedback or compensatory mechanisms that manifest in detectable differences in relative transcript abundance.

13.5 Characterizing *M. tuberculosis* Drug Resistance and Drug Tolerance

The gene expression signatures of drug-resistant and drug-sensitive *M. tuberculosis* strains have been compared successfully to highlight putative mechanisms of drug resistance. Milano and colleagues contrasted the transcriptional profiles of a spontaneous bifonazole-resistant *M. tuberculosis* mutant with sensitive wild-type *M. tuberculosis* (in the absence of drug) to reveal overexpression of the gene cluster *Rv0676c* (*mmpL5*), *Rv0677c* (*mmpS5*) and *Rv0678* in the resistant mutant. This gene cluster has been hypothesized to function as a mycobacterial efflux system. Mutations were identified in the resistant strain within and upstream of *Rv0678* which could be linked to the overexpression of these genes, thus conferring a resistant phenotype (Milano *et al.*, 2009). Interestingly, the same gene cluster was also observed to be upregulated in drug-sensitive bacilli after exposure to tetrahydrolipstatin (Waddell *et al.*, 2004) and a range of other antibiotics (Boshoff *et al.*, 2004), perhaps highlighting this transport system as a multi-solute efflux pump with a role in mediating drug tolerance in *M. tuberculosis*. Where drugs require conversion into active compounds, examining the response of resistant mutants to drug exposure may help to define the mechanism of resistance. For example, no genes were significantly differentially expressed after exposure of a catalase-negative, INH-resistant *M. tuberculosis* strain to INH (Wilson *et al.*, 1999). In contrast, a characteristic INH signature was observed after treatment of an INH-resistant *M. tuberculosis* strain with partial catalase activity with high dose INH (10 μg/ml), which was not present after exposure to low dose INH (0.2 μg/ml), reflecting the functional significance of KatG in drug activation (Fu and Shinnick, 2007).

The response of drug-sensitive bacilli to antimicrobial compounds may also be exploited to recognize processes that influence drug tolerance, mechanisms through which genetically drug-sensitive bacilli are refractory to killing. Alland *et al.* (1998) identified a cluster of genes *Rv0341–Rv0343* (*iniB/A/C*) that were induced after exposure to INH and which subsequently were demonstrated to be upregulated by multiple cell wall-targeting drugs (Wilson *et al.*, 1999; Alland *et al.*, 2000; Betts *et al.*, 2003; Boshoff *et al.*, 2004; Waddell *et al.*, 2004). Functional characterization revealed that deletion of this gene cluster, likely encoding an MDR-like pump, resulted in hypersensitivity to INH, while overexpression conferred resistance to INH and EMB (Colangeli *et al.*, 2005). Factors affecting drug tolerance are not restricted to efflux systems, but may also act by detoxifying specific compounds. For example, the gene cluster *Rv3160c–Rv3162c* (encoding a putative transcriptional regulator, probable ring dehydroxylating dioxygenase and possible membrane protein, respectively) was observed to be induced by triclosan (Betts *et al.*, 2003), SRI No 967, SRI No 9190 (Waddell *et al.*, 2004) and thioridazine (Dutta *et al.*, 2010b).

Mediators that affect global transcriptional responses have also been identified to influence the basal levels of mycobacterial tolerance to antibiotics. For example, induction of the transcriptional regulatory protein WhiB7, controlling the expression of several genes implicated in intrinsic antibiotic resistance (*Rv1258c*, *Rv1473* and *Rv1988* encoding a putative efflux pump, a probable macrolide transporter and a possible ribosomal methyltransferase, respectively), was observed after exposure of *M. tuberculosis* to sub-inhibitory concentrations of erythromycin or tetracycline (Morris *et al.*, 2005). Likewise, the gene encoding sigma factor E (which responds to cell wall-related stresses) was upregulated after peptidoglycan-targeting vancomycin treatment; furthermore, deletion of *sigE* resulted in an increased sensitivity to vancomycin (Provvedi *et al.*, 2009). The global nature of mRNA profiling was utilized by Raman and Chandra (2008), who integrated the transcriptional responses of *M. tuberculosis* after drug exposure with protein–protein interaction networks to identify novel pathways that might influence drug efficacy; for

example, identifying co-targets for drug development to help prevent the emergence of resistance to drugs targeting mycolic acid biosynthesis (RecA, Rv0823c, Rv0892 and DnaE1).

In an alternative approach to delineating *M. tuberculosis* tolerance, Tudo *et al.* (2010) mapped pathways that might be responsible for a drug-tolerant phenotype by comparing the transcriptional signatures derived from log-phase bacilli (which are effectively killed by INH) with non-replicating persistent (NRP) state 2 bacilli (which are tolerant to INH) in the presence and absence of the drug. As expected, the INH-tolerant NRP2 bacilli did not respond transcriptionally to INH treatment. Furthermore, the differential expression of genes implicated in resistance to INH (such as *inhA*, *katG*, *iniB/A/C*, *fbpC*) that might affect the action of INH could not account for the abrogation of INH-mediated killing, suggesting that the changing redox status or reduced requirement for newly synthesized mycolic acids likely influenced INH efficacy in non-replicating bacilli (Tudo *et al.*, 2010). Similarly, Karakousis and co-workers demonstrated that the INH-inducible transcriptional signature diminished in bacilli isolated from a mouse hollow fibre model representing late-stage infection. The loss of this INH signature correlated with the reduced capacity of INH to kill bacilli as infection continued, and as such may be a key indicator of drug tolerance *in vivo* (Karakousis *et al.*, 2008).

13.6 Defining Relevant *In Vitro* Models for Whole Cell Screening

Besides exploring mechanisms of drug killing and mycobacterial resistance, transcriptional profiling has been used to characterize axenic conditions modelling *in vivo* environments. These analyses serve to define and mimic the conditions that *M. tuberculosis* bacilli are exposed to during natural infection. Thus, *in vitro* culture systems have allowed the dissection of transcriptional profiles of *M. tuberculosis* isolated from intracellular or *in vivo* models of infection (Schnappinger *et al.*, 2003; Talaat *et al.*, 2004; Rachman *et al.*, 2006;

Garton *et al.*, 2008; Tailleux *et al.*, 2008). These models reveal complex patterns of divergent gene expression, reflecting changes in *M. tuberculosis* respiratory and metabolic state, recently reviewed in Waddell (2010). In a complementary approach, chemostat models have been used to capture the responses of *M. tuberculosis* bacilli to specific challenges, such as carbon starvation (Hampshire *et al.*, 2004) and low oxygen (Bacon *et al.*, 2004), while nutrient starvation (Betts *et al.*, 2002), oxygen limitation (Rustad *et al.*, 2008), phosphate depletion (Rifat *et al.*, 2009) and the transition to non-replicating persistence (Muttucumaru *et al.*, 2004; Garton *et al.*, 2008) have also been characterized by microarray analyses. In addition, multi-stress *in vitro* culture conditions (low oxygen, high CO_2, low nutrients and acidic pH) have been developed and modelled using transcriptional profiling to mimic *in vivo* conditions in axenic culture (Deb *et al.*, 2009). In this way, global RNA profiling may identify, define and then verify *in vitro* modelling conditions that imitate the stresses that bacilli experience during natural infection, enabling the development of relevant whole cell screens for novel antimycobacterial compounds. The requirement for appropriate screening conditions was highlighted recently by Pethe and colleagues, who identified inhibitors that were effective *in vitro*; with no activity in the murine model of infection, however. These novel pyrimidine-imidazole compounds targeted glycerol metabolism used by mycobacteria *in vitro*, but evidently not essential to bacterial metabolism *in vivo* (Pethe *et al.*, 2010). Therefore, transcriptional profiling offers the opportunity to recognize and characterize conditions that *M. tuberculosis* bacilli must adapt to *in vivo* which are amenable to high-throughput screening.

13.7 Transcriptomic Approaches to Target Identification

Global RNA abundance data sets provide an interpretive framework to discover, assess and rank targets in a pathway-led approach to drug development. For example, the induction of genes involved in the β-oxidation of fatty acids, glyoxylate shunt and cholesterol metabolism after macrophage infection has revealed exciting new enzymatic steps for target-based high-throughput screening (McKinney *et al.*, 2000; Schnappinger *et al.*, 2003; van der Geize *et al.*, 2007). These and similar studies, defining the adaptations of *M. tuberculosis* bacilli to intracellular and *in vivo* microenvironments, also promote the identification of novel *M. tuberculosis* targets centred on exploiting the interactions of bacilli with the host immune system (Nathan *et al.*, 2008). Beyond this, the integration of these transcriptional data sets with global gene essentiality studies (Sassetti and Rubin, 2003; Sassetti *et al.*, 2003; Dutta *et al.*, 2010a) has allowed the suitability of every enzyme in the *M. tuberculosis* genome to be evaluated, formulating hierarchies of potentially druggable targets (Raman *et al.*, 2008). Furthermore, additional key enzymatic steps that may be amenable to drug inhibition have been proposed by modelling the interactions of metabolic pathways or the changing flux of carbon after drug exposure or during infection (Raman *et al.*, 2005; Shi *et al.*, 2010).

13.8 Conclusion: Transcriptional Profiling Through the Drug Discovery Pipeline

The global response of *M. tuberculosis* to antimicrobial compounds is useful in multiple stages of the drug discovery process, illustrated in Fig. 13.3. Early in the pipeline, *in vitro* models optimized for RNA profiling are often the first opportunity to assess compound attributes such as solubility or stability outside the whole cell or high-throughput screens from which the compounds are selected. The kinetics of mycobacterial killing in relation to concentration and time may also highlight key features of drug action. Drug-specific mRNA signatures may then identify or confirm mode of action (a key step in drug development), contrasting *M. tuberculosis* responses to an interpretive transcriptional framework defining compound class or target knockdown (Boshoff *et al.*, 2004). These profiles also allow potentially problematic mutagenic or nitrosative reactions to be recognized early in the drug development process (Makarov *et al.*, 2009). Finally, as new analogues for a lead compound are developed and tested, global transcriptome analysis provides a useful checkpoint enabling target drift to be detected. This was the case in a screen of diamine analogues (modelled on the structure of EMB) that identified a number of hit compounds (including SQ109) with *M. tuberculosis*-inhibitory properties. Transcriptional profiling revealed related but distinct cell wall-targeting signatures between these diamine analogues and EMB, highlighting a shift in the mechanism of action of these new effective compounds (Boshoff *et al.*, 2004; Barry and Blanchard, 2010).

A greater understanding of drug action in *M. tuberculosis* facilitates novel chemotherapeutic approaches; for example, discovery of the mechanism of BTZ-mediated killing (Makarov *et al.*, 2009) revealed DprE1/E2 (encoded by *Rv3790/3791*) to be an excellent target that may be amenable to target-based screening (Manina *et al.*, 2010). Similarly, characterization of gene products involved in the conversion or inactivation of antimicrobial compounds that are pinpointed by transcriptional profiling may precipitate alternative therapeutic strategies. For example, demonstration that the monooxygenase EthA is required for activation of the prodrug ETA has led to the development of EthR inhibitors (which block the repression of EthA by EthR), resulting in increased efficacy of thiocarbamide derivatives (Willand *et al.*, 2009). Moreover, β-lactam antibiotics have been demonstrated to be effective against *M. tuberculosis* if combined with β-lactamase inhibitors that limit the destruction of penicillins by the hydrolysing activity of chromosomally encoded β-lactamase, *blaC* (Cynamon and Palmer, 1983; Hugonnet *et al.*, 2009).

As the drug discovery pipeline is applied increasingly to search for novel compounds to control the growing threat of MDR-TB, transcriptional profiling will continue to play an important role characterizing the complex interactions between drug action and mycobacterial physiological state.

Acknowledgements

SJW was supported by the European Commission 'New Medicines for TB – NM4TB' programme (LHSP-CT-2005-018923). PDB would like to thank the Wellcome Trust for funding the Bacterial Microarray Group at St George's (Grant Nos 062511, 080039 and 086547).

The authors declare no conflicting financial interests.

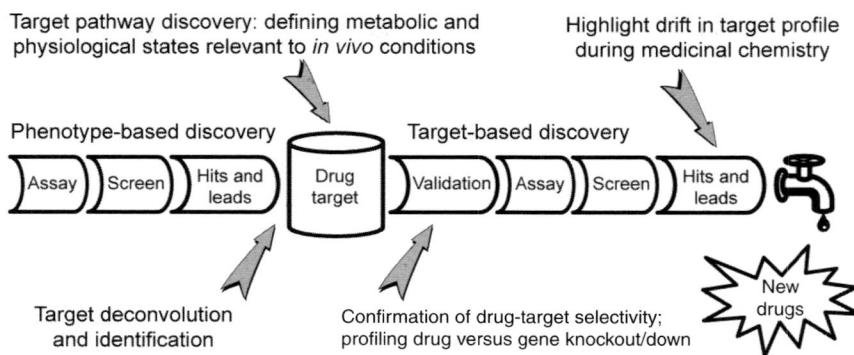

Fig. 13.3. The utility of transcriptional profiling through the drug discovery pipeline. Defining mycobacterial responses to test compounds by microarray analysis is of use at multiple stages of both phenotype and target-based screening approaches; adapted from Terstappen *et al.* (2007).

References

Alland, D., Kramnik, I., Weisbrod, T.R., Otsubo, L., Cerny, R., Miller, L.P., *et al.* (1998) Identification of differentially expressed mRNA in prokaryotic organisms by customized amplification libraries (DECAL): the effect of isoniazid on gene expression in *Mycobacterium tuberculosis*. *Proceedings of the National Academy of Sciences* 95, 13227–13232.

Alland, D., Steyn, A.J., Weisbrod, T., Aldrich, K. and Jacobs, W.R. Jr (2000) Characterization of the *Mycobacterium tuberculosis iniBAC* promoter, a promoter that responds to cell wall biosynthesis inhibition. *Journal of Bacteriology* 182, 1802–1811.

Argyrou, A., Vetting, M.W., Aladegbami, B. and Blanchard, J.S. (2006) *Mycobacterium tuberculosis* dihydrofolate reductase is a target for isoniazid. *Nature Structural and Molecular Biology* 13, 408–413.

Bacon, J., James, B.W., Wernisch, L., Williams, A., Morley, K.A., Hatch, G.J., *et al.* (2004) The influence of reduced oxygen availability on pathogenicity and gene expression in *Mycobacterium tuberculosis*. *Tuberculosis (Edinburgh)* 84, 205–217.

Barry, C.E. 3rd and Blanchard, J.S. (2010) The chemical biology of new drugs in the development for tuberculosis. *Current Opinion in Chemical Biology* 14, 456–466.

Belanger, A.E., Besra, G.S., Ford, M.E., Mikusova, K., Belisle, J.T., Brennan, P.J., *et al.* (1996) The *embAB* genes of *Mycobacterium avium* encode an arabinosyl transferase involved in cell wall arabinan biosynthesis that is the target for the antimycobacterial drug ethambutol. *Proceedings of the National Academy of Sciences* 93, 11919–11924.

Betts, J.C., Lukey, P.T., Robb, L.C., McAdam, R.A. and Duncan, K. (2002) Evaluation of a nutrient starvation model of *Mycobacterium tuberculosis* persistence by gene and protein expression profiling. *Molecular Microbiology* 43, 717–731.

Betts, J.C., McLaren, A., Lennon, M.G., Kelly, F.M., Lukey, P.T., Blakemore, S.J., *et al.* (2003) Signature gene expression profiles discriminate between isoniazid-, thiolactomycin-, and triclosan-treated *Mycobacterium tuberculosis*. *Antimicrobial Agents and Chemotherapy* 47, 2903–2913.

Boshoff, H.I., Myers, T.G., Copp, B.R., McNeil, M.R., Wilson, M.A. and Barry, C.E. 3rd (2004) The transcriptional responses of *Mycobacterium tuberculosis* to inhibitors of metabolism: novel insights into drug mechanisms of action. *The Journal of Biological Chemistry* 279, 40174–40184.

Colangeli, R., Helb, D., Sridharan, S., Sun, J., Varma-Basil, M., Hazbon, M.H., *et al.* (2005) The *Mycobacterium tuberculosis iniA* gene is essential for activity of an efflux pump that confers drug tolerance to both isoniazid and ethambutol. *Molecular Microbiology* 55, 1829–1840.

Cynamon, M.H. and Palmer, G.S. (1983) *In vitro* activity of amoxicillin in combination with clavulanic acid against *Mycobacterium tuberculosis*. *Antimicrobial Agents and Chemotherapy* 24, 429–431.

Danelishvili, L., Wu, M., Young, L.S. and Bermudez, L.E. (2005) Genomic approach to identifying the putative target of and mechanisms of resistance to mefloquine in mycobacteria. *Antimicrobial Agents and Chemotherapy* 49, 3707–3714.

Deb, C., Lee, C.M., Dubey, V.S., Daniel, J., Abomoelak, B., Sirakova, T.D., *et al.* (2009) A novel *in vitro* multiple-stress dormancy model for *Mycobacterium tuberculosis* generates a lipid-loaded, drug-tolerant, dormant pathogen. *PLoS ONE* 4, e6077.

Dutta, N.K., Mehra, S., Didier, P.J., Roy, C.J., Doyle, L.A., Alvarez, X., *et al.* (2010a) Genetic requirements for the survival of tubercle bacilli in primates. *Journal of Infectious Diseases* 201, 1743–1752.

Dutta, N.K., Mehra, S. and Kaushal, D. (2010b) A *Mycobacterium tuberculosis* sigma factor network responds to cell-envelope damage by the promising anti-mycobacterial thioridazine. *PLoS ONE* 5, e10069.

Fu, L.M. (2006) Exploring drug action on *Mycobacterium tuberculosis* using affymetrix oligonucleotide genechips. *Tuberculosis (Edinburgh)* 86, 134–143.

Fu, L.M. and Shinnick, T.M. (2007) Understanding the action of INH on a highly INH-resistant *Mycobacterium tuberculosis* strain using Genechips. *Tuberculosis (Edinburgh)* 87, 63–70.

Garton, N.J., Waddell, S.J., Sherratt, A.L., Lee, S.M., Smith, R.J., Senner, C., *et al.* (2008) Cytological and transcript analyses reveal fat and lazy persister-like bacilli in tuberculous sputum. *PLoS Medicine* 5, e75.

Hampshire, T., Soneji, S., Bacon, J., James, B.W., Hinds, J., Laing, K., *et al.* (2004) Stationary phase gene expression of *Mycobacterium tuberculosis* following a progressive nutrient depletion: a model for persistent organisms? *Tuberculosis (Edinburgh)* 84, 228–238.

Hugonnet, J.E., Tremblay, L.W., Boshoff, H.I., Barry, C.E. 3rd and Blanchard, J.S. (2009) Meropenem-clavulanate is effective against extensively drug-resistant *Mycobacterium tuberculosis*. *Science* 323, 1215–1218.

Karakousis, P.C., Williams, E.P. and Bishai, W.R. (2008) Altered expression of isoniazid-regulated genes in drug-treated dormant *Mycobacterium tuberculosis*. *Journal of Antimicrobial Chemotherapy* 61, 323–331.

McKinney, J.D., Honer zu Bentrup, K., Munoz-Elias, E.J., Miczak, A., Chen, B., Chan, W.T., *et al.* (2000) Persistence of *Mycobacterium tuberculosis* in macrophages and mice requires the glyoxylate shunt enzyme isocitrate lyase. *Nature* 406, 735–758.

Makarov, V., Manina, G., Mikusova, K., Mollmann, U., Ryabova, O., Saint-Joanis, B., *et al.* (2009) Benzothiazinones kill *Mycobacterium tuberculosis* by blocking arabinan synthesis. *Science* 324, 801–804.

Manina, G., Pasca, M.R., Buroni, S., De Rossi, E. and Riccardi, G. (2010) Decaprenylphosphoryl-beta-d-ribose 2′-epimerase from *Mycobacterium tuberculosis* is a magic drug target. *Current Medicinal Chemistry* 17, 3099–3108.

Manjunatha, U., Boshoff, H.I. and Barry, C.E. (2009) The mechanism of action of PA-824: novel insights from transcriptional profiling. *Communicative and Integrative Biology* 2, 215–218.

Milano, A., Pasca, M.R., Provvedi, R., Lucarelli, A.P., Manina, G., Ribeiro, A.L., *et al.* (2009) Azole resistance in *Mycobacterium tuberculosis* is mediated by the MmpS5-MmpL5 efflux system. *Tuberculosis (Edinburgh)* 89, 84–90.

Morris, R.P., Nguyen, L., Gatfield, J., Visconti, K., Nguyen, K., Schnappinger, D., *et al.* (2005) Ancestral antibiotic resistance in *Mycobacterium tuberculosis*. *Proceedings of the National Academy of Sciences* 102, 12200–12205.

Muttucumaru, D.G., Roberts, G., Hinds, J., Stabler, R.A. and Parish, T. (2004) Gene expression profile of *Mycobacterium tuberculosis* in a non-replicating state. *Tuberculosis (Edinburgh)* 84, 239–246.

Nathan, C., Gold, B., Lin, G., Stegman, M., De Carvalho, L.P., Vandal, O., *et al.* (2008) A philosophy of anti-infectives as a guide in the search for new drugs for tuberculosis. *Tuberculosis (Edinburgh)* 88 (Suppl 1), S25–33.

O'Sullivan, D.M., Hinds, J., Butcher, P.D., Gillespie, S.H. and McHugh, T.D. (2008) *Mycobacterium tuberculosis* DNA repair in response to subinhibitory concentrations of ciprofloxacin. *Journal of Antimicrobial Chemotherapy* 62, 1199–1202.

Pethe, K., Sequeira, P.C., Agarwalla, S., Rhee, K., Kuhen, K., Phong, W.Y., *et al.* (2010) A chemical genetic screen in *Mycobacterium tuberculosis* identifies carbon-source-dependent growth inhibitors devoid of *in vivo* efficacy. *Nature Communications* 1, 1–8.

Provvedi, R., Boldrin, F., Falciani, F., Palu, G. and Manganelli, R. (2009) Global transcriptional response to vancomycin in *Mycobacterium tuberculosis*. *Microbiology* 155, 1093–1102.

Rachman, H., Strong, M., Ulrichs, T., Grode, L., Schuchhardt, J., Mollenkopf, H., *et al.* (2006) Unique transcriptome signature of *Mycobacterium tuberculosis* in pulmonary tuberculosis. *Infection and Immunity* 74, 1233–1242.

Raman, K. and Chandra, N. (2008) *Mycobacterium tuberculosis* interactome analysis unravels potential pathways to drug resistance. *BMC Microbiology* 8, 234.

Raman, K., Rajagopalan, P. and Chandra, N. (2005) Flux balance analysis of mycolic acid pathway: targets for anti-tubercular drugs. *PLoS Computational Biology* 1, e46.

Raman, K., Yeturu, K. and Chandra, N. (2008) TargetTB: a target identification pipeline for *Mycobacterium tuberculosis* through an inter-actome, reactome and genome-scale structural analysis. *BMC Systems Biology* 2, 109.

Rifat, D., Bishai, W.R. and Karakousis, P.C. (2009) Phosphate depletion: a novel trigger for *Mycobacterium tuberculosis* persistence. *Journal of Infectious Diseases* 200, 1126–1135.

Rustad, T.R., Harrell, M.I., Liao, R. and Sherman, D.R. (2008) The enduring hypoxic response of *Mycobacterium tuberculosis*. *PLoS ONE* 3, e1502.

Sacchettini, J.C., Rubin, E.J. and Freundlich, J.S. (2008) Drugs versus bugs: in pursuit of the persistent predator *Mycobacterium tuberculosis*. *Nature Reviews Microbiology* 6, 41–52.

Sassetti, C.M. and Rubin, E.J. (2003) Genetic requirements for mycobacterial survival during infection. *Proceedings of the National Academy of Sciences* 100, 12989–12994.

Sassetti, C.M., Boyd, D.H. and Rubin, E.J. (2003) Genes required for mycobacterial growth defined by high density mutagenesis. *Molecular Microbiology* 48, 77–84.

Schnappinger, D., Ehrt, S., Voskuil, M.I., Liu, Y., Mangan, J.A., Monahan, I.M., *et al.* (2003) Transcriptional adaptation of *Mycobacterium tuberculosis* within macrophages: insights into the phagosomal environment. *The Journal of Experimental Medicine* 198, 693–704.

Shi, L., Sohaskey, C.D., Pfeiffer, C., Datta, P., Parks,

M., McFadden, J., et al. (2010) Carbon flux rerouting during Mycobacterium tuberculosis growth arrest. Molecular Microbiology 78, 1199–1215.

Slayden, R.A. and Belisle, J.T. (2009) Morphological features and signature gene response elicited by inactivation of FtsI in Mycobacterium tuberculosis. Journal of Antimicrobial Chemotherapy 63, 451–457.

Slayden, R.A., Knudson, D.L. and Belisle, J.T. (2006) Identification of cell cycle regulators in Mycobacterium tuberculosis by inhibition of septum formation and global transcriptional analysis. Microbiology 152, 1789–1797.

Tailleux, L., Waddell, S.J., Pelizzola, M., Mortellaro, A., Withers, M., Tanne, A., et al. (2008) Probing host pathogen cross-talk by transcriptional profiling of both Mycobacterium tuberculosis and infected human dendritic cells and macrophages. PLoS ONE 3, e1403.

Talaat, A.M., Lyons, R., Howard, S.T. and Johnston, S.A. (2004) The temporal expression profile of Mycobacterium tuberculosis infection in mice. Proceedings of the National Academy of Sciences 101, 4602–4607.

Terstappen, G.C., Schlupen, C., Raggiaschi, R. and Gaviraghi, G. (2007) Target deconvolution strategies in drug discovery. Nature Reviews Drug Discovery 6, 891–903.

Timmins, G.S. and Deretic, V. (2006) Mechanisms of action of isoniazid. Molecular Microbiology 62, 1220–1227.

Trefzer, C., Rengifo-Gonzalez, M., Hinner, M.J., Schneider, P., Makarov, V., Cole, S.T., et al. (2010) Benzothiazinones: prodrugs that covalently modify the decaprenylphosphoryl-beta-d-ribose 2'-epimerase DprE1 of Mycobacterium tuberculosis. Journal of the American Chemical Society 132, 13663–13665.

Tudo, G., Laing, K., Mitchison, D.A., Butcher, P.D. and Waddell, S.J. (2010) Examining the basis of isoniazid tolerance in non-replicating Mycobacterium tuberculosis using transcriptional profiling. Future Medicinal Chemistry 2, 1371–1383.

Van der Geize, R., Yam, K., Heuser, T., Wilbrink, M.H., Hara, H., Anderton, M.C., et al. (2007) A gene cluster encoding cholesterol catabolism in a soil actinomycete provides insight into Mycobacterium tuberculosis survival in macrophages. Proceedings of the National Academy of Sciences 104, 1947–1952.

Vilcheze, C. and Jacobs, W.R. Jr (2007) The mechanism of isoniazid killing: clarity through the scope of genetics. Annual Review of Microbiology 61, 35–50.

Waddell, S.J. (2010) Reprogramming the Mycobacterium tuberculosis transcriptome during host pathogenesis. Drug Discovery Today: Disease Mechanisms 7, e67–e73.

Waddell, S.J. and Butcher, P.D. (2010) Use of DNA arrays to study transcriptional responses to antimycobacterial compounds. Methods in Molecular Biology 642, 75–91.

Waddell, S.J., Stabler, R.A., Laing, K., Kremer, L., Reynolds, R.C. and Besra, G.S. (2004) The use of microarray analysis to determine the gene expression profiles of Mycobacterium tuberculosis in response to anti-bacterial compounds. Tuberculosis (Edinburgh) 84, 263–274.

Wang, F., Jain, P., Gulten, G., Liu, Z., Feng, Y., Ganesula, K., et al. (2010) Mycobacterium tuberculosis dihydrofolate reductase is not a target relevant to the antitubercular activity of isoniazid. Antimicrobial Agents and Chemotherapy 54, 3776–3782.

Willand, N., Dirie, B., Carette, X., Bifani, P., Singhal, A., Desroses, M., et al. (2009) Synthetic EthR inhibitors boost antituberculous activity of ethionamide. Nature Medicine 15, 537–544.

Wilson, M., Derisi, J., Kristensen, H.H., Imboden, P., Rane, S., Brown, P.O., et al. (1999) Exploring drug-induced alterations in gene expression in Mycobacterium tuberculosis by microarray hybridization. Proceedings of the National Academy of Sciences 96, 12833–12838.

14 Mycobacterial Lipid Bodies and Resuscitation-promoting Factor Dependency as Potential Biomarkers of Response to Chemotherapy

N.J. Garton,[1] G.V. Mukamolova[1] and M.R. Barer[1,2]

[1]Department of Infection, Immunity and Inflammation, University of Leicester College of Medicine, Biological Sciences and Psychology, Leicester, UK; [2]Department of Clinical Microbiology, University Hospitals of Leicester NHS Trust, Leicester, UK

14.1 Introduction

Current chemotherapy regimens for the treatment of tuberculosis are lengthy and generally require a combination of four antibiotics. This can lead to a breakdown in patient compliance and an increased risk of developing multidrug-resistant *Mycobacterium tuberculosis* strains. The development of new therapeutic agents and regimes with the potential to reduce the length of treatment is therefore an ongoing major focus of research. An additional goal is the identification and assessment of prognostic biomarkers of treatment response and clinical end points (Wallis *et al.*, 2010).

The current requirement for a prolonged multidrug regimen is a likely consequence of the heterogeneous physiological states of the causative *M. tuberculosis* bacilli in the infected host (Mitchison, 1979, 2004). Rapidly replicating *M. tuberculosis* bacilli are killed relatively quickly through the action of the frontline antibiotics, isoniazid (INH) and rifampicin (rifampin; RIF); however, it is believed that *M. tuberculosis* can persist in a non-replicating state in host tissues. Although genetically susceptible to antibiotics, *M. tuberculosis* bacilli in a non-replicating persistent state exhibit phenotypic antibiotic resistance (Connolly *et al.*, 2007; Dhar and McKinney, 2007), and it is this trait which complicates tuberculosis therapy. The 'persister' population in infection has never been directly identified, but is inferred from the biphasic reduction of viable counts recovered from serial sputum samples collected during therapy (Mitchison, 2004). The factors which promote *M. tuberculosis* persistence are not understood, but hostile host conditions within the caseating lung granulomas such as hypoxia, low pH and nutrient limitation may contribute. When these lesions liquefy and erode into the lower airways, cavities are formed. The cavitary lesions support rapid bacillary replication, resulting in continuous discharge of bacilli expectorated in sputum. In addition to being representative of those bacilli that go on to transmit disease, the bacilli in sputum represent a sample of those which must be eliminated by chemotherapy. The findings of our studies of the phenotypes of *M. tuberculosis* bacilli in sputum challenge the long-held belief that the bacilli are replicating rapidly; instead, available evidence supports the hypothesis that they are in a slowly growing or non-replicating state, which we have termed persister-like (Garton *et al.*, 2002, 2008; Mukamolova *et al.*, 2010). As smear-positive sputum must be populated regularly with *M. tuberculosis*, we hypothesize that at some point during the relatively short time taken for discharge from the cavity to expectoration, the bacilli adapt to a persister-like state. The environmental signals which lead to this adaptation are not known. Here, we discuss the sputum phenotypes we have identified and their potential as biomarkers for the assessment of patient response to therapy.

14.2 Sputum Phenotypes

14.2.1 Slow/non-growth

Microarray analysis of the global transcriptome of *M. tuberculosis* in sputum expectorated by four individual smear-positive patients, in comparison with that of *in vitro* aerobic log-phase growth of the *M. tuberculosis* strain H37Rv, revealed many transcript signatures suggestive of slow or non-growth (Garton *et al.*, 2008). Strikingly similar, the transcriptomes of the four *M. tuberculosis* samples had a unique profile; no single or combination of defined conditions previously reported *in vitro* or *in vivo* corresponded. Compared with the log-phase H37Rv growth, there were significant decreases in the transcription of genes required for aerobic respiration, ribosomal function and ATP synthesis, with increased expression of genes belonging to the DosR regulon, which has been widely linked to dormancy (Voskuil *et al.*, 2004). Two lines of evidence support the view that the sputum transcriptome represents a population dominated by slowly or non-replicating cells. First, the *in vitro* transcriptomes of *M. tuberculosis* in well-recognized growth arrest, those of nutrient starvation (Betts *et al.*, 2002) and the second non-replicating persistence phase

(NRP2) of the Wayne dormancy model (Wayne and Hayes, 1996; Muttucamaru *et al.*, 2004; Voskuil *et al.*, 2004) showed significant overlaps, with genes downregulated in the sputum transcriptome. Second, there were significant similarities with the transcriptome of *M. tuberculosis* during chronic murine infection, a point at which exponential bacterial replication had ceased. The *M. tuberculosis* transcripts associated with chronic murine infection reflect a shift from aerobic to anaerobic respiration (Shi *et al.*, 2005).

14.2.2 Lipid bodies

Lipid bodies (LBs) are neutral lipid-containing (triacylglycerol (TAG) and wax ester (WE)) inclusions in actinobacteria; they were recently recognized as the bacterial equivalent of the LBs that occur in eukaryotes (Wältermann and Steinbüchel, 2005). We first identified LBs by fluorescence microscopy following Nile Red staining of the rapidly growing non-pathogenic strain *M. smegmatis* and noted that the presence and appearance of LBs, and associated TAG fatty acid content, reflected the culture conditions (Garton *et al.*, 2002). By application of Nile Red in combination with auramine acid-fast staining, we observed that, in contrast to growing laboratory cultures, *M. tuberculosis* cells in sputum contained well-defined LBs at frequencies varying from 3% to 87% of the auramine-staining population (Garton *et al.*, 2002, 2008). We were able to identify an LB-positive subpopulation in most smear-positive sputum samples examined this way, a complicating factor being high Nile Red background staining of host-derived material in some samples. The same LBs can be revealed with an alternative lipophilic reagent, LipidTox red neutral lipid stain. Figure 14.1 shows LB-positive acid-fast cells revealed with LipidTox red neutral lipid labelling of a smear-positive tuberculous sample.

The transcriptome of *M. tuberculosis* in sputum revealed the upregulation of *Rv3130c* (*tgs1*) (Garton *et al.*, 2008), which encode the most active of 15 TAG synthases (Daniel *et al.*, 2004). Overexpression of *tgs1* in *M. smegmatis*

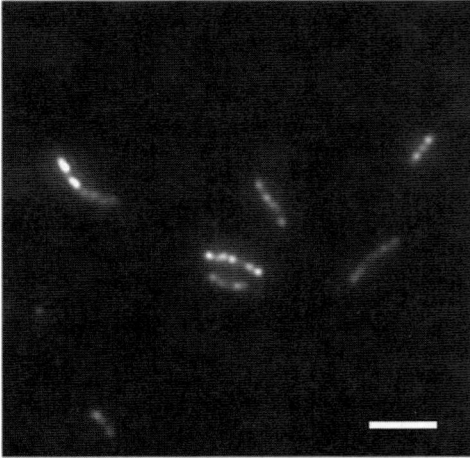

Fig. 14.1. Lipid bodies within acid-fast bacilli in an auramine/LipidTox red neutral lipid labelled, fixed tuberculous sputum smear.

and analysis of Nile Red staining of the overexpressing and plasmid control strains revealed that *tgs1* was involved in LB formation; the *tgs1* overexpressing strain contained larger, more intensely stained LBs (Garton *et al.*, 2008). A recent study aimed at identifying LB-associated proteins reported that *tgs1* in addition to *tgs2* (*Rv3734c*, the second most active TAG synthase) were both associated physically with LBs isolated from hypoxic non-replicating *M. bovis* bacillus Calmette-Guérin (BCG) (Low *et al.*, 2010).

We have so far reported inability to detect LBs in growing *M. tuberculosis* cultures *in vitro* and their induction by conditions that produce growth arrest and stimulation of the DosR regulon (of which *tgs1* is a constituent). These conditions include exposure to nitric oxide and Wayne-type non-replicating persistence (Garton *et al.*, 2008). This pattern of LB occurrence we have described has recently been substantiated in *M. bovis* BCG taken from the Wayne model (Low *et al.*, 2009, 2010). Rifat and colleagues report that phosphate limitation, a nutrient stress likely encountered by *M. tuberculosis* in macrophages, results in a dose-dependent restriction in *M. tuberculosis* growth (Rifat *et al.*, 2009). We have also identified LB-positive cells in *M. tuberculosis* biomass produced by

phosphate limitation in a chemostat (Sherrat *et al.*, unpublished results). An increasing population of LB-positive *M. tuberculosis* cells has been identified throughout the duration of a multiple-stress model of dormancy (Deb *et al.*, 2009), which involved incubation at low O_2, high CO_2, nutrient deprivation and low pH. Intriguingly, during the Deb multiple-stress model, the increase in the proportion of LB-positive cells was concomitant with a decrease in the auramine acid-fast cell population. We have made observations that are compatible with the possible presence of such cells in sputum (unpublished results) and are developing methods for quantifying the microscopically distinct sputum subpopulations accurately. Together, these results describing the LB-positive *M. tuberculosis* cells in conditions which limit growth and model persistence support our hypothesis that such persister-like cells are present in sputum (Garton *et al.*, 2008).

14.2.3 Resuscitation-promoting factor dependency

The resuscitation-promoting factor (Rpf) was first described as a protein which stimulated the growth and resuscitation of non-replicating cells of *Micrococcus luteus* (Mukamolova *et al.*, 1998). Rpf is an essential gene in *M. luteus* which is secreted into culture medium and is also detected on the surface of growing cells (Mukamolova *et al.*, 2002a). Following molecular characterization of the *M. luteus* Rpf gene, five homologues (*RpfA*, *RpfB*, *RpfC*, *RpfD* and *RpfE*) were identified in *M. tuberculosis* (Mukamolova *et al.*, 2002b). The *M. tuberculosis* recombinant Rpf proteins showed similar activity, activating growth of non-replicating cultures at picomolar concentrations. Following construction of Rpf gene knockout strains, Rpfs have been demonstrated to be important for *in vivo* persistence and reactivation of chronic infection in mice (Downing *et al.*, 2005; Tufariello *et al.*, 2006; Biketov *et al.*, 2007; Russell-Goldman *et al.*, 2008). The precise mechanism of action of these growth-stimulatory proteins is unknown, but they have been shown to possess structural motifs similar to that of lysozyme and soluble lytic transglycosylases and to possess muralytic activity (Cohen-Gonsaud *et al.*, 2004, 2005; Keep *et al.*, 2006; Mukamolova *et al.*, 2006; Kana and Mizrahi, 2010). Site-directed mutagenesis of the catalytic glutamate diminishes this activity and the ability of the proteins to stimulate growth and resuscitation, thereby suggesting that cleavage of peptidoglycan is related directly to growth stimulation and resuscitation (Mukamolova *et al.*, 2006; Telkov *et al.*, 2006). The stresses experienced by *M. tuberculosis* from the host immune system during infection are likely to result in cell wall damage and possible cell wall remodelling. Accordingly, *in vitro*, it has been shown that, following infection in macrophages, the morphology and surface properties of *M. tuberculosis* change and culturability is reduced (Biketov *et al.*, 2000). Enhanced numbers of cells were recovered following the addition of Rpf to the culture media. Similar morphological changes have been associated with the development of a population of *M. tuberculosis* which could not be cultured on agar following extended incubation in stationary phase (Shleeva *et al.*, 2002). Again, enhanced numbers of cells were recovered in liquid growth assays on the addition of Rpf to the culture media. Our interpretation of these results is that Rpf activity may be required to degrade a modified peptidoglycan (associated with the altered cell morphology) to assist cell division and regrowth. Alternatively, the degradation of peptidoglycan by Rpfs will release muropeptide fragments, which may have a role in providing a resuscitation signal via activation of a serine-threonine protein kinase signalling cascade (Jones and Dyson, 2006; Shah *et al.*, 2008; Shah and Dworkin, 2010). Evidence that these events are significant in human infection comes from the demonstration that Rpfs are expressed in *M. tuberculosis*-infected human tissues (Davies *et al.*, 2008).

Our transcriptome and LB studies of *M. tuberculosis* in sputum which provided evidence to support the presence of non-replicating *M. tuberculosis* bacilli (Garton *et al.*, 2008) led us to hypothesize that Rpf-dependent cells might be present in these samples. Sputum samples were collected from 25 smear-positive tuberculosis patients before initiation of chemotherapy and measurements of culturable cells by most probable number (MPN) assay were made with, and without, the addition of recombinant RpfE, RpfB or fresh Rpf-containing culture supernatants. Strikingly, these assays revealed that Rpf-dependent *M. tuberculosis* cells were not only present but were, in fact, the dominant population in 20 of the samples, measured at 80–99.9% of the culturable cells present (Mukamolova *et al.*, 2010). The specificity of these effects was further demonstrated by evidence that the addition of fresh culture supernatant from a quintuple *M. tuberculosis* Rpf mutant strain (Kana *et al.*, 2008) did not lead to the recovery of increased cell numbers.

Rpf dependency in sputum is a phenotypic adaptation of *M. tuberculosis* cells to specific *in vivo* signals, since it is lost after primary isolation. One possibility is that these signals are present in sputum. A candidate for such a signal was the inhibitory activity against *M. tuberculosis* growth in liquid medium we observed in sputum. Although we have been able to detect this inhibitory activity directly by the inoculation of *M. tuberculosis* H37Rv into two tuberculous sputum samples which had previously been rendered culture negative by freezing, incubation of *M. tuberculosis* in this milieu did not lead to the development of Rpf-dependent cells. With the exception of extended culture in stationary phase (Shleeva *et al.*, 2002), the only other demonstration of Rpf-dependent cells was in a population recovered from the peritoneal macrophages of *M. tuberculosis*-infected BALB/c mice (Biketov *et al.*, 2000). These observations suggest that the adaptation leading to Rpf dependence is a response to as yet unidentified environmental signals *in vivo*.

14.3 Evidence for a Relationship Between Sputum *M. tuberculosis* Phenotypes and Antibiotic Tolerance

Phenotypic antibiotic tolerance is a well-recognized microbial trait and has been recognized in many bacterial infections

(Levin and Rozen, 2006; Connolly *et al.*, 2007; Dhar and McKinney, 2007). The cidal action of many antibiotics is proportional to the growth rate of bacteria and metabolic activity; log-phase cells are killed efficiently, whereas slow-growing or non-replicating cells show phenotypic tolerance (Wallis *et al.*, 1999; Gomez and McKinney, 2004; Paramasivan *et al.*, 2005; Dhar and McKinney, 2007). *M. tuberculosis* exhibits phenotypic tolerance to various antibiotics, including the frontline agent INH, in stationary phase compared with log-phase growth (Herbert *et al.*, 1996; Paramasivan *et al.*, 2005). *M. tuberculosis* and *M. bovis* BCG conditioned in models designed to reflect the non-replicating state of the organism during latent infection, for example, Wayne's model of non-replicating persistence in which cells gradually adapt to hypoxic conditions (Wayne and Hayes, 1996; Low *et al.*, 2009) or the multiple stress model of Deb and colleagues (Deb *et al.*, 2009), are phenotypically tolerant to INH and RIF. The measured degree of tolerance to INH is greater than to RIF. However, when these mycobacteria are subject to conditions which induce a more rapid growth arrest, such as the addition of nitric oxide (NO) (Hussain *et al.*, 2009) and phosphate limitation (Rifat *et al.*, 2009), only tolerance to INH is observed. This is consistent with the target of RIF, RNA polymerase, being active during growth arrest (Wayne and Hayes, 1996; Hu *et al.*, 2000).

14.3.1 Lipid bodies

As non-replicating Wayne-type *M. tuberculosis* cultures, which show the most similar transcriptome signatures to *M. tuberculosis* in sputum and enhanced levels of LBs compared with aerobic growth, are tolerant to the action of INH and RIF (Wayne and Hayes, 1996), we have examined the action of these antibiotics against *M. tuberculosis* cultures exposed to NO. NO is an inhibitor of aerobic respiration and results in growth arrest and induction of the dormancy regulon of *M. tuberculosis* (Ohno *et al.*, 2003; Voskuil *et al.*, 2003; Daniel *et al.*, 2004). We reported initial results showing that 4 h

following NO treatment of a log-phase *M. tuberculosis* culture, the LB-positive sub-population increased to 65% compared with <1% in an untreated control. This is in accord with the reported maximal increase in TAG content 4 h following NO stimulation (Daniel *et al.*, 2004). The NO-stimulated cells sampled at this time showed nearly 50-fold greater survival following exposure to 1 µg/ml RIF than the untreated control (Garton *et al.*, 2008). A sample of the same culture 24 h after NO stimulation had a reduced LB content of 22% of the total population and approximately 10-fold greater survival following RIF treatment. This is consistent with the dissipation of NO from the culture, resulting in a resumption of growth and decrease in TAG content (Daniel *et al.*, 2004). In subsequent experiments, we have repeatedly demonstrated enhanced TAG and LB levels in NO treated cells and that these properties are associated with tolerance to INH; in contrast, results with RIF have been inconsistent (Sherratt *et al.*, unpublished results). This would suggest that although rapid growth arrest in response to NO stimulation results in an increase in LB (TAG) content of the *M. tuberculosis* (and stimulation of the dormancy regulon), additional stimuli or a more gradual adaption to slow/non-growth is required to promote tolerance to RIF in addition to INH. It is not known whether LBs are linked mechanistically to antibiotic tolerance or are a biomarker for an as yet unidentified property which would explain this. It is interesting to note, however, that the RIF tolerance of *M. tuberculosis* in the multiple-stress dormancy model reported by Deb and colleagues, was reduced, but not eliminated, in a *tgs1* mutant and restored by complementation (Deb *et al.*, 2009). This suggests that TAG content of the *M. tuberculosis* does directly influence the RIF tolerance of the cells in these stress conditions. In addition to the development of LBs, it is possible that there are associated changes, for example the accumulation of TAG, in the cell envelope, which may reduce permeability to antibiotics. In this regard, Cunningham and Spreadbury reported that *M. tuberculosis* sampled from the Wayne model, a condition in which we have demonstrated LB positivity, have thickened cell envelopes (Cunningham and Spreadbury, 1998).

It remains to be investigated whether there are any clinical correlates with the LB-positive *M. tuberculosis* population observed in the sputum of untreated tuberculosis patients. Studies to determine whether there is a relationship between the LB-positive *M. tuberculosis* population in sputum and fractional exhaled NO at the time of sputum collection are ongoing. If LB positivity is a biomarker of a non-replicating population of *M. tuberculosis* cells in a sputum sample, it would be expected that this population would become enriched in sputum during the course of treatment. In a preliminary study, assessment of sputum samples taken from seven patients prior to commencement and during chemotherapy did show a positive relationship ($R^2 = 0.53$) between LB positivity and killing (reduction of colony-forming unit (CFU) counts), which can be seen in Fig. 14.2. This supports the hypothesis that LB positivity may be predictive of treatment response; however, large-scale clinical studies are required to determine whether this observation is reproducible and whether it is reflected in clinical responses.

14.3.2 Rpf dependency

Following the demonstration that Rpf-dependent cells were a dominant population in the sputum samples of tuberculosis patients, the response of this population was monitored by assessing sputum samples collected from eight patients 7–11 days after the initiation of chemotherapy (Mukamolova *et al.*, 2010). The decrease in the viable *M. tuberculosis* counts in these samples was assessed by measuring CFUs and the Rpf-dependent population by MPN counts in the presence of fresh culture supernatant. A good correlation was found between a decline in CFU counts and the measured Rpf-dependent population. However, as would be expected if the Rpf-dependent *M. tuberculosis* cells were a non-replicating, persisting population phenotypically tolerant to antibiotics, the Rpf-dependent population was preserved relative to CFU counts in all the post-chemotherapy samples. This trend was observed to continue in samples that were collected from

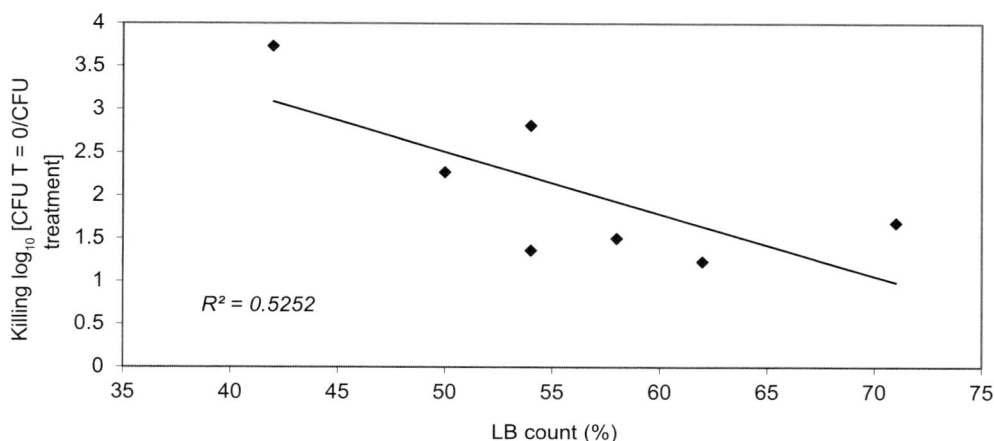

Fig. 14.2. The $\log_{10}$-fold reduction in viable counts in samples of patients' sputum following 7 or 8 days of antibiotic treatment show a correlation with the LB count of AFB in sputum samples evaluated before initiation of treatment. *M. tuberculosis* viable counts (CFU/ml) were assessed in early-morning samples of patients' sputum before the onset of treatment and at either 7 or 8 days of treatment. A separate aliquot of the pre-treatment samples were treated for LB assessment with auramine/Nile red staining.

four patients further into their treatment. At time points when no CFU assessments could be made, MPN counts were still measurable and the addition of culture supernatant revealed substantial populations of Rpf-dependent cells. These results suggest that an Rpf-dependent population present in sputum at the time of the initiation of chemotherapy are killed more slowly than a colony-forming population. However, an alternative argument that treatment induces Rpf dependence must be noted.

The addition of RIF directly to decontaminated smear-positive samples from three patients and incubation for 1 week revealed that the Rpf-dependent *M. tuberculosis* population was RIF tolerant (Mukamolova *et al.*, 2010). Although in each sample the CFU count fell below detectable levels after 7 days exposure to RIF, MPN assessment in the presence of culture supernatant revealed that the Rpf-dependent population decreased, at most, by 0.5 log. A culture of *M. tuberculosis* H37Rv which contained no Rpf-dependent cells showed a 2-log decline in the supplemented MPN count over the same duration of RIF exposure.

The demonstration of an Rpf-dependent population which appears to be relatively well conserved during treatment in samples collected during therapy and the direct measurement of RIF tolerance of Rpf-dependent cells support the hypothesis that sputum contains a population of non-replicating cells. This study highlights the potential importance of this previously overlooked population. The addition of Rpf in assessments of culturability may provide an early indication of treatment response. Furthermore, early bactericidal activity analyses of potential chemotherapeutic agents currently use CFU assessment to measure the efficacy of various agents and, therefore, such studies will not reveal the emergence of Rpf-dependent populations. There is potential for the measurement of the Rpf-dependent population to enhance such studies. A major focus of future research is to determine whether there is any relationship between the Rpf-dependent population in a patient's sputum with the clinical response during treatment and reported relapse rates.

14.4 Outstanding Questions

There remain a number of unanswered questions with regard to the *M. tuberculosis* phenotypes we have assessed in sputum. First, it is unclear whether the LB-positive cells in sputum are indeed growth arrested or slow growing. We remain unable to demonstrate convincingly LBs in growing batch cultures of *M. tuberculosis* H37Rv in rich media, but have observed LBs in *M. tuberculosis* biomass harvested from chemostat cultures under conditions of low O_2, low iron or low phosphorus (Sherratt *et al.*, unpublished results). Supplementing a growing *M. tuberculosis* batch culture with oleic acid (conditions which lead to rapid LB accumulation in *M. smegmatis*) led to an increase in TAG content but not LBs (Garton, unpublished results). This suggests that TAG may accumulate in the cell envelope until saturation is reached, at which point cytoplasmic LBs may develop. It follows that the LB-positive cell numbers may not reflect accurately total TAG accumulation in a population and we are working to develop more accurate reporters of *M. tuberculosis* lipid content. Following the identification of the sputum LB-positive *M. tuberculosis* population and the microarray study of the transcriptome, we confirmed in samples collected from nine tuberculosis patients the apparent upregulation of *tgs1* as compared with *M. tuberculosis* H37Rv aerobic growth by quantitative reverse transcription PCR (qRT-PCR) (Garton *et al.*, 2008). A larger-scale study of 30 tuberculosis patients failed to confirm an association between *tgs1* expression, as measured by qRT-PCR and LB positivity (Lee *et al.*, unpublished results). This was also the case for two other genes associated with non-replicating persistence, *hspX* and *icl1*. We do not know the age of *M. tuberculosis* cells in sputum samples, or the stability of *tgs1* transcripts *in vivo*. Daniel and colleagues reported maximal *tgs1* expression 4 h following NO stimulation of replicating *M. tuberculosis* culture; this time point was also coincidental with maximal TAG accumulation (Daniel *et al.*, 2004). Our own NO studies revealed induction of LB positivity at 4 h, followed by a threefold reduction in LB positivity 24 h post-stimulation, a point at which growth would be resumed (Garton *et al.*, 2008). High and enduring *tgs1* (and *hspX*) expression was reported throughout 30 days of the Wayne model (Voskuil *et al.*, 2004). Later studies of the expression of genes of the DosR regulon in response to a rapid transfer into hypoxia revealed that, unlike the majority of genes, the expression levels of *tgs1* and *hspX* (two of the most highly induced genes) remained high over a period of 7 days (Rustad *et al.*, 2008). Recent investigation of the stability of *M. tuberculosis* transcripts revealed an overall enhanced stability in hypoxic conditions compared with aerobic conditions (T.R. Rustad, San Diego, 2010, personal communication). In such conditions, cells which have produced LB in response to the induction of *tgs1* will retain high levels of *tgs1* transcripts. Regrowth of *M. bovis* BCG from hypoxia-induced dormancy results in the assimilation of accumulated TAG and LBs (Low *et al.*, 2009). The *M. tuberculosis* cells in sputum must, at some point, have undergone growth within the nutrient-rich environment of the patent cavity; it would be impossible to maintain ongoing smear positivity otherwise. Therefore, unless the LB-positive cells in sputum are dead or injured, we hypothesize that rather than a slow adaptation to non-replicating conditions, LB positivity is a reflection of a more rapid growth arrest in response to a change of environment. This remains to be determined, along with identification of the specific growth-arresting signal(s).

What, if any, is the relationship between the sputum *M. tuberculosis* LB-positive and Rpf-dependent populations? Although the sputum LB and Rpf-dependency sputum studies have been largely independent, it is clear that the numbers of Rpf-dependent *M. tuberculosis* can potentially be orders of magnitude higher than LB-positive cells. In the limited number of sputum samples in which LB positivity was correlated with killing as measured by a drop in the sputum CFU count following treatment (Fig. 14.2), Rpf-dependent *M. tuberculosis* cells had been identified in six out of seven samples. Larger-scale studies are required to determine whether there is any significant connection

between LB and Rpf-dependent sputum *M. tuberculosis* populations.

14.5 Conclusions

LB positivity and Rpf dependency are two quantifiable phenotypes which, in addition to the transcriptome signatures, provide evidence for the presence of non-replicating *M. tuberculosis* cells in sputum. Although our knowledge of the biological and clinical significance of these phenotypes is limited and remains to be developed, both LB positivity and Rpf dependence can be linked to phenotypic antibiotic tolerance. The evidence to support the view that one or either of these measurable phenotypes may constitute a potential biomarker for treatment response is gathering. Large-scale clinical studies are required to test this hypothesis and to determine any clinical correlates of these phenotypes. In the laboratory, greater understanding of the stimuli leading to the development of these sputum phenotypes will allow us to develop *in vitro* conditions in which we can study the adaption in *M. tuberculosis*. In combination, these studies will provide exciting new opportunities to address the problem of persisters in the treatment of tuberculosis.

References

Betts, J.C., Lukey, P.T., Robb, L.C., McAdam, R.A. and Duncan, K. (2002) Evaluation of a nutrient starvation model of *Mycobacterium tuberculosis* persistence by gene and protein expression profiling. *Molecular Microbiology* 43, 717–731.

Biketov, S., Mukamolova, G.V., Potapov, V., Gilenkov, E., Vostroknutova, G., Kell, D.B., *et al.* (2000) Culturability of *Mycobacterium tuberculosis* cells isolated from murine macrophages: a bacterial growth factor promotes recovery. *FEMS Immunology and Medical Microbiology* 29, 233–240.

Biketov, S., Potapov, V., Ganina, E., Downing, K., Kana, B.D. and Kaprelyants, A. (2007) The role of resuscitation promoting factors in pathogenesis and reactivation of *Mycobacterium tuberculosis* during intra-peritoneal infection in mice. *BMC Infectious Diseases* 7, 146.

Cohen-Gonsaud, M., Keep, N.H., Davies, A.P., Ward, J., Henderson, B. and Labesse, G. (2004)

Resuscitation-promoting factors possess a lysozyme-like domain. *Trends in Biochemical Sciences* 29, 7–10.

Cohen-Gonsaud, M., Barthe, P., Bagneris, C., Henderson, B., Ward, J., Roumestand, C., *et al.* (2005) The structure of a resuscitation-promoting factor domain from *Mycobacterium tuberculosis* shows homology to lysozymes. *Nature Structural and Molecular Biology* 12, 270–273.

Connolly, L.E., Edelstein, P.H. and Ramakrishnan, L. (2007) Why is long-term therapy required to cure tuberculosis? *PLoS Medicine* 4, e120.

Cunningham, A.F. and Spreadbury, C.L. (1998) Mycobacterial stationary phase induced by low oxygen tension: cell wall thickening and localization of the 16-kilodalton alpha-crystallin homolog. *Journal of Bacteriology* 180, 801–808.

Daniel, J., Deb, C., Dubey, V.S., Sirakova, T.D., Abomoelak, B., Morbidoni, H.R., *et al.* (2004) Induction of a novel class of diacylglycerol acyltransferases and triacylglycerol accumulation in *Mycobacterium tuberculosis* as it goes into a dormancy-like state in culture. *Journal of Bacteriology* 186, 5017–5030.

Davies, A.P., Dhillon, A.P., Young, M., Henderson, B., McHugh, T.D. and Gillespie, S.H. (2008) Resuscitation-promoting factors are expressed in *Mycobacterium tuberculosis*-infected human tissue. *Tuberculosis (Edinburgh)* 88, 462–468.

Deb, C., Lee, C.M., Dubey, V.S., Daniek, J., Abomoelak, B., Sirakova, T.D., *et al.* (2009) A novel *in vitro* multiple-stress dormancy model for *Mycobacterium tuberculosis* generates a lipid-loaded, drug-tolerant, dormant pathogen. *PLoS One* 4, e6077.

Dhar, N. and McKinney, J.D. (2007) Microbial phenotypic heterogeneity and antibiotic tolerance. *Current Opinion in Microbiology* 10, 30–38.

Downing, K.J., Mischenko, V.V., Shleeva, M.O., Young, D.I., Young, M., Kaprelyants, A.S., *et al.* (2005) Mutants of *Mycobacterium tuberculosis* lacking three of the five Rpf-like genes are defective for growth *in vivo* and for resuscitation *in vitro*. *Infection and Immunity* 73, 3038–3043.

Garton, N.J., Christensen, H., Minnikin, D.E., Adegbola, R.A. and Barer, M.R. (2002) Intracellular lipophilic inclusions of mycobacteria *in vitro* and in sputum. *Microbiology* 148, 2951–2958.

Garton, N.J., Waddell, S.J., Sherratt, A.L., Lee, S.M., Smit, R.J., Senner, C., *et al.* (2008) Cytological and transcript analyses reveal fat and lazy persister-like bacilli in tuberculous sputum. *PLoS Medicine* 5, e75.

Gomez, J.E. and McKinney, J.D. (2004) *Mycobacterium tuberculosis* persistence, latency, and drug tolerance. *Tuberculosis (Edinburgh)* 84, 29–44.

Herbert, D., Paramasivan, C.N., Venkatesan, P., Kubendiran, G., Prabhakar, R. and Mitchson, D.A. (1996) Bactericidal action of ofloxacin, sulbactam-ampicillin, rifampin, and isoniazid on logarithmic- and stationary-phase cultures of *Mycobacterium tuberculosis*. *Antimicrobial Agents and Chemotherapy* 40, 2296–2299.

Hu, Y., Mangan, J.A., Dhillon, J., Sole, K.M., Mitchison, D.A., Butcher, P.D., *et al.* (2000) Detection of mRNA transcripts and active transcription in persistent *Mycobacterium tuberculosis* induced by exposure to rifampin or pyrazinamide. *Journal of Bacteriology* 182, 6358–6365.

Hussain, S., Malik, M., Shi, L., Gennaro, M.L. and Drlica, K. (2009) *In vitro* model of mycobacterial growth arrest using nitric oxide with limited air. *Antimicrobial Agents and Chemotherapy* 53, 157–161.

Jones, G. and Dyson, P. (2006) Evolution of transmembrane protein kinases implicated in coordinating remodeling of Gram-positive peptidoglycan: inside versus outside. *Journal of Bacteriology* 188, 7470–7476.

Kana, B.D. and Mizrahi, V. (2010) Resuscitation-promoting factors as lytic enzymes for bacterial growth and signaling. *FEMS Immunology and Medical Microbiology* 58, 39–50.

Kana, B.D., Gordhan, B.G., Downing, K.J., Sung, N., Vostroktunova, G., Machowski, E.E., *et al.* (2008) The resuscitation-promoting factors of *Mycobacterium tuberculosis* are required for virulence and resuscitation from dormancy but are collectively dispensable for growth *in vitro*. *Molecular Microbiology* 67, 672–684.

Keep, N.H., Ward, J.M., Cohen-Gonsaud, M. and Henderson, B. (2006) Wake up! Peptidoglycan lysis and bacterial non-growth states. *Trends in Microbiology* 14, 271–276.

Levin, B.R. and Rozen, D.E. (2006) Non-inherited antibiotic resistance. *Nature Reviews. Microbiology* 4, 556–562.

Low, K.L., Rao, P.S., Shui, G., Bendt, A.K., Pethe, K., Dick, T., *et al.* (2009) Triacylglycerol utilization is required for regrowth of *in vitro* hypoxic nonreplicating *Mycobacterium bovis* bacillus Calmette–Guerin. *Journal of Bacteriology* 191, 5037–5043.

Low, K.L., Shui, G., Natter, K., Yeo, W.K., Kohlwein, S.D., Dick, T., *et al.* (2010) Lipid droplet-associated proteins are involved in the biosynthesis and hydrolysis of triacylglycerol in

Mycobacterium bovis bacillus Calmette–Guerin. *Journal of Biological Chemistry* 285, 21662–21670.

Mitchison, D.A. (1979) Basic mechanisms of chemotherapy. *Chest* 76, 771–781.

Mitchison, D.A. (2004) The search for new sterilizing anti-tuberculosis drugs. *Frontiers of Bioscience* 9, 1059–1072.

Mukamolova, G.V., Yanopolskaya, N.D., Kell, D.B. and Kaprelyants, A.S. (1998) On resuscitation from the dormant state of *Micrococcus luteus*. *Antonie Van Leeuwenhoek* 73, 237–243.

Mukamolova, G.V., Turapov, O.A., Kazarian, K., Telkov, M., Kaprelyants, A.S., Kell, D.B., and Young, M. (2002a) The Rpf gene of *Micrococcus luteus* encodes an essential secreted growth factor. *Molecular Microbiology* 46, 611–621.

Mukamolova, G.V., Turapov, O.A., Young, D.I., Kaprelyants, A.S., Kell, D.B. and Young, M. (2002b) A family of autocrine growth factors in *Mycobacterium tuberculosis*. *Molecular Microbiology,* 46, 623-35.

Mukamolova, G.V., Murzin, A.G., Salina, E.G., Demina, G.R., Kell, D.B., Kaprelyants, A.S., *et al.* (2006) Muralytic activity of *Micrococcus luteus* Rpf and its relationship to physiological activity in promoting bacterial growth and resuscitation. *Molecular Microbiology* 59, 84–98.

Mukamolova, G.V., Turapov, O., Malkin, J., Woltmann, G. and Barer, M.R. (2010) Resuscitation-promoting factors reveal an occult population of tubercle bacilli in sputum. *American Journal of Respiratory and Critical Care Medicine* 181, 174–180.

Muttucamaru, D.G., Roberts, G., Hinds, J., Stabler, R.A. and Parish, T. (2004) Gene expression profile of *Mycobacterium tuberculosis* in a non-replicating state. *Tuberculosis (Edinburgh)* 84, 239–246.

Ohno, H., Zhu, G., Mohan, V.P., Chu, D., Kohno, S., Jacobs, W.R. Jr, *et al.* (2003) The effects of reactive nitrogen intermediates on gene expression in *Mycobacterium tuberculosis*. *Cellular Microbiology* 5, 637–648.

Paramasivan, C.N., Sulochana, S., Kubendiran, G., Venkatesan, P. and Mitchison, D.A. (2005) Bactericidal action of gatifloxacin, rifampin, and isoniazid on logarithmic- and stationary-phase cultures of *Mycobacterium tuberculosis*. *Antimicrobial Agents and Chemotherapy* 49, 627–631.

Rifat, D., Bishai, W.R. and Karkousis, P.C. (2009) Phosphate depletion: a novel trigger for *Mycobacterium tuberculosis* persistence. *Journal of Infectious Diseases* 200, 1126–1135.

Russell-Goldman, E., Xu, J., Wang, X., Chan, J. and Tufariello, J.M. (2008) A *Mycobacterium tuberculosis* Rpf double-knockout strain exhibits profound defects in reactivation from chronic tuberculosis and innate immunity phenotypes. *Infection and Immunity* 76, 4269–4281.

Rustad, T.R., Harrell, M.I., Liao, R. and Sherman, D.R. (2008) The enduring hypoxic response of *Mycobacterium tuberculosis*. *PLoS One* 3, e1502.

Shah, I.M. and Dworkin, J. (2010) Induction and regulation of a secreted peptidoglycan hydrolase by a membrane Ser/Thr kinase that detects muropeptides. *Molecular Microbiology* 75, 1232–1243.

Shah, I.M., Laaberki, M.H., Popham, D.L. and Dworkin, J. (2008) A eukaryotic-like Ser/Thr kinase signals bacteria to exit dormancy in response to peptidoglycan fragments. *Cell* 135, 486–496.

Shi, L., Sohaskey, C.D., Kana, B.D., Dawes, S., North, R.J., Mizrahi, V., *et al.* (2005) Changes in energy metabolism of *Mycobacterium tuberculosis* in mouse lung and under in vitro conditions affecting aerobic respiration. *Proceedings of the National Academy of Sciences* 102, 15629–15634.

Shleeva, M.O., Bagramyan, K., Telkov, M.V., Mukamolova, G.V., Young, M., Kell, D.B., *et al.* (2002) Formation and resuscitation of 'non-culturable' cells of *Rhodococcus rhodochrous* and *Mycobacterium tuberculosis* in prolonged stationary phase. *Microbiology* 148, 1581–1591.

Telkov, M.V., Demina, G.R., Voloshin, S.A., Salina, E.G., Dudik, T.V., Stekhanova, T.N., *et al.* (2006) Proteins of the Rpf (resuscitation promoting factor) family are peptidoglycan hydrolases. *Biochemistry (Moscow)* 71, 414–422.

Tufariello, J.M., Mi, K., Xu, J., Manabe, Y.C., Kesavan, A.K., Drumm, J., *et al.* (2006) Deletion of the *Mycobacterium tuberculosis* resuscitation-promoting factor Rv1009 gene results in delayed reactivation from chronic tuberculosis. *Infection and Immunity* 74, 2985–2995.

Voskuil, M.I., Schnappinger, D., Visconti, K.C., Harrell, M.I., Dolganov, G.M., Sherman, D.R., *et al.* (2003) Inhibition of respiration by nitric oxide induces a *Mycobacterium tuberculosis* dormancy program. *Journal of Experimental Medicine* 198, 705–713.

Voskuil, M.I., Visconti, K.C. and Schoolnik, G.K. (2004) *Mycobacterium tuberculosis* gene expression during adaptation to stationary phase and low-oxygen dormancy. *Tuberculosis (Edinburgh)* 84, 218–227.

Wallis, R.S., Patil, S., Cheon, S.H., Edmonds, K., Phillips, M., Perkins, M.D., *et al.* (1999) Drug tolerance in *Mycobacterium tuberculosis*. *Antimicrobial Agents and Chemotherapy* 43, 2600–2606.

Wallis, R.S., Pai, M., Menzies, D., Doherty, T.M., Walzl, G., Perkins, M.D., *et al.* (2010) Biomarkers and diagnostics for tuberculosis: progress, needs, and translation into practice. *The Lancet* 375, 1920–1937.

Wältermann, M. and Steinbüchel, A. (2005) Neutral lipid bodies in prokaryotes: recent insights into structure, formation, and relationship to eukaryotic lipid depots. *Journal of Bacteriology* 187, 3607–3619.

Wayne, L.G. and Hayes, L.G. (1996) An *in vitro* model for sequential study of shiftdown of *Mycobacterium tuberculosis* through two stages of nonreplicating persistence. *Infection and Immunity* 64, 2062–2069.

Part IV

Treatment Strategies

15 Clinical Trials in Tuberculosis Chemotherapy: The Challenges

Stephen H. Gillespie

Sir James Black Professor of Medicine, The Bute Medical School, St Andrews University, Scotland, UK

15.1 Introduction

The first antibiotics, penicillins and sulfonamides, were not active against *Mycobacterium tuberculosis* and some commentators at the time considered the organism might be beyond the reach of chemotherapy (Ryan, 1992; Dormandy, 1999). Selman Waksman did not take that view and rather considered the closely related organisms might produce antibiotics that would inhibit mycobacteria, an idea that might have come from his medical student son (Daniel, 2005). His PhD student, Albert Schatz, was given a culture of *Streptomyces griseus* that had been isolated from a chicken and he isolated the compound that became known as streptomycin (SM) – a revolution in anti-tuberculosis chemotherapy and one which opened the floodgates for isoniazid (INH), pyrazinamide (PZA), para-amino-salicylic acid and eventually rifampicin (RIF) (Ryan, 1992; Dormandy, 1999).

When SM became available, it was rushed into use in the USA, where it had first been produced. In the UK, a small amount was imported and given to the Medical Research Council (MRC), who formed a trials committee. There was not enough of this wonder drug to treat all of the patients. The MRC sponsored a study to evaluate the use of SM and allocated patients randomly to receive the current best treatment with or without SM. The initial results showed significant benefit for the patients who had received SM, but found evidence of toxicity and development of drug resistance (MRC, 1948). At 5 years follow-up, the benefit of the added antibiotic had disappeared as the organisms had developed resistance and infection had relapsed. This trial and its results were seminal in several ways. Not only was it the first randomized placebo controlled clinical trial in medical history but also it was a pioneering study that established the way new drugs were developed. It also demonstrated the importance of long-term follow-up in tuberculosis clinical trials (McDermott, 1960; Fox and Mitchison, 1975; Fox *et al.*, 1999).

In subsequent years, a series of trials were performed that evaluated each new anti-tuberculosis drug as it became ready for introduction in clinical practice. INH's potent bactericidal activity was realized, and when RIF was introduced and was used in a three-drug regimen with SM, treatment duration dropped from 24 to 9 months (EABMR Council, 1973; Grosset, 1978). In the late 1970s, PZA was re-evaluated in anti-tuberculosis regimens. It had been developed at the same time as INH, but it was withdrawn from therapy due to toxicity. The later trials used a lower dose, and a series of trials sponsored by the MRC and the British Thoracic Society showed that treatment was possible in 6 months (EACA/BMR Councils, 1986). Trials to shorten treatment further resulted in unacceptable rates of relapse, and the duration of treatment using an optimal regimen was fixed at 6 months. Other regimens in resource-poor settings using less potent agents needed a treatment duration of at least 8 months. The success of anti-tuberculosis chemotherapy was deemed complete and many countries with efficient treatment and control pro- grammes did witness a year-on-year decline in the prevalence of tuberculosis. This rosy picture neglected several important problems: in many countries there was no effective control programme and tuberculosis raged unchecked. When Human Immunodeficiency Virus appeared, it formed a malignant alliance with the tubercle bacillus, reversing the favourable trend in countries that had seen success. Importantly, for patients infected with bacteria that had become resistant or that were not able to tolerate the current regimen, there were few alternative regimens available.

The Cape Town Conference, held in Somerset West, South Africa, in 2000, addressed the pressing need to develop shorter treatment regimens and new drugs for resistant disease. Global bodies formed the Global Alliance for TB Drug Development to address the paucity of alternative anti- tuberculosis drugs (Pablos-Mendez, 2000). The spotlight that this has thrown on tubercu- losis drug development means that there are now many new drugs in development, although only a few have reached the clinical trials stage (Duncan and Barry, 2004; Ginsberg, 2010). This immediately poses the question of how, 60 years after the first golden age, will the tuberculosis community manage the clinical evaluation of new drugs for tuberculosis?

15.2 Tuberculosis Clinical Trials

Tuberculosis clinical trials differ from those for other indications as, at the first stage after Phase I studies are completed, what are often

described as 'early bactericidal studies' are performed where the new drug is given as monotherapy for a short period (Jindani et al., 1980, 2003; Gillespie et al., 2002). Since the drug is novel and the duration of therapy is short, there is little chance that this will result in the emergence of resistance (Gillespie et al., 2002; Gosling, 2003a,b). This phenomenon of the higher activity of INH in the first 2 days of therapy was named 'early bactericidal activity', which is somewhat of a misnomer (Jindani et al., 1980, 2003) as subsequent studies with other drugs did not find the same characteristic. Thus, these studies should, more properly, be described as monotherapy studies. They have considerable benefits in the drug development process, as they provide the first indication of whether the new drug is active in killing tubercle bacilli in the human host. It also provides the opportunity to identify a dose that is likely to be effective (Rustomjee et al., 2008a). Some authors also suggest that it may be possible to evaluate combinations in regimens but, in combinations with RIF and INH, the effect size of the established drugs are usually too large to see the contribution of the novel agent reliably (Gillespie, 2005). Moreover, regimen building is more complex and depends on the pharmacokinetic interaction between all of the drugs in the regimens. Finding a solution to evaluate combinations rapidly, reliably and cheaply is a major challenge. Once this stage is complete, more conventional Phase II studies can be devised, but tuberculosis poses particular challenges of its own, as set out in the paragraphs below.

15.2.1 Additive or substitutive

It is essential that the treatment of tuberculosis is with a multiple drug regimen, because *M. tuberculosis* develops resistance rapidly through mutation of chromosomal genes (Gillespie, 2002). Although this occurs at a relatively low rate among the majority of the most effective drugs (e.g. once in a billion cell divisions for RIF), the large number of bacilli in the body would mean that monotherapy inevitably would result in resistance emerg- ing (Shimao, 1986). This is solved by using multiple-drug regimens, which means that the risk of a bacterium being spontaneously resistant to three of the agents in the regimen is essentially nil. The added advantage is that the various drugs target the bacteria in different ways and have differing pharmacokinetics, reducing the risk that a metabolically inactive bacterium in a hard-to-reach site, such as an empyema, would elude therapy.

How should new drugs be evaluated in the context of a multiple-drug regimen? Should they be added to the regimen or should one of the current drugs be substituted?

Adding a new agent to a three- or four-drug regimen has a number of difficulties. The more drugs that are present, the higher the risk of pharmacokinetic interaction or adverse events. Care must also be taken to ensure that combining drugs with a given mode of action is rational. It has been shown for other organisms that agents which suppress protein synthesis can inhibit the activity of agents that depend on protein synthesis for their mechanism of action. Careful mind experiments and *in vitro* synergy studies supplemented by mouse interaction studies might be used to select the components of novel regimens.

There is some experience of additive regimens: a trial of levofloxacin added to conventional anti-tuberculosis failed to show benefit because the standard regimen was already sufficiently effective (el-Sadr *et al.*, 1998).

An alternative approach is to substitute the new agent with established members of the regimen. This is a more attractive proposition, as several of the components of standard anti-tuberculosis chemotherapy are toxic. In a series of *in vitro* and mouse experiments, it was shown that substituting the new fluoroquinolone, moxifloxacin, for either ethambutol or INH in the regimen resulted in a stable cure more rapidly than with standard therapy (Nuermberger *et al.*, 2004a,b). This prompted the series of clinical trials in the evaluation of moxifloxacin and gatifloxacin in which these various substitutions were trialled in Phase IIb and Phase III trials (Burman *et al.*, 2006; Rustomjee *et al.*,

2008b; Dorman *et al.*, 2009). This represents a model for the tuberculosis drug development pathway (Nunn *et al.*, 2008b).

15.3 Trial Design

Although we know that the control of tuberculosis globally will require improved treatment that is shorter and easier to tolerate, when designing tuberculosis clinical trials we are confronted with the fact that, for susceptible disease, currently recommended regimens have more than 95% efficacy under controlled clinical trial conditions (Fox *et al.*, 1999; Nunn *et al.*, 2008b). It is very unlikely that a better result could be achieved with one or a combination of new drugs. Thus, clinical trials of new drugs must focus on developing a regimen that is shorter in duration. In order for any proposed regimen to be licensed, it will have to prove that it is comparable to the existing regimen in terms of its efficacy. Although this issue has occasionally proved controversial, future trials of treatment in susceptible disease will have a non-inferiority design (Nunn *et al.*, 2008a,b). In planning such studies, considerable care must be taken to choose and justify the choice of the margin of non-inferiority, which should be justified both statistically and, in terms of the impact, clinically and programmatically. The trial methodology must be rigorous, with the effective recruitment and retention of patients. If there are substantial losses to follow-up or unsatisfactory laboratory procedures, non-inferiority could be concluded falsely. The sample size should be calculated carefully to ensure that the study has sufficient power to answer the clinical question posed (Nunn *et al.*, 2008b).

15.3.1 Multiple drug-resistant tuberculosis

Multiple drug-resistant (MDR-TB) and extensively drug-resistant tuberculosis (XDR-TB) pose unique challenges for clinical trials (Sacks and Behrman, 2008; WHO, 2008). Although a growing problem, patients are scattered, with few clinical centres having a large number of cases or, alternatively, the number of sites with a large number of MDR-/XDR-TB cases is small and the multiplicity of sites enhances the complexity of running clinical trials in order to ensure uniform clinical and laboratory practice. Moreover, although there are clear definitions of MDR- and XDR-TB, the susceptibility pattern of individual strains differs significantly, with the effect that a 'standard' regimen cannot be established easily for comparison. Alternative approaches include the use of the best available regimen, as defined by WHO guidelines, compared to this regimen plus the new drug (WHO, 2008). This approach is expected to work well, as the activity of many second- or third-line regimens is modest and the addition of a potent novel agent may have a significant impact (Sacks and Behrman, 2008). Trials that have taken this approach have been able to yield a positive outcome with modest numbers of patients, for example TMC207, which was shown to have only modest activity in the first monotherapy trial, made a very significant impact when tested in MDR. The addition of TMC207 to standard therapy for MDR-TB reduced the time to conversion to a negative sputum culture, as compared with placebo (hazard ratio, 11.8; 95% confidence interval, 2.3–61.3; $P = 0.003$ by Cox regression analysis) and increased the proportion of patients with conversion of sputum culture (48% versus 9%) (Diacon et al., 2009, 2010).

15.3.2 End points

For the early stage/Phase II clinical trial, the usual end point is defined as the proportion of patients who are deemed culture negative after 2 months of therapy (Fox et al., 1999). Although this has become a standard approach, the reasoning behind may not be as sound. A series of studies have indicated that there is an association between the 2-month culture negativity rate and relapse (Aber and Nunn, 1978). In this statement, there are a number of assumptions: that the laboratory methods are the same as in the studies that identified the relationship and that the post 2-month therapy is appropriate.

These basic constraints on the relationship are often forgotten. Clearly, a patient who is rendered culture negative by an effective regimen and then goes on to a less satisfactory regimen for the remainder of the treatment period or who stops therapy for whatever reasons will have a poorer outcome than an individual on an effective consolidation regimen taken completely. The importance of this relationship was demonstrated in 'Study A', organized by the International Union against Tuberculosis and Lung Disease, in which an inadequate consolidation regimen resulted in an excess of relapses in the 8-month regimen against the standard 6-month regimen, even though there was no significant difference in culture negativity data at 2 months (Jindani et al., 2004).

In tuberculosis clinical trials, the conventional end point for a Phase III study is combined bacteriological failure at the end of treatment and relapse in the 2 years following. In practice, most of the relapses occur within the first year of treatment completion. In a review of 15 treatment trials, 68% of relapses occurred within 6 months and 91% within 1 year (Nunn et al., 2010). Also, the availability of highly discriminatory typing methods have shown that many of the cases that were thought to be relapses were, in fact, new infections with different strains (Verver et al., 2005; van Helden et al., 2008). There is increasing evidence that the risk of reinfection is related to the incidence of disease in the community (van Helden et al., 2008). In other words, in areas where rates of transmission are high, the proportion of reinfections to relapses increases. Thus, a relapse can be identified only if the strain has been subjected to a modern typing technique such as IS6110 RFLP (restrictive fragment length polymorphism) analysis, MIRU (mycobacterial intergenic repeat unit) typing or whole genome sequencing that demonstrates that the initial and relapse strain are indistinguishable (Nunn et al., 2008b).

15.4 Subjects and Locations

For a clinical trial to be truly useful, it should be representative of the human population.

For reasons of practicality and applicability, it is more efficient to perform clinical trials in areas where tuberculosis is a common diagnosis. This is often a country that is resource poor, both financially and in terms of community medical facilities. This poses its own challenges for the management of Phase III clinical trials.

To ensure patient safety and to detect mycobacteria safely to perform susceptibility tests and provide a full range of safety, blood test and electrocardiographic and radiology facilities are necessary. This limits the sites in which trials can be performed and recent studies have shown that the number of suitable sites is relatively limited (van Niekerk and Ginsberg, 2009). Beyond the basic physical infrastructure, the differences between the approach for clinical practice and the constraints essential for a clinical trial can be a challenge for many sites in resource-poor settings where the large patient burden means that diagnosis and treatment are stripped down to their bare essentials. Accreditation and quality assurance of clinical and laboratory facilities can be a major challenge in any setting. For a location to be suitable for a Phase III clinical trial, the site must be highly committed to developing and adapting their processes to the constraints of the clinical trial paradigm. Central to the success of this programme is the effective training of staff, not only in the requirements of Good Clinical Practice and Good Laboratory Clinical Practice but also to understand the nature of the disease and the research being undertaken (Perrin and Gillespie, 2006). Short cuts taken in the training aspects of trial development will result in unreliable data.

It might be argued that tuberculosis is a disease of poverty. It is important, therefore, that care is taken with the recruitment of patients who are clinically and financially vulnerable. It is essential that patients entering a pivotal Phase III study should give fully informed consent. This means that the risks of participation should be explained clearly and simply, using non-specialist language. Ideally, consent should be taken by someone who is not directly involved in the study and who is supported by trained counsellors. In any international study, there will be a challenge of languages, so it is essential that the informed consent documents are translated into the relevant local languages and then translated back into the original language, to ensure that the meaning has been rendered accurately. Participation in the trial should not be an added financial burden for the patient, but investigators should ensure that payments are appropriate and do not, in themselves, provide an inducement to participate (Perrin and Gillespie, 2006).

15.5 Laboratory Methodology

Since the series of trials performed by the MRC and the US Public Health Service, there has been a revolution in mycobacterial laboratory methods. The trials were conducted when diagnosis was defined by examination of Zhiel–Neelsen stained smears and cultivation of the organism on Löwenstein–Jensen (LJ) slopes (Fox *et al.*, 1999). Modern mycobacteriology includes liquid culture and automates susceptibility testing, molecular susceptibility testing and molecular typing (Wallis *et al.*, 2010).

Modern liquid culture is monitored continuously, signalling positive when changes in CO_2 concentration generated by metabolizing bacteria pass a critical threshold, sensed by the machine. The machine is monitored constantly: this shortens the time to diagnosis, as solid cultures are only monitored intermittently. A positive result can be expected approximately 2 weeks quicker than could be achieved using LJ slopes (Rusch-Gerdes *et al.*, 1999; Hillemann *et al.*, 2006; Chihota *et al.*, 2010). In addition, liquid culture is significantly more sensitive than solid culture: the effect of this is that a positive culture on an LJ slope and in a liquid culture flask relate to a different number of organisms in the specimen (Nunn *et al.*, 2008). In effect, a patient will become culture negative more quickly if the measure is LJ culture than if it were liquid culture. Thus, it is essential that laboratories use a single method for determining culture positivity in the protocol, but since all of the data that we have to date are based on solid culture, it would be prudent to have both methods running in parallel. This is the approach that is being used in the current REMoxTB clinical trial (Bateson *et al.*, 2011).

It is also important to recognize that liquid culture is more susceptible to growth of non-tuberculosis organisms, resulting in the loss of that data point (Chihota *et al.*, 2010). This should be tackled by ensuring that the decontamination process is controlled carefully and adjusted to ensure standard performance. It also means that additional samples may be necessary to ensure that data are available for the crucial post-treatment end points.

Liquid-based susceptibility testing means that patients that have resistances can be removed from a trial of susceptible disease rapidly and classified as a late protocol exclusion. The availability of rapid molecular hybridization-based methods means that it is now possible to identify patients with MDR-TB within a few hours and exclude them from the trial. This is especially important when performing trials of susceptible disease in areas where the rate of drug resistance is high (Boehme *et al.*, 2010; Kiet *et al.*, 2010).

Smear diagnosis remains a cornerstone of the recruitment process, as demonstrating that a patient is smear positive increases the likelihood, in a high-burden country, that the patient has tuberculosis (Bonnet *et al.*, 2010). Modern molecular methods based on a number of different techniques allow for smear-positive samples to be screened to exclude non-tuberculosis mycobacteria (NTM), which are being recognized increasingly in high-burden countries. NTM can be identified more frequently when liquid culture is used. This is important if patients are found to revert from smear negativity to positivity later in the trial or their liquid culture is positive with an acid-fast bacterium. In these situations, it is important to perform a test to ensure that a positive result comes from *M. tuberculosis* and not from an NTM (Boehme *et al.*, 2010); Bateson *et al.*, 2011).

Questions are raised frequently about patients who stop producing sputum towards the end of or after treatment. There is a linger-ing concern that they may not be culture negative, a question that is left tantalizingly out of sight as their sputum samples are often contaminated with other organisms. The question is often raised whether sputum should be induced to identify cryptic positive patients. The evidence that is available does suggest that those patients who have reverted to sputum negativity rarely yield a positive culture following sputum induction, which suggests that treated patients who have difficulty producing sputum should be classed a treatment successes (Perrin *et al.*, 2009).

15.6 Conclusion

There is encouraging news that there are a large number of new anti-tuberculosis drugs in development. This brings the challenge that we need to expand the number of sites that are capable of performing high-quality studies internationally. Further work is required to understand the impact of new laboratory technology on clinical trials design. Importantly, we need to harmonize the methodologies that are used in trials to ensure that results are reliable and that they can be translated in other environments.

References

Aber, V.R. and Nunn, A.J. (1978) Short term chemotherapy of tuberculosis. Factors affecting relapse following short term chemotherapy. *Bulletin of the International Union against Tuberculosis* 53(4), 276–280.

Bateson, A.L., Batt, S., Betteridge, M., Bongard, E., Ciesielczuk, H., Gillespie, S.H., *et al.* (2011) *REMoxTB Laboratory Manual* (http://www.ucl.ac.uk/infection-immunity/research/res_ccm/ccm_files/CCM_REMox, accesssed 4 October 2012).

Boehme, C.C., Nabeta, P., Hillemann, D., Nicol, M.P., Shenai, S., Krapp, F., *et al.* (2010) Rapid molecular detection of tuberculosis and rifampin resistance. *New England Journal of Medicine* 363(11), 1005–1015.

Bonnet, M., Tajahmady, A., Hepple, P., Ramsay, A., Githui, W., Gagdnidze, L., *et al.* (2010) Added value of bleach sedimentation microscopy for diagnosis of tuberculosis: a cost-effectiveness study. *International Journal for Tuberculosis and Lung Disease* 14(5), 571–577.

Burman, W.J., Goldberg, S., Johnson, J.L., Muzanye, G., Engle, M., Mosher, A.W., *et al.* (2006) Moxifloxacin versus ethambutol in the first 2 months of treatment for pulmonary tuberculosis. *American Journal of Respiratory and Critical Care Medicine* 174(3), 331–338.

Chihota, V.N., Grant, A.D., Fielding, K., Ndibongo, B., van Zyl, A., Muirhead, D., *et al.* (2010) Liquid vs. solid culture for tuberculosis: performance and cost in a resource-constrained setting. *International Journal for Tuberculosis and Lung Disease* 14(8), 1024–1031.

Daniel, T.M. (2005) Selman Abraham Waksman and the discovery of streptomycin. *International Journal for Tuberculosis and Lung Disease* 9(2), 120–122.

Diacon, A.H., Pym, A., Grobusch, M., Patientia, R., Rustomjee, R., Page-Shipp, L., *et al.* (2009) The diarylquinoline TMC207 for multidrug-resistant tuberculosis. *New England Journal of Medicine* 360(23), 2397–2405.

Diacon, A.H., Dawson, R., Hanekom, M., Narunsky, K., Maritz, S.J., Venter, A., *et al.* (2010) Early bactericidal activity and pharmacokinetics of PA-824 in smear-positive tuberculosis patients. *Antimicrobial Agents and Chemotherapy* 54(8), 3402–3407.

Dorman, S.E., Johnson, J.L., Goldberg, S., Muzanye, G., Padayatchi, N., Bozeman, L., *et al.*, the Tuberculosis Trials Consortium (2009) Substitution of moxifloxacin for isoniazid during intensive phase treatment of pulmonary tuberculosis. *American Journal of Respiratory and Critical Care Medicine* 180(3), 273–280.

Dormandy, T. (1999) *The White Death: A History of Tuberculosis.* Hambleton Press, London.

Duncan, K. and Barry, C.E. 3rd (2004) Prospects for new antitubercular drugs. *Current Opinion in Microbiology* 7(5), 460–465.

EABR Council (1973) Controlled clinical trial of four short-course (6-month) regimens of chemotherapy for treatment of pulmonary tuberculosis. Second report. *The Lancet* 1(7816), 1331–1338.

EACA/BMR Councils (1986) Controlled clinical trial of 4 short-course regimens of chemotherapy (three 6-month and one 8-month) for pulmonary tuberculosis: final report. East and Central African/British Medical Research Council Fifth Collaborative Study. *Tubercle* 67(1), 5–15.

el-Sadr, W.M., Perlman, D.C., Matts, J.P., Nelson, E.T., Cohn, D.L., Salomon, N., *et al.* (1998) Evaluation of an intensive intermittent-induction regimen and duration of short-course treatment for human immunodeficiency virus-related pulmonary tuberculosis. Terry Beirn Community Programs for Clinical Research on AIDS (CPCRA) and the AIDS Clinical Trials Group (ACTG). *Clinical Infectious Diseases* 26(5), 1148–1158.

Fox, W. and Mitchison, D.A. (1975) Short-course chemotherapy for pulmonary tuberculosis. *American Review of Respiratory Disease* 111(3), 325–353.

Fox, W., Ellard, G.A. and Mitchison, D.A. (1999) Studies on the treatment of tuberculosis undertaken by the British Medical Research Council tuberculosis units, 1946–1986, with relevant subsequent publications. *International Journal for Tuberculosis and Lung Disease* 3(10 Suppl 2), S231–279.

Gillespie, S.H. (2002) Evolution of drug resistance in *Mycobacterium tuberculosis*: clinical and molecular perspective. *Antimicrobial Agents and Chemotherapy* 46(2), 267–274.

Gillespie, S.H. (2005) Early bactericidal activity of a moxifloxacin and isoniazid combination in smear-positive pulmonary tuberculosis. *Journal of Antimicrobial Chemotherapy* 56(6), 1169–1171.

Gillespie, S.H., Gosling, R.D. and Charalambous, B.M. (2002) A reiterative method for calculating the early bactericidal activity of antituberculosis drugs. *American Journal of Respiratory and Critical Care Medicine* 166(1), 31–35.

Ginsberg, A.M. (2010) Tuberculosis drug development: progress, challenges, and the road ahead. *Tuberculosis (Edinburgh)* 90(3), 162–167.

Gosling, R.D. (2003a) A multicentre comparison of a novel surrogate marker for determining the specific potency of anti-tuberculosis drugs. *Journal of Antimicrobial Chemotherapy* 52(3), 473–476.

Gosling, R.D. (2003b) The bactericidal activity of moxifloxacin in patients with pulmonary tuberculosis. *American Journal of Respiratory and Critical Care Medicine* 168(11), 1342–1345.

Grosset, J. (1978) The sterilizing value of rifampicin and pyrazinamide in experimental short-course chemotherapy. *Bulletin of the International Union Against Tuberculosis* 53(1), 5–12.

Hillemann, D., Richter, E. and Rüsch-Gerdes, S. (2006) Use of the BACTEC Mycobacteria Growth Indicator Tube 960 automated system for recovery of mycobacteria from 9,558 extrapulmonary specimens, including urine samples. *Journal of Clinical Microbiology*

44(11), 4014–4017.

Jindani, A., Aber, V.R., Edwards, E.A. and Mitchison, D.A. (1980) The early bactericidal activity of drugs in patients with pulmonary tuberculosis. *American Review of Respiratory Disease* 121(6), 939–949.

Jindani, A., Dore, C.J. and Mitchison, D.A. (2003) Bactericidal and sterilizing activities of antituberculosis drugs during the first 14 days. *American Journal of Respiratory and Critical Care Medicine* 167(10), 1348–1354.

Jindani, A., Nunn, A.J. and Enarson, D. (2004) Two 8-month regimens of chemotherapy for treatment of newly diagnosed pulmonary tuberculosis: international multicentre randomised trial. *The Lancet* 364(9441), 1244–1251.

Kiet, V.S., Lan, N.T.N., An, D.D., Dung, N.H., Hoa, D.V., van Vinh Chau, N., *et al.* (2010) Evaluation of the MTBDRsl test for detection of second-line-drug resistance in *Mycobacterium tuberculosis*. *Journal of Clinical Microbiology* 48(8), 2934–2939.

McDermott, W. (1960) Antimicrobial therapy of pulmonary tuberculosis. *Bulletin of the World Health Organization* 23(4–5), 427–461.

MRC (1948) Streptomycin in the treatment of pulmonary tuberculosis. *British Medical Journal* ii, 769–783.

Niekerk, C. van and Ginsberg, A. (2009) Assessment of global capacity to conduct tuberculosis drug development trials: do we have what it takes? *International Journal for Tuberculosis and Lung Disease* 13(11), 1367–1372.

Nuermberger, E.L., Yoshimatsu, T., Tyagi, S., O'Brien, R.J., Vernon, A.N., Chaisson, R.E., *et al.* (2004a) Moxifloxacin-containing regimen greatly reduces time to culture conversion in murine tuberculosis. *American Journal of Respiratory and Critical Care Medicine* 169(3), 421–426.

Nuermberger, E.L., Yoshimatsu, T., Tyagi, S., Williams, K., Rosenthal, I., O'Brien, R.J., *et al.* (2004b) Moxifloxacin-containing regimens of reduced duration produce a stable cure in murine tuberculosis. *American Journal of Respiratory and Critical Care Medicine* 170(10), 1131–1134.

Nunn, A.J., Meredith, S.K., Spigelman, M.K., Ginsberg, A.M. and Gillespie, S.H. (2008a) The ethics of non-inferiority trials. *The Lancet* 371(9616), 895; author reply 896–897.

Nunn, A.J., Phillips, P.P. and Gillespie, S.H. (2008b) Design issues in pivotal drug trials for drug sensitive tuberculosis (TB). *Tuberculosis (Edinburgh)* 88(Suppl 1), S85–92.

Nunn, A.J., Phillips, P.P. and Mitchison, D.A. (2010)

Timing of relapse in short-course chemotherapy trials for tuberculosis. *International Journal for Tuberculosis and Lung Disease* 14(2), 241–242.

Pablos-Mendez, A. (2000) Working alliance for TB drug development, Cape Town, South Africa, February 8th, 2000. *International Journal for Tuberculosis and Lung Disease* 4(6), 489–490.

Perrin, F.M. and Gillespie, S.H. (2006) A new world approach to an old disease. *Good Clinical Practice* 8, 18–21.

Perrin, F.M., Breen, R.A., McHugh, T.D., Gillespie, S.H. and Lipman, M.C.I. (2009) Are patients on treatment for pulmonary TB who stop expectorating sputum genuinely culture negative? *Thorax* 64(11), 1009–1010.

Rusch-Gerdes, S., Domehl, C., Nardi, G., Gismondo, M.R., Welscher, H.M. and Pfyffer, G.E. (1999) Multicenter evaluation of the mycobacteria growth indicator tube for testing susceptibility of *Mycobacterium tuberculosis* to first-line drugs. *Journal of Clinical Microbiology* 37(1), 45–48.

Rustomjee, R., Diacon, A.H., Allen, J., Venter, A., Reddy, C., Patientia, R.F., *et al.* (2008a) Early bactericidal activity and pharmacokinetics of the diarylquinoline TMC207 in treatment of pulmonary tuberculosis. *Antimicrobial Agents and Chemotherapy* 52(8), 2831–2835.

Rustomjee, R., Lienhardt, C., Kanyok, T., Davies, G.R., Levin, J., Mthiyane, T., *et al.* (2008b) A Phase II study of the sterilising activities of ofloxacin, gatifloxacin and moxifloxacin in pulmonary tuberculosis. *International Journal for Tuberculosis and Lung Disease* 12(2), 128–138.

Ryan, F. (1992) *The Forgotten Plague: How the Battle Against Tuberculosis Was Won and Lost.* Little Brown, Boston, Massachusetts.

Sacks, L.V. and Behrman, R.E. (2008) Developing new drugs for the treatment of drug-resistant tuberculosis: a regulatory perspective. *Tuberculosis (Edinburgh)* 88(Suppl 1), S93–100.

Shimao, T. (1986) Review of tuberculosis control programmes in the Far East Region of the International Union Against Tuberculosis. *Bulletin of the International Union Against Tuberculosis* 61(1–2), 7–27.

van Helden, P.D., Warren, R.M. and Uys, P. (2008) Predicting reinfection in tuberculosis. *Journal of Infectious Disease* 197(1), 172–173; author reply 173–174.

Verver, S., Warren, R.M., Beyers, N., Richardson, M., van der Spuy, G.D., Borgdorff, M.W., *et al.* (2005) Rate of reinfection tuberculosis after successful treatment is higher than rate of new tuberculosis. *American Journal of Respiratory and Critical Care Medicine* 171(12), 1430–1435.

Wallis, R.S., Pai, M., Menzies, D., Doherty, T.M., Walzl, G., Perkins, M.D., *et al.* (2010) Biomarkers and diagnostics for tuberculosis: progress, needs, and translation into practice. *The Lancet* 375(9729), 1920–1937.

WHO (2008) *Guidelines for the Programmatic Management of MDRTB Emergency Update 2008.* WHO, Geneva, Switzerland.

16 The Identification of 2-Aminothiazole-4-carboxylates (ATCs) as a New Class of Tuberculosis Agent: A Lesson in 'HIT' Identification

Geoff Coxon

Strathclyde Institute of Pharmacy and Biomedical Sciences, University of Strathclyde, Glasgow, UK

16.1 Introduction: Strategies to Find New Tuberculosis Drug Scaffolds

So, how and where does one begin when looking for a new class of anti-*Mycobacterium tuberculosis* drug? This is a question asked by many a scientist looking for new therapeutic interventions to eradicate diseases of all types and one to which there is no single, or simple, answer. Finding the answer can be achieved using a number of methods and technologies and can be split broadly into two categories (Balganesh *et al.*, 2004, 2008).

The first method or classical approach to finding compounds with anti-tubercular activity involves taking a compound or mixture of compounds and assessing their ability to inhibit the growth of the pathogen (in this case, mycobacteria) at given, or a series of, concentrations. This is often referred to as the phenotypic approach, as the inhibition of growth is the phenotypic result of the action of the compound against one or more gene products in the organism.

A more modern approach, and one which has been used most over the last decade since the complete sequencing of the *M. tuberculosis* genome, is to target the gene products directly and use them as templates to design new inhibitors or ligands. The expectation using this approach is that the discovered compound will confer a similar effect to the organism as observed during the genetic validation experiments which were used to identify the target. Known as the target or genetic-based approach, this technique, as yet, has not afforded the plethora of new chemical entities that were expected from its exploitation (Projan, 2003; Payne *et al.*, 2007; Barry, 2009). Nevertheless, this approach still receives much attention and has received some credit in the antibiotic drug discovery field in the pharmaceutical industry (Lerner *et al.*, 2007).

The result of these assessments usually yields a quantitative indication of how the three-dimensional structural features of the compound(s) affect its activity. In the case of the phenotypic approach, this is normally expressed as the minimum concentration required to inhibit the growth of mycobacteria (MIC) or, in the target-based approach, the concentration required to reduce the turnover of an enzymatic reaction by 50% (IC_{50}).

It is the role of the medicinal chemist to interpret these data and develop structure–

activity relationships (SARs) from which an iterative modification process may increase the potency of inhibition of the target enzyme or mycobacterial growth. Of course, this is only the start of the process and the medicinal chemist must ensure that selectivity over the host cells and good physico-chemical properties are not sacrificed in the pursuit of potency in order to retain good drug-like characteristics.

16.2 Validated Drug Targets for Mycobacterial Killing

Our research began looking for validated drug targets and possible mechanisms of action that would lead to mycobacterial killing action. It is known that the cell wall of *M. tuberculosis* is rich with many unique key structural components that are necessary for the mycobacteria to survive and grow within the human host, and has long been a target for anti-*M. tuberculosis* drug development (Fig. 16.1). Essential to the cell wall are the mycolic acids, which are high molecular weight 2-alkyl, 3-hydroxy fatty acids that

exist in several forms of differing chemical functionality. Indeed, the first-line anti-tubercular drug, isoniazid (INH), works by inhibiting their biosynthesis. The complete sequencing of the *M. tuberculosis* genome (Cole *et al.*, 1998) has revealed significant biochemical and genetic insight into mycolic acid biosynthesis that will aid the search for new druggable targets. These unique lipids are biosynthesized by both fatty acid synthase enzyme systems I and II (FAS-I and FAS-II) to produce C_{56-64} meromycolic acids and the C_{26} α-branch (Portevin *et al.*, 2004; Takayama *et al.*, 2005) after a series of biotransformations (Yuan *et al.*, 1995; Takayama *et al.*, 2005).

The logical step at this stage was to search the literature for known inhibitors of this pathway to exploit this biochemical knowledge. In looking for compounds that will inhibit an enzyme as part of a series of biochemical steps, it is best to target validated enzymes early in the sequence. As part of our investigations, we were fortunate that the naturally occurring antibiotic, thiolactomycin 1 (TLM; Fig. 16.2), had already been identified as such an inhibitor. This compound, a secondary metabolite produced by the

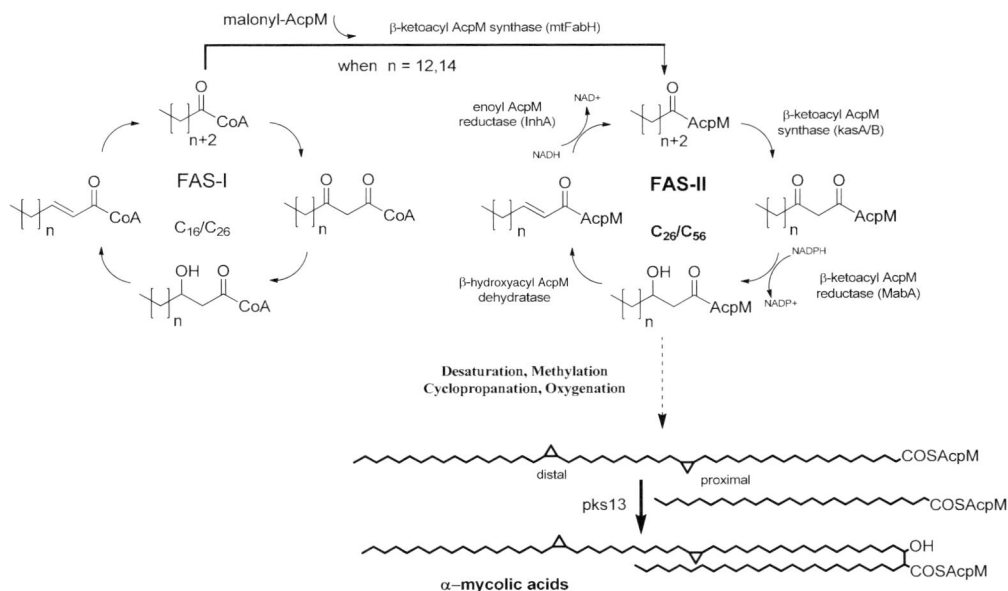

Fig. 16.1. Mycolic acid biosynthesis as a target for anti-*M. tuberculosis* drug design.

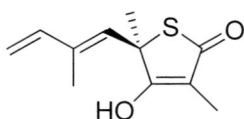

Fig. 16.2. The structure of thiolactomycin (TLM).

soil-dwelling *Nocardia* sp. (Slayden *et al.*, 1996) acts primarily by inhibiting the FAS-II β-ketoacyl-ACP synthase-condensing enzymes, halting mycolic acid biosynthesis and subsequently leading to *M. tuberculosis* cell death (Choi *et al.*, 2000; Kremer *et al.*, 2000; Schaeffer *et al.*, 2001; Kremer *et al.*, 2002).

Importantly, TLM is also orally available and non-toxic in the mouse model, which makes it an attractive compound for development. However, one of the disadvantages of this compound in this regard is that the chemical scaffold of TLM possesses a chiral centre at the 5-position. This structural feature makes the synthesis of a series of TLM analogues lengthy and costly, and complicates the optimization process. When one considers the target product profile of a drug to treat tuberculosis, a key feature is affordability, as no commercial market exists to sustain the development and subsequent distribution of drugs at the clinic. With the current cost of the drugs required to treat the disease being very low, and in some cases free, a simple molecular scaffold for development is vital.

In recent years, this issue of synthetic tractability has focused researchers' efforts towards the synthesis of either racemic analogues or derivatives of TLM that contain simple modifications and has yielded limited improvements in activity against *M. tuberculosis* and modest activity against mtFabH (Douglas *et al.*, 2002; Senior *et al.*, 2003, 2004; Kamal *et al.*, 2005; Kim *et al.*, 2006; Bhowruth *et al.*, 2007). Instead, we focused on identifying alternative, easily accessible 5-membered ring isosteres potentially to generate large compound libraries targeted against the condensing enzyme mtFabH and *M. tuberculosis*, and our attention, after reviewing the literature, focused on the thiazole ring as a template for exploitation.

The following section of this chapter will detail the rationale, design and synthesis of the thiazole ring scaffold which led to the identification of methyl 2-amino-5-benzyl-thiazole-4-carboxylate (Fig. 16.3) and methyl 2-(2-bromoacetamido)-5-(3-chlorophenyl) thiazole-4-carboxylate (Fig. 16.4). The compound in Fig. 16.3 was discovered to be a potent inhibitor of *M. tuberculosis* $H_{37}R_v$ with an MIC of 0.06 µg/ml (0.24 µm), which was more effective than both TLM and the first-line drug INH (MICs of 13 µg/ml (62.5 µm) and 0.25 µg/ml (1.8 µm), respectively) (Kamal *et al.*, 2005). The compound in Fig. 16.4 was found to inhibit mtFabH with an IC_{50} of 0.95 µg/ml (2.43 µm), which compares well with TLM and its most potent racemic analogue in Fig. 16.5 (IC_{50} values of 16 µg/ml (75 µm) and 1.1 µg/ml (3.0 µm), respectively) (Bhowruth *et al.*, 2007).

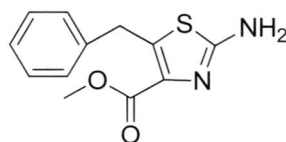

Fig. 16.3. The structure of methyl 2-amino-5-benzylthiazole-4-carboxylate.

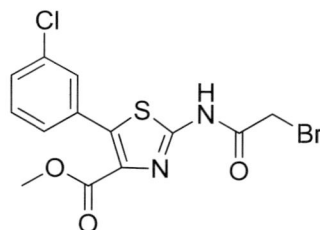

Fig. 16.4. The structure of methyl 2-(2-bromoacetamido)-5-(3-chlorophenyl)thiazole-4-carboxylate.

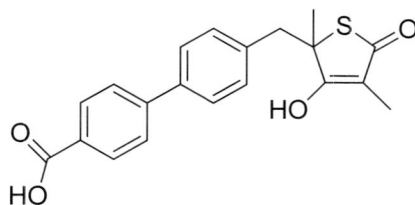

Fig. 16.5. The structure of 4′ ((3-hydroxy-2,4-dimethyl-5-oxo-2,5-dihydrothiophen-2-yl)methyl)-[1,1′-biphenyl]-4-carboxylic acid.

16.2.1 The target-based approach using mtFabH

Ligand design

Our strategy was based initially on the active site geometry and mechanism of action of mtFabH, a homodimer (PDB: 1M1M) that converts C_{12-20} acyl-CoA substrates to the corresponding β-ketoacyl-AcpM product after reaction with mal-AcpM in a two-step process (Brown *et al.*, 2005) (Figs 16.6a and b).

At the molecular level, the acyl-CoA substrate enters an L-shaped binding pocket consisting of a lateral and longitudinal channel, with the active site catalytic triad of Cys112-His244-Asn274 located at the junction. Transacylation of the Cys122 residue occurs when the adjacent His244 deprotonates the thiol group (directly or via a molecule of water, as postulated by Brown *et al.* (2005)) to generate a thiolate nucleophile that attacks the carbonyl group of the acyl chain occupying the longitudinal channel and releases CoA-SH from the lateral channel through which the substrate entered. The second substrate, mal-AcpM, then enters the lateral channel and is decarboxylated by the catalytic residues, His244 and Asn274, and condensed with the thioester formed at Cys112 to generate the β-ketoacyl-AcpM, which also dissociates via the lateral channel. Recently, however, Sachdeva *et al.* have postulated that the overall reaction may occur simultaneously in both active sites of the dimer (Sachdeva and Reynolds, 2008; Sachdeva *et al.*, 2008a,b).

As no inhibitor-mtFabH co-crystal structures had been solved, we investigated the binding pattern of TLM with the closely related analogue ecFabB from *Escherichia coli* (Price *et al.*, 2001). TLM inhibits ecFabB reversibly by forming a number of non-covalent interactions: the methyl group at carbon 3 of TLM is positioned in a hydrophobic pocket defined by residues Phe229 and Phe392; the 5-isoprenoid moiety is wedged between two peptide bonds – from above by residues Val271 and Phe272 and from below by Gly391 and Phe392, which are important for specificity (Brown *et al.*, 2005); the carbonyl oxygen forms two H-bonds with the two histidines in the active site; the

4-hydroxyl group H-bonds to the carbonyl oxygen of Val270 and the amide NH of Gly305 through a lattice of three water molecules; and the sulfur is adjacent to the active site Cys residue, although without any obvious interaction. The strong H-bonding between the active site His residues of ecFabB and the TLM carbonyl group is believed to be crucial for effective inhibitory activity against this enzyme. Based on this analysis, we postulated that the closely related active site of mtFabH could be expected to form an equivalent H-bonding network with TLM, and any new isosteric scaffold would need to maintain many of these important interactions. The equivalent condensing enzyme from *E. coli* (ecFabH) is also closely related to mtFabH, and has been co-crystallized with the very potent inhibitor, 2-hydroxy-6-(3-phenoxy-4-phenyl-benzamido) benzoic acid (Ashek and Cho, 2006). This complex reveals an important role for a carboxylic acid moiety in the ligand, as it forms specific interactions in the active site with the His250 residue from ecFabH (Ashek and Cho, 2006). We considered inclusion of this moiety to be important for our inhibitors and proposed the achiral 2-aminothiazole-5-carboxylate scaffold as an alternative to the TLM substructure to combine pharmacodynamic potency with essential pharmacokinetic considerations such as solubility. Finally, synthetic tractability and subsequent diverse library generation were considered possible by exploiting this scaffold.

Using the molecular modelling software package, GOLD, docking studies were performed to investigate the poses for our scaffold in the mtFabH active site (Jones *et al.*, 1995; Al-Balas *et al.*, 2009). We observed that the carboxyl group of the thiazole ring formed H-bonds with the NH of Cys112, while the NH_2 was proximal to and H-bonds with the imidazole ring of His244. This allowed us to generate a hypothetical template for the development of inhibitors of mtFabH (Fig. 16.7a). Further docking studies were carried out with phenyl, *m*-chlorophenyl (Fig. 16.7b) and benzyl substituents in the 5-position, as both the 4-methyl ester and free acid forms of the thiazoles. In these cases, the

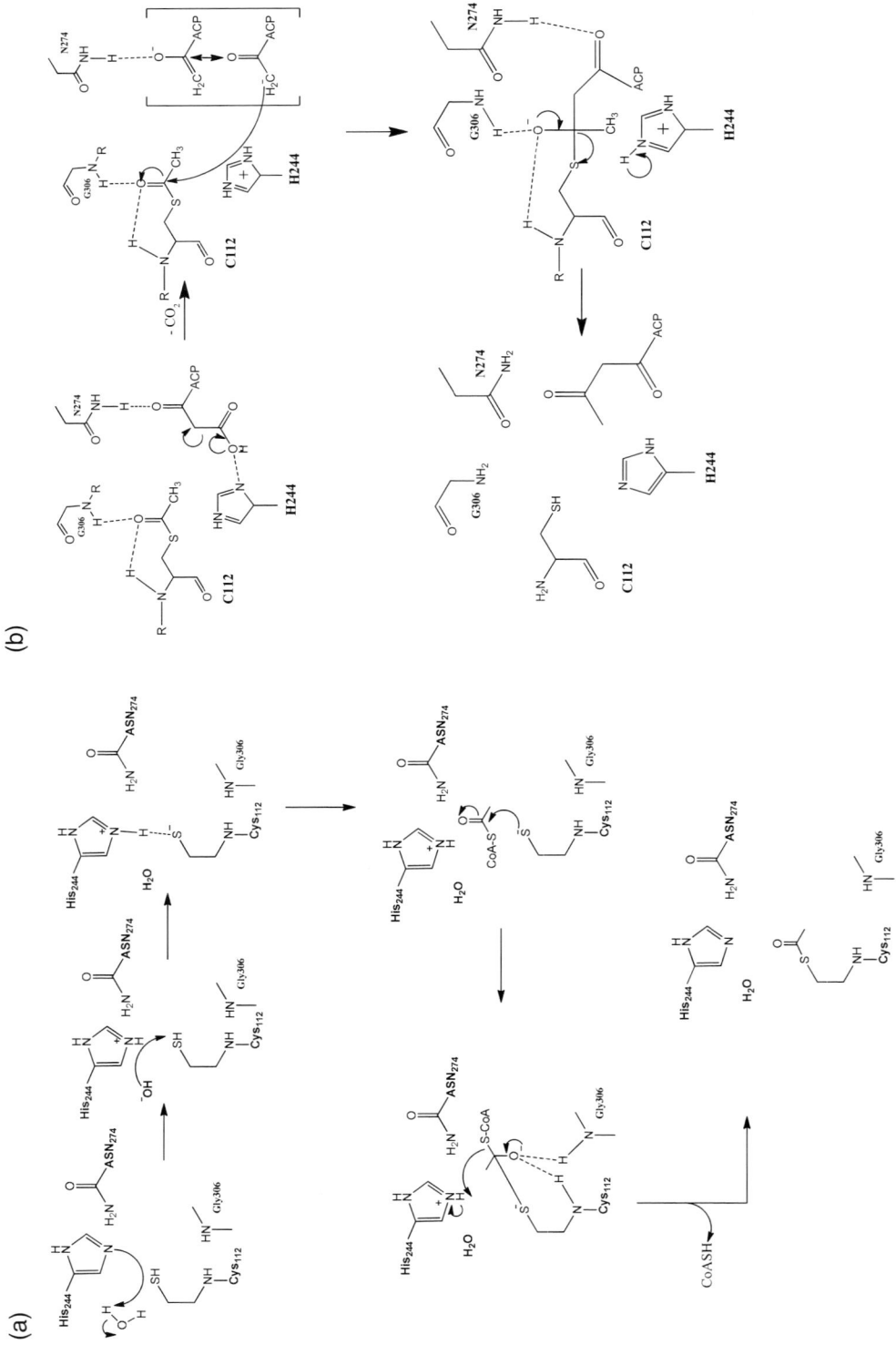

Fig. 16.6. (a) Transacylation mechanism in mtFabH, as proposed by Brown et al. (2005); (b) proposed scheme for the decarboxylation and condensation mechanism in mtFabH.

longitudinal channel appears to be the pre-ferred residence for the 5 substituents, while the 2-amino group and potentially amide derivatives thereof could be accommodated in the lateral channel. We also noted that a 2-bromoacetamido substituent in this posi-tion would place the thiol group of Cys112 in a position to become alkylated via a nucleophilic S_N2 reaction, and could lead to irreversible inhibition of the enzyme (Fig. 16.7c). While such a strategy normally would be performed once a selective and relatively potent inhibitor had been found, we postu-lated that it would be reasonable at this early stage of inhibitor design to attempt this in order to establish if ligand inhibition was at all possible before addressing selectivity in later rounds of ligand optimization. Based on this rationale, we decided to prepare a series of thiazoles that included the substituents studied for evaluation against the enzyme and *M. tuberculosis*.

Chemical synthesis

When reviewing the literature to identify suitable 5-membered ring isosteres of TLM, the flexible synthetic procedure described by Barton *et al.* was identified (Barton *et al.*, 1982). This would facilitate the flexibility

required to build large numbers of com-pounds with structural diversity required to build SARs, while retaining the potential to yield a candidate drug which would meet the cost specifications of the TTP.

The synthesis of our initial fragment-sized (Mwt <250) analogues (Fig. 16.8) was achieved starting with the Darzens reaction between methyl dichloroacetate **5** and the appropriate aldehyde. This afforded a mix-ture of the α-chloro glycidic ester and β-chloro α-oxoester, which was extracted with diethylether and reacted immediately with thiourea dissolved in methanol to generate the methyl ester thiazoles **2, 6–8**. To investigate whether a free carboxylic acid functionality would increase binding within the active site through facilitating electrostatic interactions proposed by the modelling studies, we hydrolysed the esters with 0.1 M sodium hydroxide solution followed by work-up with dilute hydrochloric acid to generate compounds **9–12**. In order to generate 2-bromoacetamido analogues, the free amines **2, 6–12** were reacted with 2-bromoacetylchloride in anhydrous tetra-hydrofuran at 0°C to afford the amides **3, 13–15**. As described previously, hydrolysis with 0.1 M sodium hydroxide gave the correspond-ing carboxylic acids **16–19** for comparison.

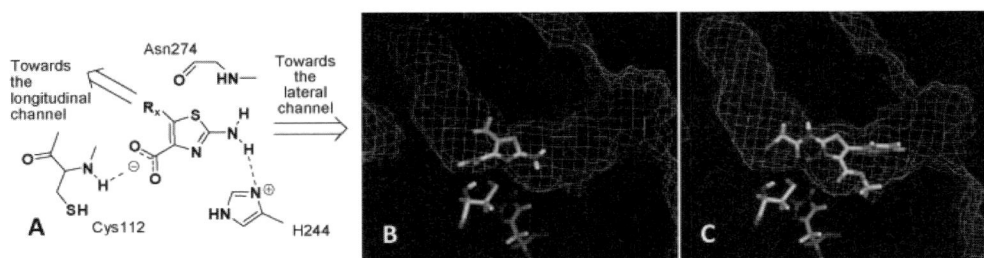

Fig. 16.7. The modelling studies of the 2-aminothiazole-4-carboxylate analogues with mtFabH. (a) The hypothetical template of the 2-aminothiazole-4-carboxylates for mtFabH inhibitor development. This illustrates the key H-bonding interactions with the catalytic triad amino acid residues. (b) The binding pose of methyl 2-amino-5-methylthiazole-4-carboxylate in the active site of mtFabH showing the NH₂ group proximal to His244 and directed towards the lateral channel, with the 5-methyl group directed towards the longitudinal channel. (c) The binding pose of methyl 2-(2-bromoacetamido)-5-(3-chlorophenyl)thiazole-4-carboxylate with the bromomethylene portion in the vicinity of the Cys112 thiol group.

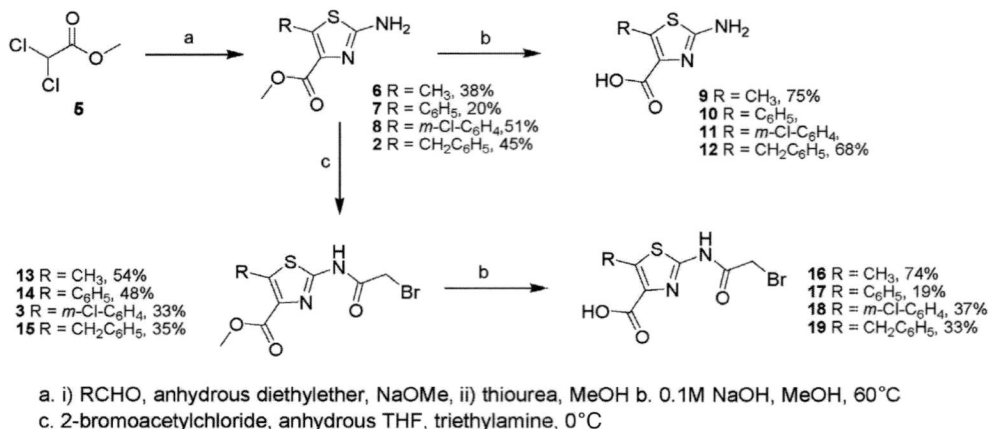

a. i) RCHO, anhydrous diethylether, NaOMe, ii) thiourea, MeOH b. 0.1M NaOH, MeOH, 60°C
c. 2-bromoacetylchloride, anhydrous THF, triethylamine, 0°C

Fig. 16.8. The flexible synthetic route to the ATCs.

16.2.2 Enzymatic assay versus whole cell assay conflict observed in the development of *in vitro* SARs

The compounds were first assessed against the target enzyme mtFabH using the procedure developed by Brown *et al.* (Brown *et al.*, 2005). Despite many of them not demonstrating any inhibitory activity at a concentration of 200 µg/ml, it was pleasing to see the bromoacetamido analogues that were prepared to facilitate an S_N^2 type substitution between the ligand and the Cys112 residue were active. The bromoacetamido esters 3, 14 and 15 inhibited the enzyme with IC_{50} values of 0.95 ± 0.05 µg/ml (2.43 ± 0.13 µm), 1.1 ± 0.1 µg/ml (3.22 ± 0.29 µm) and 59 ± 1.1 µg/ml (159.8 ± 3.0 µm), respectively, while the corresponding carboxylic acid 19 inhibited the enzyme at 225 ± 2.81 µg/ml (718 ± 8.97 µm). Interestingly, the ester 13 and carboxylic acids 16, 17 and 18 failed to inhibit the enzyme.

It is clear that while the electrophilic bromomethyl substituent establishes activity against the enzyme, its effect is modified by different substituents at the 4- and 5-positions. Assuming that the inhibition observed involves reaction with the Cys112 residue, then the ligands must be situated in the vicinity of the catalytic triad. As the longitudinal and lateral tunnels are composed of lipophilic amino acid residues, we suggest that 13 and 16, which possess methyl groups at position 5,

are unable to maximize the hydrophobic interactions with these channels necessary to facilitate enzyme inhibition. However, inserting a phenyl group at position 5 and augmenting it with an *m*-Cl, as in 14 and 3, respectively, allows the appropriate hydrophobic interactions with the enzyme to occur and enables effective inhibition. The flexibility of the ligand also appears to be an important factor; the *m*-Cl phenyl carboxylic acid analogue 18 is inactive, whereas its 5-benzyl counterpart 19, which is less lipophilic, inhibits the enzyme with an IC_{50} of 225 ± 2.81 µg/ml (718 ± 8.97 µm). Comparison with its benzyl ester 15, which inhibits mtFabH with an IC_{50} of 59 ± 1.1 µg/ml (159.8 ± 3.0 µm) suggests that both hydrophobicity and flexibility at the 5 position of the thiazole ring are instrumental in orientating the ligand to achieve effective inhibition. It is interesting that 13 fails to inhibit mtFabH, as it appears that the free acids are weaker inhibitors than the esters. This may be accounted for by the molecule possessing a methyl group at position 5, which does not enable it to maximize the hydrophobic interactions necessary to bind to the enzyme. Conversely, such interactions may be permitted by the flexible benzyl substituent on the free acid 19, which enables weak inhibition.

While it was encouraging to find that a small number of compounds inhibited the target enzyme, it was important to know if this activity would lead to inhibition of the whole cell organism. From the data obtained, it was clear that all of the bromoacetamido analogues failed to inhibit *M. tuberculosis* $H_{37}R_v$ (Table 16.1). We did not know whether these compounds did not inhibit the myco- bacteria through an inability to access the target enzyme due to inappropriate physico- chemical properties or because the bromo- methyl moiety was inactivated chemically or metabolically by the mycobacterium.

Table 16.1. The *in vitro* activity and molecular properties of the 2-aminothiazole-4-carboxylates. [a,b]Compounds regarded as not active (N/A) if no inhibition is observed at 200 µg/ml. [c]FAS-I/II assay conducted at 200 µg/ml and compounds regarded as not active is <50% inhibition observed. [d]AlogP and logD calculated using Pipeline Pilot (SciTegic) software. [e]From Makarov *et al.*, 2009. [f]From Projan, 2003.

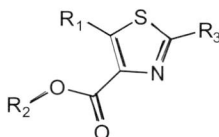

	MWt	R_1	R_2	R_3	mtFabH IC_{50} µg/ml (mM)[a]	TB MIC µg/ml (mM)[b]	FAS-I[c]	FAS-II[c]	AlogP[d] (logD)[d]
1 (TML)	210.29	–	–	–	16 (75)[e]	13 (62.5)[f]	N/A[e]	Active[e]	2.62 (1.94)
2	248.3	$C_6H_5CH_2$	CH_3	NH_2	N/A	0.06 (0.24)	N/A	N/A	2.20 (2.21)
3	389.65	*m*-Cl- C_6H_5	CH_3	$NHCOCH_2Br$	0.95 ± 0.05 (2.43 ± 0.13)	N/A	N/A	Active	3.38 (3.38)
6	172.2	CH_3	CH_3	NH_2	N/A	16 (93)	N/A	N/A	0.51 (0.51)
7	234.27	C_6H_5	CH_3	NH_2	N/A	N/A	N/A	N/A	2.17 (2.17)
8	268.72	*m*-Cl- C_6H_5	CH_3	NH_2	N/A	N/A	N/A	N/A	2.84 (2.84)
9	158.1	CH_3	H	NH_2	N/A	0.06 (0.35)	N/A	N/A	0.28 (−1.18)
10	220.25	C_6H_5	H	NH_2	N/A	N/A	N/A	N/A	1.95 (1.82)
11	254.69	*m*-Cl- C_6H_5	H	NH_2	N/A	32 (125)	N/A	N/A	2.61 (2.48)
12	234.27	$C_6H_5CH_2$	H	NH_2	N/A	N/A	N/A	N/A	1.98 (0.83)
13	293.13	CH_3	CH_3	$NHCOCH_2Br$	N/A	N/A	Active	Active	1.05 (1.05)
14	355.21	C_6H_5	CH_3	$NHCOCH_2Br$	1.1 ± 0.1 (3.22 ± 0.29)	N/A	N/A	Active	2.72 (2.72)
15	369.23	$C_6H_5CH_2$	CH_3	$NHCOCH_2Br$	59 ± 1.1 (159.8 ± 3.0)	N/A	N/A	N/A	2.75 (2.78)
16	279.11	CH_3	H	$NHCOCH_2Br$	N/A	N/A	N/A	Active	0.83 (−0.56)
17	341.18	C_6H_5	H	$NHCOCH_2Br$	N/A	N/A	Active	Active	2.49 (2.46)
18	375.63	*m*-Cl- C_6H_5	H	$NHCOCH_2Br$	N/A	N/A	Active	N/A	3.16 (3.13)
19	355.21	$C_6H_5CH_2$	H	$NHCOCH_2Br$	225 ± 2.81 (718 ± 8.97)	N/A	Active	Active	2.56 (1.38)

In contrast to the 2-bromoacetamido analogues, four of the free amine compounds (**2**, **6**, **9** and **11**) inhibited *M. tuberculosis* $H_{37}R_v$ with MIC values of 0.06, 16, 0.06 and 32 µg/ml (0.24, 93, 0.35 and 125 µm), respectively, while the other analogues of this group showed no activity. Given that these compounds did not inhibit mtFabH, their mechanism of action must involve other targets within the organism.

Although these compounds exhibit excellent activity, in the absence of any recognizable trends in the series, it is difficult to ascertain clear SARs. The best activity was obtained with **2**, with a benzyl group in the 5-position and a methyl ester in the 4-position, whereas the carboxylic acid analogue was shown to be inactive. The opposite observations were seen with the inactive methyl ester analogue **8** possessing an *m*-Cl phenyl group at the 5-position and the corresponding active acid **11**. A similar trend was observed for the 5-methyl analogues **9** and **6**, with MIC values of 0.06 and 16 µg/ml (0.35 and 93 µm), respectively. We speculate that these observations may result from the compounds' ability to enter the cell. In all cases, the primary amine at the 2-position would be associated with a dissociation equilibrium at physiological pH which could penetrate cellular membranes in the unionized state. Compounds **9** and **11**, on the other hand, with both carboxylic acid and amino substituents, would exist as zwitterions and would not normally be expected to penetrate the lipophilic cell wall. The uptake of these compounds could involve a cellular uptake mechanism, such as mycobacterial porins that the inactive zwitterionic compounds **10** and **12** are not substrates for. However, we postulate that the inactivity of the 2-amino analogue **7** is more likely, due to its inability to interact structurally with the target in the organism.

16.2.3 Specificity and selectivity of the 2-aminothiazole-4-carboxylates

It is of key importance that when one designs a series of molecules in a compound class, they confer a high degree of specificity. This is vitally important and ensures that the compound will not be potentially toxic in the patient and assists with complicated regulatory issues associated with progressing the class of compounds through the later stages of drug development.

It is important to recall that the intended site of action of the ATCs is the enzyme mtFabH, which provides the pivotal link in the mycobacterial FAS-II system. It was thus important that selectivity over the related mammalian FAS-I system was achievable. To examine selectivity, the compounds were assessed using the procedures of Slayden *et al.* (1996) and Brown *et al.* (2005).

When studying the SAR in this regard, no inhibition of the FAS enzymes was observed, either as the acid or ester, when the 2-position was the free amine (Table 16.1). These data support the possibility that activity against *M. tuberculosis* $H_{37}R_v$ of compounds **2**, **6**, **9** and **11** involves a target other than mtFabH, or indeed the other FAS-II enzymes. However, with the exception of **15**, all of the compounds possessing the bromoacetamido group at the 2-position showed activity against the FAS enzymes, although no obvious trends were observed across this series. This is perhaps not surprising, as these compounds may be inhibiting other enzymes in the FAS-II system or indeed at different sites in the multifunctional FAS-I complex. However, it was evident from the data that the phenyl **14** and *m*-Cl-phenyl **3** analogues were the only compounds active against mtFabH and selective against FAS-II. The mtFabH inhibitor **19** inhibited both FAS-I and FAS-II, whereas **16** inhibited only FAS-II and **18** FAS-I. Intriguingly, compound **15** failed to inhibit the FAS enzymes, although inhibited mtFabH with an IC_{50} of 59 ± 1.1 µg/ml (159.8 ± 3.0 µm). While 15 may have shown activity against purified mtFabH, its inhibitory potential against mtFabH in the crude FAS-II assay may be difficult to detect, as the related enzyme KasA (present in the crude reaction mix) has been shown to have FabH-type activity and could have had a compensatory effect (Kremer *et al.*, 2002).

Having demonstrated that the killing action of the ATCs against *M. tuberculosis* was clearly not via fatty acid metabolism, it was critical to establish that the compounds would not confer toxicity against mammalian cells. To ascertain this knowledge, and thus understand if this class of compounds still warranted further investigation in future studies, cytoxicity was evaluated against human foreskin fibroblast HS-27 cells (Fig. 16.9) to establish toxicity profiles for our compounds. It was reassuring to find that none of the 2-amino analogues or the free carboxylic analogues of the bromoacetamido compounds showed significant cytotoxicity at a concentration of 100 μg/ml. Conversely, the carboxylic esters of the bromoacetamido compounds **3**, **13**, **14** and **15** all showed signs of significant cytotoxicity. We speculate that this may be due to the indiscriminate alkylation of essential cellular components rather than the increased ability of these esters to penetrate the cells over the carboxylic acids. This is supported by the fact that the non-cytotoxic acids **17**, **18** and **19** have comparable logD values to those of the cytotoxic esters **13**, **14** and **15**, and thus possess similar physicochemical characteristics.

16.3 Conclusions and Future Direction

Although a promising new scaffold has been identified with excellent *in vitro* activity against *M. tuberculosis* and promising selectivity versus mammalian cells, there remains much work to be done in the development of these compounds. In doing so, care must be taken to retain the non-toxic and oral bioavailability properties of the molecule. However, while the zwitterionic, low molecular weight compound **9** has a structure that is highly hydrophilic, which has implications for both absorption and excretion by patients, this should be viewed in the context of INH, a successful and routinely administered antituberculosis drug, which also has a low molecular weight and a logP value of –1.1.

Further information is needed regarding how these compounds work. For example, it is clear it is more advantageous that the action of the compounds is to destroy the mycobacteria outright rather than simply inhibit its growth. Similarly, it is important to understand if the activity of these compounds in a multi-drug regime with existing antitubercular drugs such as INH or rifamipicin provide an additive, synergistic or antagonistic effect.

Pharmacodynamic (PD) and pharmacokinetic (PK) considerations also require investigation. Early, *in vitro* PD can be investigated quickly in the mouse macrophage model, where one would hope to see similar killing action against the mycobacteria as observed *in vitro*, and also evidence of SARs is required in order to optimize activity. Critical information about the initial PK drivers, or routes of metabolism, for these compounds may be obtained using HPLC,

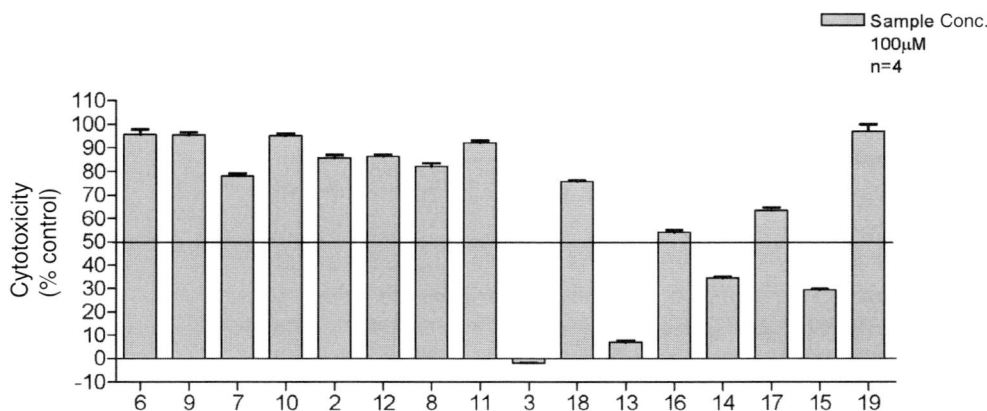

Fig. 16.9. The cytotoxic effects of the compounds against HS-27 human fibroblast cells.

MS and NMR methodology following incubation of the compounds in rat hepatocyte or microsomal assays. Information about the potential formation of reactive metabolites may also be generated using similar experiments where levels of glutathione are monitored and structural elucidation of the formed metabolites is performed. Hepatic cytotoxicity may also be established and comparison of this data in the presence of a blanket Cyp450 inhibitor will indicate whether toxicity is a phenomenon of the intrinsic structure of the compound or its metabolite(s). All of these data can help determine the progression of a chemical series.

Of course, obtaining *in vivo* data is critical and a murine model may be used in the first instance to understand acute toxicity, initial PK and then efficacy. However, being labour- and time-intensive and requiring significant resources, there are a number of *in vitro* experiments which may be further used to 'triage' promising compounds. These include plasma stability models, which give an indication of structural stability in the presence of plasma esterase that may hydrolyse ester groups. This is, of course, important if the retention of ATC ester functionality is critical for activity.

Plasma protein binding should also be measured *in vitro*. Compounds can bind to albumin (HAS), α_1-acid glycoprotein (AGP) or lipoproteins in the blood, and this reduces the amount of free drug in solution for penetration into tissue to reach the therapeutic target or to the liver and kidney for elimination. As the ATCs feature acid and basic moieties in their structure, this is an important experiment as these features may be expected to lead to binding to HAS (potential 2-amino and 4-carboxyl group binding) and AGP (potential 2-amino binding), and the extent of this binding needs to be identified.

The permeability properties of the ATCs may be evaluated *in vitro* by two possible methods, by using a parallel artificial membrane permeability assay (PAMPA) or Caco-2 methods. This will give important information about the potential of the molecules' ability to move across the gut and into the bloodstream and may be used along with physico-chemical knowledge (pKa, logD, polar surface area) and could be used to select compounds for *in vivo* work. As many of the ATCs have polarizable groups, and in some cases are zwitterionic, then these may not be expected to have good passive diffusion properties. However, it is possible that an active uptake mechanism may help adsorb highly charged molecules through the gut wall and thus the Caco-2 model may be an appropriate experiment.

Of course, further preclinical development will be more time-consuming and resource-intensive and thus knowledge of the mechanism of action of the compounds, which is a regulatory requirement, should be gained before embarking on further development. To address this, in a similar strategy used to identify the target of the benzothiazinones, mutants may be selected and comparison of their DNA wild-type sequences performed (Makarov *et al.*, 2009).

It is clear that the development of the ATCs is at an early stage. However, they are very active against *M. tuberculosis*, simple to make and are non-toxic against human cell lines. Moreover, important lessons have been learned during their discovery in that while a single or multiple target approach may be used as a template for ligand design, this often does not correlate with whole cell activity. Additionally, it can be hard to develop meaningful SARs from a small set of compounds and thus a synthesis of larger libraries of the same structural class with increased structural diversity may be required. There is no doubt, however, that the basic ATC scaffold yields promise for further investigation as a potential new tuberculosis drug.

References

Al-Balas, Q., Anthony, N.G., Al-Jaidi, B., Alnimr, A., Abbott, G., Brown, A.K., *et al.* (2009) Identification of 2-aminothiazole-4-carboxylate derivatives active against *Mycobacterium tuberculosis* H37Rv and the beta-ketoacyl-ACP synthase mtFabH. *PLoS One* 4(5), e5617.

Ashek, A. and Cho, S.J. (2006) A combined approach of docking and 3D QSAR study of beta-ketoacyl-acyl carrier protein synthase III

(FabH) inhibitors. *Bioorganic and Medicinal Chemistry* 14(5), 1474–1482.

Balganesh, T.S., Balasubramanian, V. and Kumar, S.A. (2004) Drug discovery for tuberculosis: bottlenecks and path forward. *Current Science* 86(1), 167–176.

Balganesh, T.S., Alzari, P.M. and Cole, S.T. (2008) Rising standards for tuberculosis drug development. *Trends in Pharmacological Sciences* 29(11), 576–581.

Barry, C.E. 3rd (2009) Unorthodox approach to the development of a new antituberculosis therapy. *New England Journal of Medicine* 360(23), 2466–2467.

Barton, A., Breukelman, S.P., Kaye, P.T., Meakins, G.D. and Morgan, D.J. (1982) The preparation of thiazole-4-carboxylates and thiazole-5-carboxylates, and an infrared study of their rotational isomers. *Journal of the Chemical Society, Perkin Transactions* 1(1), 159–164.

Bhowruth, V., Brown, A.K., Senior, S.J., Snaith, J.S. and Besra, G.S. (2007) Synthesis and biological evaluation of a C5-biphenyl thiolactomycin library. *Bioorganic and Medicinal Chemistry Letters* 17(20), 5643–5646.

Brown, A.K., Sridharan, S., Kremer, L., Lindenberg, S., Dover, L.G., Sacchettini, J.C., *et al.* (2005) Probing the mechanism of the *Mycobacterium tuberculosis* beta-ketoacyl-acyl carrier protein synthase III mtFabH: factors influencing catalysis and substrate specificity. *Journal of Biological Chemistry* 280(37), 32539–32547.

Choi, K.H., Kremer, L., Besra, G.S. and Rock, C.O. (2000) Identification and substrate specificity of beta-ketoacyl (acyl carrier protein) synthase III (mtFabH) from *Mycobacterium tuberculosis*. *Journal of Biological Chemistry* 275(36), 28201–28207.

Cole, S.T., Brosch, R., Parkhill, J., Garnier, T., Churcher, C., Harris, D., *et al.* (1998) Deciphering the biology of *Mycobacterium tuberculosis* from the complete genome sequence. *Nature* 393(6685), 537–544.

Douglas, J.D., Senior, S.J., Morehouse, C., Phetsukiri, B., Campbell, I.B., Besra, G.S., *et al.* (2002) Analogues of thiolactomycin: potential drugs with enhanced anti-mycobacterial activity. *Microbiology* 148(Pt 10), 3101–3109.

Jones, G., Willett, P. and Glen, R.C. (1995) Molecular recognition of receptor sites using a genetic algorithm with a description of desolvation. *Journal of Molecular Biology* 245(1), 43–53.

Kamal, A., Shaik, A.A., Sinha, R., Yadav, J.S. and Arora, S.K. (2005) Antitubercular agents. Part 2: new thiolactomycin analogues active against *Mycobacterium tuberculosis*. *Bioorganic and Medicinal Chemistry Letters* 15(7), 1927–1929.

Kim, P., Zhang, Y.M., Shenoy, G., Nguyen, Q.A., Boshoff, H.I., Manjunatha, U.H., *et al.* (2006) Structure–activity relationships at the 5-position of thiolactomycin: an intact (5R)-isoprene unit is required for activity against the condensing enzymes from *Mycobacterium tuberculosis* and *Escherichia coli*. *Journal of Medicinal Chemistry* 49(1), 159–171.

Kremer, L., Douglas, J.D., Baulard, A.R., Morehouse, C., Guy, M.R., Alland, D., *et al.* (2000) Thiolactomycin and related analogues as novel anti-mycobacterial agents targeting KasA and KasB condensing enzymes in *Mycobacterium tuberculosis*. *Journal of Biological Chemistry* 275(22), 16857–16864.

Kremer, L., Dover, L.G., Carrere, S., Nampoothiri, K.M., Lesjean, S., Brown, A.K., *et al.* (2002) Mycolic acid biosynthesis and enzymic characterization of the beta-ketoacyl-ACP synthase A-condensing enzyme from *Mycobacterium tuberculosis*. *Biochemical Journal* 364(Pt 2), 423–430.

Lerner, C.G., Hajduk, P.J., Wagner, R., Wagenaar, F.L., Woodall, C., Gu, Y.G., *et al.* (2007) From bacterial genomes to novel antibacterial agents: discovery, characterization, and antibacterial activity of compounds that bind to HI0065 (YjeE) from *Haemophilus influenzae*. *Chemical Biology and Drug Design* 69(6), 395–404.

Makarov, V., Manina, G., Mikusova, K., Mollmann, U., Ryabova, O., Saint-Joanis, B., *et al.* (2009) Benzothiazinones kill *Mycobacterium tuberculosis* by blocking arabinan synthesis. *Science* 324(5928), 801–804.

Payne, D.J., Gwynn, M.N., Holmes, D.J. and Pompliano, D.L. (2007) Drugs for bad bugs: confronting the challenges of antibacterial discovery. *Nature Reviews Drug Discovery* 6(1), 29–40.

Portevin, D., De Sousa-D'Auria, C., Houssin, C., Grimaldi, C., Chami, M., Daffe, M., *et al.* (2004) A polyketide synthase catalyzes the last condensation step of mycolic acid biosynthesis in mycobacteria and related organisms. *Proceedings of the National Academy of Sciences* 101(1), 314–319.

Price, A.C., Choi, K.H., Heath, R.J., Li, Z., White, S.W. and Rock, C.O. (2001) Inhibition of beta-ketoacyl-acyl carrier protein synthases by thiolactomycin and cerulenin. Structure and mechanism. *Journal of Biological Chemistry* 276(9), 6551–6559.

Projan, S.J. (2003) Why is big Pharma getting out of antibacterial drug discovery? *Current Opinion in Microbiology* 6(5), 427–430.

Sachdeva, S. and Reynolds, K.A. (2008) *Mycobacterium tuberculosis* beta-ketoacyl acyl carrier protein synthase III (mtFabH) assay: principles and method. *Methods in Molecular Medicine* 142, 205–213.

Sachdeva, S., Musayev, F., Alhamadsheh, M.M., Neel Scarsdale, J., Tonie Wright, H. and Reynolds, K.A. (2008a) Probing reactivity and substrate specificity of both subunits of the dimeric *Mycobacterium tuberculosis* FabH using alkyl-CoA disulfide inhibitors and acyl-CoA substrates. *Bioorganic Chemistry* 36(2), 85–90.

Sachdeva, S., Musayev, F.N., Alhamadsheh, M.M., Scarsdale, J.N., Wright, H.T. and Reynolds, K.A. (2008b) Separate entrance and exit portals for ligand traffic in *Mycobacterium tuberculosis* FabH. *Chemistry and Biology* 15(4), 402–412.

Schaeffer, M.L., Agnihotri, G., Volker, C., Kallender, H., Brennan, P.J. and Lonsdale, J.T. (2001) Purification and biochemical characterization of the *Mycobacterium tuberculosis* beta-ketoacyl-acyl carrier protein synthases KasA and KasB. *Journal of Biological Chemistry* 276(50), 47029–47037.

Senior, S.J., Illarionov, P.A., Gurcha, S.S., Campbell, I.B., Schaeffer, M.L., Minnikin, D.E., *et al.* (2003) Biphenyl-based analogues of thiolactomycin, active against *Mycobacterium tuberculosis* mtFabH fatty acid condensing enzyme. *Bioorganic and Medicinal Chemistry Letters* 13(21), 3685–3688.

Senior, S.J., Illarionov, P.A., Gurcha, S.S., Campbell, I.B., Schaeffer, M.L., Minnikin, D.E., *et al.* (2004). Acetylene-based analogues of thiolactomycin, active against *Mycobacterium tuberculosis* mtFabH fatty acid condensing enzyme. *Bioorganic and Medicinal Chemistry Letters* 14(2), 373–376.

Slayden, R.A., Lee, R.E., Armour, J.W., Cooper, A.M., Orme, I.M., Brennan, P.J., *et al.* (1996) Antimycobacterial action of thiolactomycin: an inhibitor of fatty acid and mycolic acid synthesis. *Antimicrobial Agents and Chemotherapy* 40(12), 2813–2819.

Takayama, K., Wang, C. and Besra, G.S. (2005) Pathway to synthesis and processing of mycolic acids in *Mycobacterium tuberculosis*. *Clinical Microbiology Reviews* 18(1), 81–101.

Yuan, Y., Lee, R.E., Besra, G.S., Belisle, J.T. and Barry, C.E. 3rd (1995) Identification of a gene involved in the biosynthesis of cyclopropanated mycolic acids in *Mycobacterium tuberculosis*. *Proceedings of the National Academy of Sciences* 92(14), 6630–6634.

17 Rifamycins Revisited

Martin J. Boeree

Radboud University Nijmegen Medical Centre, Nijmegen, The Netherlands

17.1 Introduction

In 1957, Sensi and co-workers at Group Lepetit SpA Laboratories in Milan, Italy, isolated a new drug with antibiotic properties which they named rifomycin (Sensi *et al.*, 1959); the name was later changed to rifamycin. The rifamycins are a member of the ansamycin family of antibiotics. Rifamycin was extracted from fermentation cultures of *Amycolatopsis rifamycinica* (previously *Streptomyces mediterranei*). It actually consisted of seven substances and therefore was renamed rifamycin A, B, C, D, E, S and SV. These substances were poorly absorbed and were first developed as parenteral agents. Rifamycin B was the most stable, least toxic and active against a broad spectrum of bacteria, mainly Gram-positive cocci and *Mycobacterium tuberculosis* (Lester, 1972; Sensi, 1983). Peculiarly, the name rifamycin was dedicated to the popular 1955 French 'film noir' movie, Rififi (see Fig. 17.1) (Sensi, 1983). Rifamycin B was not much used clinically in tuberculosis treatment, because of its toxicity and parenteral administration. In the years to follow, the Sensi group tried to synthesize an oral equivalent with good intestinal absorption. In 1965, rifampicin, a hydrazone of a rifamycin B derivate with *N*-amino-*N′*-methylpiperazine, showed to be well absorbed orally and, moreover, was still highly bactericidal (Maggi *et al.*, 1966; Lester, 1972; Sensi, 1983). With rifampicin (RIF or R) available, the use of rifamycin B was almost fully abolished, although it remained available for use in some (mainly European) countries (van Ingen *et al.*, 2011b).

After the introduction of RIF, optimism came into the tuberculosis scientific society and tuberculosis control institutions. The possibility of elimination was even becoming a feasible target. This led to several years of relative apathy in tuberculosis drug discovery. Yet several derivatives of RIF were synthesized and tested for clinical use in search for even more efficiency in terms of duration, dosing intervals and tolerability. Rifapentine (RPT) (2008d) was approved for use in humans in 1998. It is attractive because of its long half-life. It needs to be dosed once weekly, or even once fortnightly. Rifalazil (2008b) has an equally long half-life, but never made it to registration because of adverse events. Rifabutin (RBT) (2008a) was first released in 1983 on a compassionate use basis for the treatment of disseminated *M. avium* infection. It is not registered for use in tuberculosis (Davies *et al.*, 2007). RBT is probably as equally efficient as RIF, has more adverse events but has favourable pharmacological properties to use concurrently with antiretroviral drugs.

All rifamycins express their anti-tubercu-

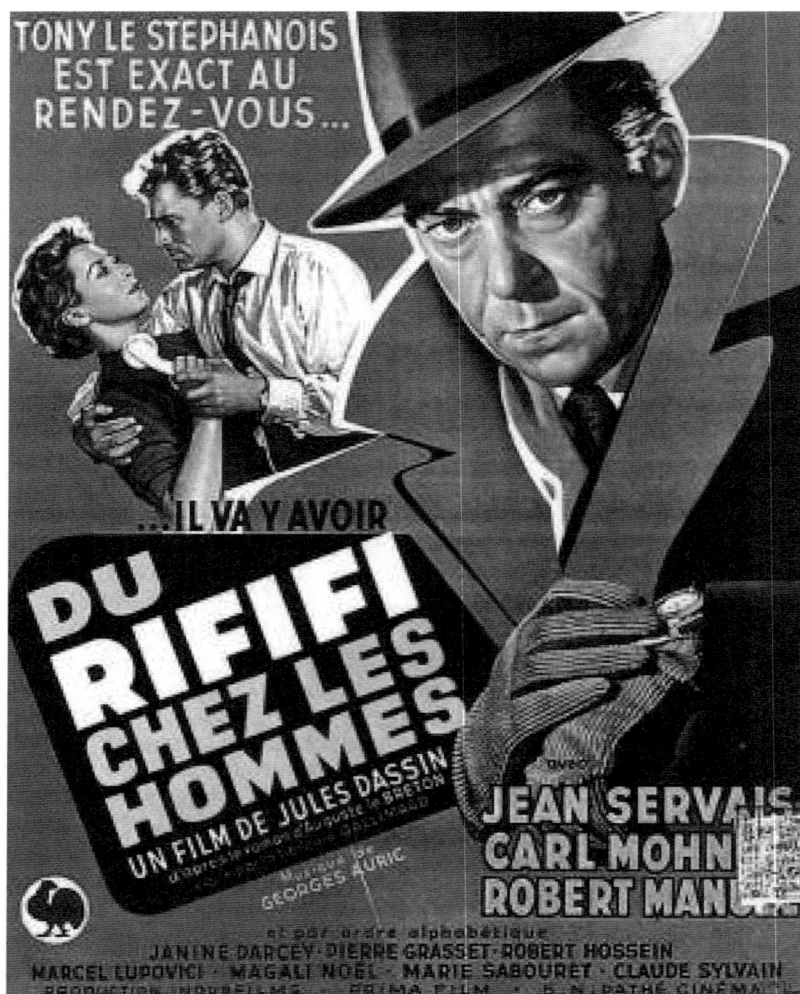

Fig. 17.1. The Rififi film poster, French version. The rifamycins were named after the novel and film.

losis activity by inhibiting the essential β-subunit of RNA polymerase (RNAP) by binding to it. This subunit is produced by the *rpoB* gene (2008c). In addition, the rifamycins may act bactericidally by activating the 'suicide gene module', *mazEF*, and hence inducing apoptosis of the mycobacteria. A vexing problem in tuberculosis treatment with all currently used tuberculosis drugs is the rapid emergence of resistance, especially if used in monotherapy. The existing rifamycins are no exception. Drug resistance for

the rifamycins works in >97% of cases, through mutations in the RIF resistance-determining region (RRDR) around amino acids 513–531 of the *rpoB* gene (Huitric *et al.*, 2006). Some mutations, especially in codon 531, cause resistance to all rifamycins and some mutations in codons 511 and 516 result in resistance specific to RIF and RPT, but not to RBT.

In this chapter, the several rifamycins will be reviewed, with a special emphasis on rifampicin, its chosen dosage, the potential role of rifapentine, the place rifabutin has taken and the rifamycins that have not yet made it to clinical use.

17.2 Rifampicin

17.2.1 History

Rifampicin (also rifampin, rifamycin AMP or rifaldazine, abbreviated RIF, RMP or R; Fig. 17.2) was registered by the FDA in 1971 (Sensi, 1983). By this time, several trials and case series had established efficacy for RIF-containing regimens in tuberculosis treatment (Maggi *et al.*, 1966; De *et al.*, 1968; Gyselen *et al.*, 1968; Newman *et al.*, 1971; Nitti *et al.*, 1971; Constans *et al.*, 1972; Corpe and Sanchez, 1972; Davidson *et al.*, 1972; Favez *et al.*, 1972). Originally, RIF was reserved to be a second-line drug, since first-line triple therapy (streptomycin (S or SM), isoniazid (INH or H) and para-amino-salicylic acid (PAS or P)) was already highly effective and RIF was considered to be too dire (Citron, 1972). An editorial in the *British Medical Journal* stated that the price for 10 g of sodium PAS was £02.5, 1 g of ethambutol was £0.22 and 600 mg of RIF was £0.68 (1973) (the latter comparable to £3.79 or US$6.05 today). The British Medical Research Council (BMRC) preferred INH and pyrazinamide (PZA or Z) regimens over equally active INH–RIF regimens, as RIF cost over £110 for 6 months, more than four times the cost of PZA. In a respected review on tuberculosis treatment, Fox *et al.* repeatedly remind us that the first short-course therapy trials were designed 'to use the minimum amount of expensive rifampicin' (in East Africa) or did not include RIF because of the

high cost (Hong Kong and Singapore) (Fox *et al.*, 1999). At the same time, the introduction of RIF containing first-line regimens was advocated for four reasons: easier administration, less toxicity, faster conversion and – the most important – a shorter duration of therapy. The shortening of treatment would therefore justify (and, in part, make up for) the expense (Houk, 1972). In the second half the 1970s, RIF gained a foothold as a first-line drug, at least for countries that could afford its use (McConville and Rapoport, 1976; Angel, 1977; Robinson, 1978). The body of evidence to support the use of RIF and introduce successful treatment with 6-month short-course regimens overruled the associated cost (McConville and Rapoport, 1976; Angel, 1977; Long *et al.*, 1979). Still, use of this costly drug was, at times, met with controversy (Gosling *et al.*, 2003). Eventually, RIF treatment made its way into tuberculosis treatment guidelines, but it did so in the lowest effective dosage of 10 mg/kg (Angel, 1977; Fox *et al.*, 1999). RIF had been shown to be efficient, expressed by favourable cure rates and low relapse rates, with a considerable shorter duration of the standard treatment of at least 12–18 months. Hence, these RIF-containing regimens of short duration were called – at present, paradoxically – short-course chemotherapy.

17.2.2 Microbiological activity

RIF has potent antibiotic activity against *M. tuberculosis*. *In vitro*, the minimum inhibitory concentration (MIC) against the laboratory strain H37Rv is 0.1–0.4 μg/ml (Rastogi *et al.*, 1996). The MIC_{90} (the MIC in which 90% of the bacterial population is inhibited) is 0.25 μg/ml. RIF also acts as exposure dependent in macrophages and other cells (Jayaram *et al.*, 2003). RIF is heavily protein bound (83%), which leads to increased MIC in serum. It is bactericidal. There are *in vitro* synergies with several quinolones, macrolides, ethambutol and streptomycin (Bhusal *et al.*, 2005). Recently, a synergy with the efflux pump inhibitor, thioridazine, has been demonstrated (see Chapter 18). For INH, there is no synergy observed. In the animal model, RIF has

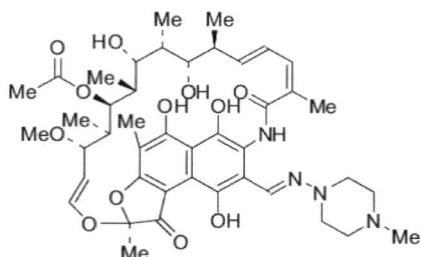

Fig. 17.2. Rifamycin.

shown its sterilizing efficacy repeatedly, and in the mouse model, it has demonstrated its sterilizing activity repeatedly. In one study, there was a complete sterilization of the mice given INH 25 mg/kg and RIF 25 mg/kg for 9 months. If RIF was withdrawn in the last 3 months, there was a 20% relapse rate. The existing evidence shows that there is a dose relation; in the extreme, a complete steriliza-tion was achieved in the infected mice in 6 days with a dose of 810 mg/kg (2008c).

17.2.3 Clinical efficacy

RIF is an efficient drug against drug-sensitive tuberculosis in humans. In a combination regimen with INH and PZA for 2 months in an intensive phase, followed by a continuation phase of 4 months, cure rates are high: in programme conditions, 85% is considered to be realistic and in the early trials, cure rates are >95% at a dose of 10 mg/kg (Long et al., 1979). In the studies that showed efficacy for RIF, eventually a daily dosage of 10 mg/kg was chosen, for several reasons (1972; Gyselen et al., 1968; Newman et al., 1971; Nitti et al., 1971; Constans et al., 1972; Corpe and Sanchez, 1972; Davidson et al., 1972). Whether this was the right choice is currently being debated: there are several arguments to assume that the dosage is at the lower end of the dose–response curve. Higher dosages of RIF are currently being investigated for their potential to shorten the duration of tubercu-losis treatment. Van Ingen et al., 2011b) have performed a literature search focusing on the dosing question, reviewing papers published in the first two decades after the development of RIF. The most explicit comment came from Richard O'Brien and Andrew Vernon, who, in their 1998 editorial (O'Brien and Vernon, 1998), stated that determination of the optimal dose of RIF 'was done by the United States Public Health Service (USPHS) Tuberculosis Study 19 from 1979 which established 600 mg as the optimal dose for most adults'. Study 19 evaluated a daily dosage of 450 (7.5 mg/kg), 600 (10 mg/kg) and 750 mg (12.5 mg/kg) of RIF with a fixed dose of INH and observed no significant difference in sputum conversion or relapse between the

600 mg and 750 mg arms. The regimen containing 450 mg was significantly less effective than the other two regimens, with a lower rate of sputum conversion and a higher rate of treatment failures (Long et al., 1979). Interestingly, the 600 mg dose had become standard practice even before the FDA's approval of RIF for tuberculosis treatment in 1971, and it is still recommended as the maximum daily dose (World Health Organization, 2009). Other trials had studied doses other than 600 mg, but the differences were either small (±150 mg in the USPHS study) or were part of regimens that deviated so far from common practice that it was difficult to single out the effect of RIF. An important example is the study by Kreis et al., published in 1976, which tested two 3-month regimens of high-dose RIF (1200 mg daily or every other day) combined with high daily doses of INH and S. These regimens had almost 100% sputum culture conversion, but 16% of patients relapsed after 12–24 months (Kreis et al., 1976). From today's perspective, the most likely contributor to the high initial cure rate achieved is the high dose of RIF. This also makes the daily dose of 600 mg RIF worth being reconsidered. More importantly, what renders a dose 'optimal' from today's point of view? According to current stand-ards, the optimal dose of RIF would be derived from the relationships between dos-ing, drug exposure achieved and desirable and undesirable responses in Phase I and II studies with clearly differing doses of RIF, followed by pivotal Phase III studies of regimens. No such studies have been done. In 2010, 2011 and 2012 three Phase II trials were executed in Africa to establish a more accurate maximum tolerated dose with a proof a concept for more efficacy in terms of shorter duration of treatment.

17.2.4 Pharmacokinetics

Early pharmacokinetic studies showed that a single daily dose of 600 mg of RIF resulted in serum concentrations of 7.0 µg/ml 90 min after ingestion, or 8.80–12.0 µg/ml after 2 h, i.e. well above 0.2 µg/ml, the mean MIC of *M. tuberculosis* (Furesz et al., 1967; Verbist and

Gyselen, 1968; Nitti *et al.*, 1972). Higher doses were explored and showed significantly higher serum concentrations and half-life, suggesting a non-linear association (Constans *et al.*, 1968; Acocella *et al.*, 1971; Ruslami *et al.*, 2006); one early study in France applied 900 mg RIF once daily and found average serum concentrations of 16.2 µg/ml 3 h after intake (Constans *et al.*, 1968). Since peak serum concentrations (C_{max}) are reached 2 h after intake (Acocella *et al.*, 1971; Nitti *et al.*, 1972; Ruslami *et al.*, 2006), the C_{max} was likely to be higher. A year later, Furesz and co-workers measured peak serum concentrations (after 2 h) of 20.87 ± 3.25 after a single 750 mg dose and 27.70 ± 4·16 µg/ml after administration of 900 mg of RIF in healthy volunteers. Yet they stated that the 600 mg doses already ensured therapeutic (i.e. equal to or above MIC) blood levels for 24 h after administration (Furesz *et al.*, 1967). Although this pharmacokinetic argument is compelling, it is based on the assumption that RIF is active when serum concentrations exceed the MIC throughout the dosing interval, which means that the ratio of the trough concentration (C_{min}) to MIC is the relevant pharmacodynamic index ('time-dependent inhibition') (Pallanza *et al.*, 1967; Verbist and Gyselen, 1968; Favez *et al.*, 1972; Lester, 1972). Similar reasoning is illustrated by the statement of Constans *et al.* that the 900 mg dose applied in a pilot of their trial was 'unnecessarily high' (Constans *et al.*, 1972).

In the years following, this assumption changed into the view that the efficacy of RIF was concentration dependent, i.e. correlating with peak plasma concentration (C_{max}) divided by the MIC (Pallanza *et al.*, 1967; Nuermberger and Grosset, 2004). This view was based on the intracellular mode of action of RIF; other drugs with intracellular targets, such as aminoglycosides and fluoroquinolones, were shown to have concentration-dependent activity. Concentration-dependent activity and the associated post-antibiotic effect also explained the efficacy of RIF better when it was administered intermittently (Pallanza *et al.*, 1967; Nuermberger and Grosset, 2004). Recent studies have challenged this assumption again and established that the activity of RIF is more exposure

dependent; in other words, the area under the concentration–time curve (AUC) divided by the MIC correlates better with killing than C_{max}/MIC (Burman *et al.*, 2001; Peloquin, 2001; Jayaram *et al.*, 2003; Nuermberger and Grosset, 2004; Gumbo *et al.*, 2007).

Pharmacokinetic studies generally have been based on serum assays. *M. tuberculosis* is predominantly an intracellular organism, so serum may not be the right compartment. A few studies have examined RIF concentrations in alveolar macrophages and epithelial lining fluid (ELF) (Ziglam *et al.*, 2002; Goutelle *et al.*, 2009). RIF concentrations in ELF and bronchial biopsies are slightly below those in serum, whereas those in alveolar macrophages are over ten times higher (Ziglam *et al.*, 2002). As a result, AUC/MIC or C_{max}/MIC ratios compatible with bacterial killing are generally achievable in serum and alveolar macrophages, but not in ELF. The use of a 1200 mg RIF dose improved significantly the attainment of AUC/MIC or C_{max}/MIC ratios compatible with bacterial killing (Goutelle *et al.*, 2009). Importantly, if the 600 mg dose was applied, RIF concentrations attained at the site of infection were too low. Recently, Gumbo *et al.* showed – as in serum – that exposure to higher concentrations of RIF might lead to a non-linear increase in RIF concentrations inside the bacteria. The exact mechanism is not known; it may be related to saturation of bacterial efflux pumps (Ruslami *et al.*, 2006; Gumbo *et al.*, 2007). The question is whether increasing the concentrations in the bacillus and at the site of infection actually improves killing and improves treatment outcome. Studies of higher doses of RIF and other rifamycins are therefore important and are being performed at the time of writing of this chapter.

In conclusion, the current dose of RIF used in internationally recommended regimens has not been based on careful evaluation of the relationships between dosing, drug exposure achieved at the site of infection and desirable and undesirable responses. By the time of the introduction of the drug, and because of its success, a proper dose-escalating study had not been performed. Recent studies suggest that the current dose of RIF is at the lower end of the dose–response curve (Mitchison, 2000; Jayaram et al., 2003; Peloquin, 2003), as suggested already by the study of Kreis et al. mentioned previously (Kreis et al., 1976). The probable non-linear increase of RIF concentrations means that a relatively small increase in dose is associated with a more than proportional increase in RIF AUC. Clearly, this characteristic should be assessed further in future studies that explore the utility of higher doses of RIF.

17.2.5 Adverse events

Most frequently and remarkably, RIF causes a red-orange staining of all body fluids. Other adverse effects of RIF are mainly gastro-intestinal discomfort (nausea, vomiting, diarrhoea) and, more infrequently, hepatitis and hypersensitivity reactions such as thrombocytopaenia, haemolytic anaemia and interstitial nephritis. Quite rare side effects include hypotension and shock, shortness of breath, organic brain syndrome and per-ipheral neuropathy.

One argument for not using higher doses of RIF is that of these feared side effects. There is little evidence that higher daily doses lead to increased toxicity, which may also be expected because of the non-linear increase of pharmacokinetic (PK) parameters. However, this has not been observed in the few studies that have looked at higher doses of RIF. The few that have been performed report little or no safety and toxicity data (Constans et al., 1968; Acocella et al., 1971; Favez et al., 1972; Kreis et al., 1976; Ruslami et al., 2006). In the study with 900 mg of RIF, Constans and co-workers said that this was 'liable to induce slight disorders', without providing additional data (Constans et al., 1972); Favez and co-workers drew similar conclusions (Favez et al., 1972). In the USPHS Study 19, drug-induced hepatitis frequency did not differ between patients who were given 450, 600 or 750 mg of RIF (Long et al., 1979). Recent studies of higher RIF doses (13 mg/kg and 20 mg/kg) did not report increased hepatotoxicity or other adverse effects (Ruslami et al., 2006; Diacon et al., 2007). The patient numbers of the studies were small. In contrast, inter-

mittent therapy with high doses of RIF (once or twice weekly) has been associated with increased toxicity (Poole et al., 1971; Peloquin, 2001, 2003; Ruslami et al., 2006). Poole and co-authors noted that intermittent high doses of RIF (1200 mg twice weekly with 900 mg INH) led to RIF sensitization and antibody for-mation; 11 (22%) of the 49 patients dis-continued treatment after developing mostly fever, thrombocytopaenia or renal failure, designated as the 'flu-like syndrome'. The high incidence of flu-like syndrome has been ascribed to the intermittency of dosing rather than the height of the dose. Nevertheless, this experience resulted in an end to clinical trials with high-dose RIF. In retrospect, it appears that this was an overreaction that might have prevented the research community identify-ing the correct dosage regimen for RIF. It has been said that the 'baby was thrown out with the bath water'. It is notable that higher doses of RIF (900–2400 mg) have been used in other diseases, for example brucellosis, osteo-myelitis and leishmaniasis, without signifi-cant tolerability problems. In these contexts, RIF is co-administered with less toxic drugs such as co-trimoxazole, and it is used for weeks rather than months (Solera et al., 1995; Kochar et al., 2000).

RIF may not be the most toxic drug in the multi-drug regimen currently used for tuberculosis. In studies of 4-month RIF monotherapy for latent tuberculosis, hepato-toxicity was rare compared with its frequency in RIF–PZA treatment. This may be due to the PZA or to drug interactions rather than to RIF itself (Ziakas and Mylonakis, 2009). The arrival of novel anti-tuberculosis drugs and novel combinations may shed more light on this issue and allow higher doses of RIF to be used safely.

17.3 Rifapentine

17.3.1 History

In 1975, the same LePetit group from Milan who discovered RIF developed a new derivative with a long half-life: DL 473, later called rifapentine (cyclopentylrifamycin, RPT;

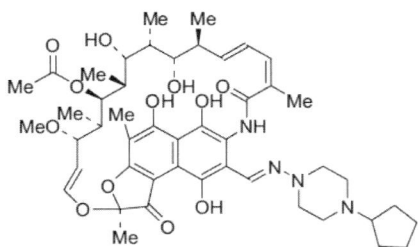

Fig. 17.3. Rifapentine.

Fig. 17.3) (Arioli *et al.*, 1981). RPT was approved by the FDA in 1993 for the treatment of tuberculosis. The long half-life permitted RPT to be dosed once or twice weekly.

17.3.2 Microbiological activity

RPT has the same mechanism of action as RIF. *In vitro*, the MIC against the *M. tuberculosis* strain H37Rv is 0.031 µg/ml and is about tenfold lower than RIF (2008d). There are post-antibiotic effects measured with RPT, especially with INH and moxifloxacin. In the mouse model, RPT was clearly efficient, especially in higher doses (10–15 mg/kg). RPT was not able to sterilize the mice completely, but did so in combination with INH and PZA (Daniel *et al.*, 2000). In another experiment, the activity of RPT was especially enhanced when INH was added in the same weekly dose frequency (Chapuis *et al.*, 1994). Also, a combination with moxifloxacin showed good sterilizing activity, though only when MOX was dosed on a daily basis (Veziris *et al.*, 2005). In a series of experiments, it was shown that the duration of treatment could be reduced considerably by higher doses of RPT in mice (Rosenthal *et al.*, 2006, 2007).

17.3.3 Clinical efficacy

The registration for RPT is restricted for use in HIV-negative patients who are sputum negative at 2 months treatment. This is based on clinical data from the Tuberculosis Trials Consortium (TBTC) Study 25 in 35 patients, in which three doses of RPT once weekly, combined with INH of 15 mg/kg, were evaluated (Weiner *et al.*, 2004). Similarly, it was demonstrated that low INH caused an unacceptable failure rate in the HIV-positive population. The current role for RPT has been assessed recently in a systematic review (Gao *et al.*, 2009). Based on nine evaluable clinical trials, they concluded that once or twice weekly RPT and daily RIF had a similar outcome on cure rates and safety for the treatment of HIV-negative pulmonary tuberculosis, but once-weekly or less frequent use of RPT increased the risk of bacteriological relapse. Additionally, they observed that the risk of resistance to RIF in HIV-positive patients was increased. The hope for a role for RPT in the treatment in drug-sensitive tuberculosis is being focused on its potential to shorten treatment with higher dosages, based mainly on the exciting mouse experiments of Grosset's group (Rosenthal *et al.*, 2006, 2007). There are several ongoing trials by various research groups, such as the TBTC and InterTB, to investigate this concept. Very recently, RPT in combination with INH for 3 months was shown to be non-inferior to 9 months of INH alone in the treatment of latent tuberculosis infection (Sterling and TBTC, 2011).

17.3.4 Pharmocokinetics

RPT was introduced as a more potent and longer-acting rifamycin. The notable characteristic of RPT is its high ratio of protein binding (97%), with a long half-life as result. Bioavailability is about 70%. Tissue levels are generally higher than in plasma concentrations (Burman *et al.*, 2001). Like RIF, there is a long post-antibiotic effect (75 h) (Chan *et al.*, 2004). The other PK characteristics are outlined in Table 17.1.

17.3.5 Adverse events

The adverse events profile very much resembles that of RIF. Hepatitis is as frequent

Table 17.1. PK parameters of rifapentine.

Species	Half-life (h)	AUC (mg/h/l)	C_{max} (µg/ml)	Volume distribution (l/kg)	Clearance (l/h)	PK methodology
Mouse	–	309 ± 35.5[a]	11.1 ± 3.09[a]	–	–	Single dose of MOXI 100 mg/kg in mice of [a]10 mg/kg and [b]15 mg/kg.
		474 ± 5.8[b]	16.7 ± 1.1[b]			
Human	13.18 ± 7.38	319.54 ± 91.52	15.05 ± 4.62	–	2.03 ± 0.6	Dose 300 mg/day. PK determined at day 10.
25-deactyl RIFAP metabolite	13.35 ± 2.67	215.88 ± 86	6.26 ± 2.06	–	–	

Notes: [a]10 mg/kg; [b]15 mg/kg.

as for RIF. There is a difference in the occurrence of the flu-like syndrome, as seen in intermittent admission of higher doses of RIF. For RPT, this phenomenon is observed infrequently.

17.4 Rifabutin

17.4.1 History

In the search for better and safer rifamycin derivatives, Marsili – again, from Milan – described a spiropiperidyl derivative of rifamycin S in 1981 (Marsili *et al.*, 1981). It was called ansamycine LM 427 and later rifabutin (RBT) or mycobutin (Fig. 17.4). The drug had good properties against mycobacteria, especially against *M. avium*, and was initially for compassionate use in disseminated *M. avium* infection in HIV patients (O'Brien *et al.*, 1987).

17.4.2 Microbiological activity

RBT works similarly to RIF and RPT. *In vitro*, the MIC against *M. tuberculosis* strain H37Rv is <0.015 µg/ml (2008a). In the mouse model, RBT was clearly efficient, comparable with RPT, though pharmacokinetically the C_{max}

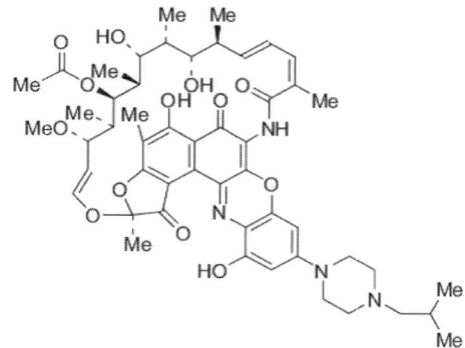

Fig. 17.4. Rifabutin.

and half-life were lowest (Ji *et al.*, 1993). *M. tuberculosis* may retain sensitivity to RBT in 30% of the strains resistant to RIF, because of a point mutation at a different codon in the *rpoB* gene.

17.4.3 Clinical efficacy

In clinical trials investigating the clinical efficacy of RBT, there were no significant differences between RBT and RIF in curing tuberculosis and preventing relapse. However, higher doses of RBT may be associated with more adverse effects and discontinuation.

RBT is a considerably weaker inducer of the CYP450 system and therefore has less influence on the concentration of other drugs. This makes it especially suitable for use in HIV. It can be combined better with anti-retroviral drugs, especially with the class of protease inhibitors (PIs). Consequently, RBT is now reserved specifically for use in HIV patients. In a recent Cochrane review, Davies *et al.* conclude that 'RBT containing regimens perform as well as RIF-containing regimen … There is no evidence currently to support the replacement of RIF by RBT for the treatment of new cases of tuberculosis on the basis of efficacy….' (Davies *et al.*, 2007).

17.4.4 Pharmocokinetics

RBT was very promising in terms of its PK profile: a relatively high C_{max} and AUC. The C_{max}/MIC ratio is lower than for RIF (7.5 versus 67), but protein binding is less than RIF (85%) and RPT (98%) with 70%, and there is a relatively long half-life. It accumulates better in the cell than RIF. There is no food effect, though bioavailability is only 20%. For an overview of the PK characteristics of RBT, see Table 17.2 (2008a).

17.4.5 Adverse events

The adverse events profile of RBT resembles that of RIF: hepatitis, gastrointestinal symptoms and, rarely, cardiovascular, respiratory and neurological events. Hypersensitivity reactions are also reported, as is the flu-like syndrome. Unusual RBT-specific toxicity with myositis and uveitis is reported; this is dose related (2008a).

17.5 Rifalazil

Recently, rifalazil (KRM-1648 or ABI-1648) was developed by Kaneka Corp, Japan. Its MIC for *M. tuberculosis* was considerably lower than for other rifamycins (MIC 0.0125). It had more potential than RIF. Unfortunately, its development had to be suspended because of the side effects in clinical trials (Aristoff *et al.*, 2010).

17.6 Conclusions and Looking Forward

It is important to engage with the question of the optimal dose of RIF and RPT and, in addition, the potential of newer rifamycins. The tuberculosis pandemic is still uncontrolled; there is a pressing need to improve the treatment of tuberculosis, to render patients smear and culture negative as quickly as possible. There is a need to shorten the duration of treatment, ideally to 3 months or even less. In the future, treatment will be of short duration, while some patients may be identified with biomarkers that predict failure or relapse. These patients can then receive a tailor-made treatment, probably of longer duration.

First, in small-scale studies, high (20 mg/kg) doses of RIF have already been shown to have bactericidal activity up to twice that of the 600 mg (10 mg/kg) dose (Gosling *et al.*, 2003; Diacon *et al.*, 2007). In addition, RIF has a sterilizing effect, i.e. the capacity to kill the remaining mycobacteria that undergo sporadic metabolism and that remain after the initial phase of treatment (Jindani *et al.*, 2003). This provides the most exciting reason to address this issue: if higher doses of RIF

Table 17.2. PK parameters of rifabutin.

Species	Half-life (h)	AUC (mg/h/l)	C_{max} (µg/ml)	Volume distribution (l/kg)	Clearance (l/h/kg)	PK methodology
Human	45 ± 17 (range 16–69)	–	375 ± 267	–	0.69 ± 0.32	300 mg single oral dose to healthy volunteers

and RPT are safe and well tolerated, and kill tubercle bacilli more rapidly, we may be able to shorten tuberculosis treatment further. This will have an immediate effect on completion and cure rates. The original dose has helped to reduce treatment duration of the multi-drug regimen to 6 months but has failed to reduce the duration of treatment to 4 months, as 5–15% of the patients experienced bacteriological relapses in the BMRC Study 4 trials (Fox *et al.*, 1999). A further reduction should still be our goal. In addition, faster smear and culture conversion decreases the size of the infectious pool of patients in the community and can reduce further transmission of tuberculosis. Second, higher doses of RIF and RPT may expose the bacteria to AUC/MIC values that prevent the emergence of resistance or, according to the concept of mutant prevention concentration (MPC), raise concentrations to a level that prevents the emergence of RIF-resistant mutants, and thus risk of the emergence of MDR-TB. Third, there is a recent report that higher-dose RIF may have a role in infections caused by low-level resistant strains (i.e. MICs of 1–2 mg/l, just above the 1 mg/l breakpoint concentration). Such resistance may be overcome by applying higher doses of RIF (van Ingen *et al.*, 2011a). If higher doses prove to be more efficacious and tolerable, a new regimen could be implemented quickly. Finally, financial restrictions are no longer warranted; the price of a complete treatment regimen for a single patient, based on the 2HRZE4HR regimen, is now US$38.15 through the Stop TB Partnerships' Global Drug Facility. This price equals the price of 1 week of RIF monotherapy in 1973.

Since the development of the rifamycins in the 1950s and 1960s, and especially in the last decades, there are several groups who have developed new rifamycin derivatives with potentially better properties (Aristoff *et al.*, 2010). Ideally, new rifamycins need to be able to: (i) shorten treatment; (ii) be effective against MDR-TB; and (iii) be effective against latent tuberculosis. Researchers have expanded on the structure of RIF. On the basis of such studies, RPT was developed; later azinomethylrifamycins such as FCE 22250 and rifametane were promising

derivatives in terms of *in vitro* MICs. Unfortunately, the bactericidal activity was inferior to RIF. A promising development in the search for better rifamycin derivatives is the synthesis of crystal structures of inhibitors with RNAP, which in theory may block RNA polymerase and will not be sensitive to point mutations in the *rpoB* gene (Ho *et al.*, 2009). Consequently, resistance will not emerge through this pathway. In fact, it may be possible to develop inhibitors that bind tighter to a resistant mutant than to a wild-type RNAP (Barluenga *et al.*, 2006). These are rifamycin derivatives with a C3/C4 tail (in contrast with RIF and RPT, which have C3 tails). RBT and rifalazil are examples of such derivatives. Rifalazil derivatives such as ABI-0418, 0299, 11331 and 0043, all from scientists at ActivBiotics (Tucker, Georgia, USA), are described in a series of patent applications (Murphy *et al.*, 2007). Finally, researchers at Cumbre Pharmaceuticals (Dallas, Texas, USA) have prepared novel rifamycin–quinolone hybrids (the lead component being CBR-2092) that are very active against *S. aureus* (Robertson *et al.*, 2008).

References

(1972) Controlled clinical trial of short-course (6-month) regimens of chemotherapy for treatment of pulmonary tuberculosis. *The Lancet* 2(7760), 1079–1085.

(1973) Editorial: Rifampicin or ethambutol in the routine treatment of tuberculosis. *British Medical Journal* 4(5892), 568.

(2008a) Rifabutin. *Tuberculosis (Edinburgh)* 88(2), 145–147.

(2008b) Rifalazil. *Tuberculosis (Edinburgh)* 88(2), 148–150.

(2008c) Rifampin. *Tuberculosis (Edinburgh)* 88(2), 151–154.

(2008d) Rifapentine. *Tuberculosis (Edinburgh)* 88(2), 155–158.

Acocella, G., Pagani, V., Marchetti, M., Baroni, G.C. and Nicolis, F.B. (1971) Kinetic studies on rifampicin. I. Serum concentration analysis in subjects treated with different oral doses over a period of two weeks. *Chemotherapy* 16(6), 356–370.

Angel, J.H. (1977) Short-course chemotherapy in pulmonary tuberculosis. *Journal of Antimicrobial Chemotherapy* 3(4), 290–294.

Arioli, V., Berti, M., Carniti, G., Randisi, E., Rossi, E. and Scotti, R. (1981) Antibacterial activity of DL 473, a new semisynthetic rifamycin derivative. *Journal of Antibiotics (Tokyo)* 34(8), 1026–1032.

Aristoff, P.A., Garcia, G.A., Kirchhoff, P.D. and Hollis Showalter, H.D. (2010) Rifamycins – obstacles and opportunities. *Tuberculosis (Edinburgh)* 90(2), 94–118.

Barluenga, J., Aznar, F., Garcia, A.B., Cabal, M.P., Palacios, J.J. and Menendez, M.A. (2006) New rifabutin analogs: synthesis and biological activity against *Mycobacterium tuberculosis. Bioorganic and Medicinal Chemistry Letters* 16(22), 5717–5722.

Bhusal, Y., Shiohira, C.M. and Yamane, N. (2005) Determination of *in vitro* synergy when three antimicrobial agents are combined against *Mycobacterium tuberculosis. International Journal of Antimicrobial Agents* 26(4), 292–297.

Burman, W.J., Gallicano, K. and Peloquin, C. (2001) Comparative pharmacokinetics and pharmaco-dynamics of the rifamycin antibacterials. *Clinical Pharmacokinetics* 40(5), 327–341.

Chan, C.Y., Au-Yeang, C., Yew, W.W., Leung, C.C. and Cheng, A.F. (2004) In vitro post-antibiotic effects of rifapentine, isoniazid, and moxifloxacin against *Mycobacterium tuberculosis. Antimicrobial Agents and Chemotherapy* 48(1), 340–343.

Chapuis, L., Ji, B., Truffot-Pernot, C., O'Brien, R.J., Raviglione, M.C. and Grosset, J.H. (1994) Preventive therapy of tuberculosis with rifapentine in immunocompetent and nude mice. *American Journal of Respiratory and Critical Care Medicine* 150(5, Pt 1), 1355–1362.

Citron, K.M. (1972) Tuberculosis – chemotherapy. *British Medical Journal* 1(5797), 426–428.

Constans, P., Saint-Paul, M., Morin, Y., Bonnaud, G. and Bariety, M. (1968) Rifampicin: initial study of plasma levels during prolonged treatment of pulmonary tuberculosis patients. *Reviews in Tuberculosis and Pneumology (Paris)* 32(8), 991–1006.

Constans, P., Baron, A., Parrot, R. and Coury, C. (1972) A study of 200 cases of active, recent pulmonary tuberculosis treated with rifampin-isoniazid. A follow-up history of one and one-half to three years. *Chest* 61(6), 539–549.

Corpe, R.F. and Sanchez, E.S. (1972) Rifampin in initial treatment of advanced pulmonary tuberculosis. *Chest* 61(6), 564–573.

Daniel, N., Lounis, N., Ji, B., O'Brien, R.J., Vernon, A., Geiter, L.J., *et al.* (2000) Antituberculosis activity of once-weekly rifapentine-containing regimens in mice. Long-term effectiveness with 6- and 8-month treatment regimens. *American*

Journal of Respiratory and Critical Care Medicine 161(5), 1572–1577.

Davidson, P.T., Goble, M. and Lester, W. (1972) The antituberculosis efficacy of rifampin in 136 patients. *Chest* 61(6), 574–578.

Davies, G., Cerri, S. and Richeldi, L. (2007) Rifabutin for treating pulmonary tuberculosis. *Cochrane Database Systematic Reviews* 4, CD005159.

De, M.G., Iodice, F. and Lappa, B. (1968) Preliminary observations on the therapeutic effect of rifampycin associated with streptomycin or isoniazid. *Archivio di Tisiologia e delle Malatie dell'Apparato Respiratorio* 23(5), 377–386.

Diacon, A.H., Patientia, R.F., Venter, A., van Helden, P.D., Smith, P.J., McIlleron, H., *et al.* (2007) Early bactericidal activity of high-dose rifampin in patients with pulmonary tuberculosis evidenced by positive sputum smears. *Antimicrobial Agents and Chemotherapy* 51(8), 2994–2996.

Favez, G., Chiolero, R. and Willa, C. (1972) Rifampin-isoniazid compared with streptomycin-isoniazid in the original treatment of infectious pulmonary tuberculosis. Results of a controlled study. *Chest* 61(6), 583–586.

Fox, W., Ellard, G.A. and Mitchison, D.A. (1999) Studies on the treatment of tuberculosis undertaken by the British Medical Research Council tuberculosis units, 1946–1986, with relevant subsequent publications. *International Journal of Tuberculosis and Lung Disease* 3(10, Suppl 2), S231–S279.

Furesz, S., Scotti, R., Pallanza, R. and Mapelli, E. (1967) Rifampicin: a new rifamycin. 3. Absorption, distribution, and elimination in man. *Arzneimittelforschung* 17(5), 534–537.

Gao, X.F., Li, J., Yang, Z.W. and Li, Y.P. (2009) Rifapentine vs. rifampicin for the treatment of pulmonary tuberculosis: a systematic review. *International Journal of Tuberculosis and Lung Disease* 13(7), 810–819.

Gosling, R.D., Heifets, L. and Gillespie, S.H. (2003) A multicentre comparison of a novel surrogate marker for determining the specific potency of anti-tuberculosis drugs. *Journal of Antimicrobial Chemotherapy* 52(3), 473–476.

Goutelle, S., Bourguignon, L., Maire, P.H., Van, G.M., Conte, J.E. Jr and Jelliffe, R.W. (2009) Population modeling and Monte Carlo simulation study of the pharmacokinetics and antituberculosis pharmacodynamics of rifampin in lungs. *Antimicrobial Agents and Chemotherapy* 53(7), 2974–2981.

Gumbo, T., Louie, A., Deziel, M.R., Liu, W., Parsons, L.M., Salfinger, M., *et al.* (2007) Concentration-dependent *Mycobacterium tuberculosis* killing and prevention of resistance by rifampin. *Antimicrobial Agents and Chemotherapy* 51(11), 3781–3788.

Gyselen, A., Verbist, L., Cosemans, J., Lacquet, L.M. and Vandenbergh, E. (1968) Rifampin and ethambutol in the retreatment of advanced pulmonary tuberculosis. *American Review of Respiratory Diseases* 98(6), 933–941.

Ho, M.X., Hudson, B.P., Das, K., Arnold, E. and Ebright, R.H. (2009) Structures of RNA polymerase-antibiotic complexes. *Current Opinion in Structural Biology* 19(6), 715–723.

Houk, A.N. (1972) Rifampin: its role in the treatment of tuberculosis. *Chest* 61(6), 518–519.

Huitric, E., Werngren, J., Jureen, P. and Hoffner, S. (2006) Resistance levels and rpoB gene mutations among *in vitro*-selected rifampin-resistant *Mycobacterium tuberculosis* mutants. *Antimicrobial Agents and Chemotherapy* 50(8), 2860–2862.

Jayaram, R., Gaonkar, S., Kaur, P., Suresh, B.L., Mahesh, B.N., Jayashree, R., *et al.* (2003) Pharmacokinetics–pharmacodynamics of rifampin in an aerosol infection model of tuberculosis. *Antimicrobial Agents and Chemotherapy* 47(7), 2118–2124.

Ji, B., Truffot-Pernot, C., Lacroix, C., Raviglione, M.C., O'Brien, R.J., Olliaro, P., *et al.* (1993) Effectiveness of rifampin, rifabutin, and rifapentine for preventive therapy of tuberculosis in mice. *American Review of Respiratory Diseases* 148(6, Pt 1), 1541–1546.

Jindani, A., Dore, C.J. and Mitchison, D.A. (2003) Bactericidal and sterilizing activities of anti-tuberculosis drugs during the first 14 days. *American Journal of Respiratory and Critical Care Medicine* 167(10), 1348–1354.

Kochar, D.K., Aseri, S., Sharma, B.V., Bumb, R.A., Mehta, R.D. and Purohit, S.K. (2000) The role of rifampicin in the management of cutaneous leishmaniasis. *Quarterly Journal of Medicine* 93(11), 733–737.

Kreis, B., Pretet, S., Birenbaum, J., Guibout, P., Hazeman, J.J., Orin, E., *et al.* (1976) Two three-month treatment regimens for pulmonary tuberculosis. *Bulletin of the International Union Against Tuberculosis* 51(1), 71–75.

Lester, W. (1972) Rifampin: a semisynthetic derivative of rifamycin – a prototype for the future. *Annual Reviews of Microbiololgy* 26, 85–102.

Long, M.W., Snider, D.E. Jr and Farer, L.S. (1979) U.S. Public Health Service Cooperative trial of three rifampin–isoniazid regimens in treatment of pulmonary tuberculosis. *American Review of Respiratory Diseases* 119(6), 879–894.

McConville, J.H. and Rapoport, M.I. (1976) Tuberculosis management in the mid-1970s. *Journal of the American Medical Association* 235(2), 172–176.

Maggi, N., Pasqualucci, C.R., Ballotta, R. and Sensi, P. (1966) Rifampicin: a new orally active rifamycin. *Chemotherapy* 11(5), 285–292.

Marsili, L., Pasqualucci, C.R., Vigevani, A., Gioia, B., Schioppacassi, G. and Oronzo, G. (1981) New rifamycins modified at positions 3 and 4. Synthesis, structure and biological evaluation. *Journal of Antibiotics (Tokyo)* 34(8), 1033–1038.

Mitchison, D.A. (2000) Role of individual drugs in the chemotherapy of tuberculosis. *International Journal of Tuberculosis and Lung Disease* 4(9), 796–806.

Murphy, C.K., Karginova, E., Sahm, D. and Rothstein, D.M. (2007) *In vitro* activity of novel rifamycins against gram-positive clinical isolates. *Journal of Antibiotics (Tokyo)* 60(9), 572–576.

Newman, R., Doster, B., Murray, F.J. and Ferebee, S. (1971) Rifampin in initial treatment of pulmonary tuberculosis. A U.S. Public Health Service tuberculosis therapy trial. *American Review of Respiratory Diseases* 103(4), 461–476.

Nitti, V., Catena, E., Delli, V.F., De, M.G. and Marra, A. (1971) Rifampin in association with isoniazid, streptomycin, and ethambutol, respectively, in the initial treatment of pulmonary tuberculosis. *American Review of Respiratory Diseases* 103(3), 329–337.

Nitti, V., Delli, V.F., Ninni, A. and Meola, G. (1972) Rifampicin blood serum levels and half-life during prolonged administration in tuberculous patients. *Chemotherapy* 17(2), 121–129.

Nuermberger, E. and Grosset, J. (2004) Pharmaco-kinetic and pharmacodynamic issues in the treatment of mycobacterial infections. *European Journal of Clinical Microbiology and Infectious Diseases* 23(4), 243–255.

O'Brien, R.J. and Vernon, A.A. (1998) New tuberculosis drug development. How can we do better? *American Journal of Respiratory and Critical Care Medicine* 157(6, Pt 1), 1705–1707.

O'Brien, R.J., Lyle, M.A. and Snider, D.E. Jr (1987) Rifabutin (ansamycin LM 427): a new rifamycin-S derivative for the treatment of mycobacterial diseases. *Reviews in Infectious Diseases* 9(3), 519–530.

Pallanza, R., Arioli, V., Furesz, S. and Bolzoni, G. (1967) Rifampicin: a new rifamycin. II. Laboratory studies on the antituberculous activity and preliminary clinical observations. *Arzneimittelforschung* 17(5), 529–534.

Peloquin, C.A. (2001) Pharmacological issues in the treatment of tuberculosis. *Annals of the New York Academy of Science* 953, 157–164.

Peloquin, C. (2003) What is the 'right' dose of rifampin? *International Journal of Tuberculosis and Lung Disease* 7(1), 3–5.

Poole, G., Stradling, P. and Worlledge, S. (1971) Potentially serious side-effects of high-dose twice-weekly rifampicin. *Postgraduate Medical Journal* 47(553), 727–747.

Rastogi, N., Labrousse, V. and Goh, K.S. (1996) In vitro activities of fourteen antimicrobial agents against drug susceptible and resistant clinical isolates of *Mycobacterium tuberculosis* and comparative intracellular activities against the virulent H37Rv strain in human macrophages. *Current Microbiology* 33(3), 167–175.

Robertson, G.T., Bonventre, E.J., Doyle, T.B., Du, Q., Duncan, L., Morris, T.W., *et al.* (2008) In vitro evaluation of CBR-2092, a novel rifamycin-quinolone hybrid antibiotic: microbiology profiling studies with staphylococci and streptococci. *Antimicrobial Agents and Chemotherapy* 52(7), 2324–2334.

Robinson, D. (1978) Treatment of tuberculosis. *British Medical Journal* 1(6119), 1053–1054.

Rosenthal, I.M., Williams, K., Tyagi, S., Peloquin, C.A., Vernon, A.A., Bishai, W.R., *et al.* (2006) Potent twice-weekly rifapentine-containing regimens in murine tuberculosis. *American Journal of Respiratory and Critical Care Medicine* 174(1), 94–101.

Rosenthal, I.M., Zhang, M., Williams, K.N., Peloquin, C.A., Tyagi, S., Vernon, A.A., *et al.* (2007) Daily dosing of rifapentine cures tuberculosis in three months or less in the murine model. *PLoS Medicine* 4(12), e344.

Ruslami, R., Nijland, H., Aarnoutse, R., Alisjahbana, B., Soeroto, A.Y., Ewalds, S., *et al.* (2006) Evaluation of high- versus standard-dose rifampin in Indonesian patients with pulmonary tuberculosis. *Antimicrobial Agents and Chemotherapy* 50(2), 822–823.

Sensi, P. (1983) History of the development of rifampin. *Reviews of Infectious Diseases* 5 (Suppl 3), S402–S406.

Sensi, P., Margalith, P. and Timbal, M.T. (1959) Rifomycin, a new antibiotic; preliminary report. *Farmaco Sci* 14(2), 146–147.

Solera, J., Rodriguez-Zapata, M., Geijo, P., Largo, J., Paulino, J., Saez, L., *et al.* (1995) Doxycycline-rifampin versus doxycycline-streptomycin in treatment of human brucellosis due to Brucella melitensis. The GECMEI Group.

Grupo de Estudio de Castilla-la Mancha de Enfermedades Infecciosas. *Antimicrobial Agents and Chemotherapy* 39(9), 2061–2067.

Sterling, T.R., Villarino, M.E., Borisov, A.S., Shang, N., Gordin, F., Bliven-Sizemore, E., *et al.* (2011) Three months of rifapentine and isoniazid for latent tuberculosis infection. *New England Journal of Medicine* 365(23), 2155–2166.

van Ingen, J., Aarnoutse, R., de Vries, G., Boeree, M.J. and van Soolingen, D. (2011a) Low-level rifampicin-resistant *Mycobacterium tuberculosis* strains raise a new therapeutic challenge. *International Journal of Tuberculosis and Lung Disease* 15(7), 990–992.

van Ingen, J., Aarnoutse, R.E., Donald, P.R., Diacon, A.H., Dawson, R., Plemper van, B.G., *et al.* (2011b) Why do we use 600 mg of rifampicin in tuberculosis treatment? *Clinical Infectious Diseases* 52(9), e194–e199.

Verbist, L. and Gyselen, A. (1968) Antituberculous activity of rifampin in vitro and in vivo and the concentrations attained in human blood. *American Review of Respiratory Diseases* 98(6), 923–932.

Veziris, N., Lounis, N., Chauffour, A., Truffot-Pernot, C. and Jarlier, V. (2005) Efficient intermittent rifapentine-moxifloxacin-containing short-course regimen for treatment of tuberculosis in mice. *Antimicrobial Agents and Chemotherapy* 49(10), 4015–4019.

Weiner, M., Bock, N., Peloquin, C.A., Burman, W.J., Khan, A., Vernon, A., *et al.* (2004) Pharmaco-kinetics of rifapentine at 600, 900, and 1,200 mg during once-weekly tuberculosis therapy. *American Journal of Respiratory and Critical Care Medicine* 169(11), 1191–1197.

World Health Organization, S.T.D. (2009) *Treatment of Tuberculosis: Guidelines*, 4th edn. WHO, Geneva, Switzerland.

Ziakas, P.D. and Mylonakis, E. (2009) 4 months of rifampin compared with 9 months of isoniazid for the management of latent tuberculosis infection: a meta-analysis and cost-effectiveness study that focuses on compliance and liver toxicity. *Clinical Infectious Diseases* 49(12), 1883–1889.

Ziglam, H.M., Baldwin, D.R., Daniels, I., Andrew, J.M. and Finch, R.G. (2002) Rifampicin concentrations in bronchial mucosa, epithelial lining fluid, alveolar macrophages and serum following a single 600 mg oral dose in patients undergoing fibre-optic bronchoscopy. *Journal of Antimicrobial Chemotherapy* 50(6), 1011–1015.

18 Therapy of the XDR-TB Patient with Thioridazine – An Old Drug with New Applications

Leonard Amaral,[1,2,3] Marta Martins,[1,2,4] Isabel Couto[1,5] and Miguel Viveiros[1,3]

[1]Unit of Mycobacteriology and [2]UPMM, Instituto de Higiene e Medicina Tropical, Universidade Nova de Lisboa (IHMT/UNL), Lisbon, Portugal; [3]Cost Action BM0701 (ATENS) of Cost Action of the European Commission; [4]UCD Centre for Food Safety, School of Agriculture, Food Science and Veterinary Medicine, University College Dublin, Ireland; [5]Centro de Recursos Microbiológicos (CREM), Faculdade de Ciências e Tecnologia, UNL, Caparica, Portugal

18.1 Introduction

Pulmonary tuberculosis produced by the human bacterial pathogen *Mycobacterium tuberculosis* has plagued modern man since he moved from foraging and gathering to becoming one dependent on agricultural and animal husbandry as sources of food. Nevertheless, with the advent of antibiotics such as isoniazid (INH) and rifampicin (RIF), and their availability throughout the Western world, with few exceptions, it seemed possible that this essentially lethal infection could be eradicated (Martins *et al.*, 2008b). However, because the cost of these antibiotics was beyond the means of most of the world's population, the number of new cases of tuberculosis remained high in sub-Saharan Africa, South and Latin America, South-east Asia, Eastern Europe, India and Portugal (Amaral *et al.*, 2001a). Moreover, conditions which predispose the spread of the infection, such as war, poverty, overcrowding, famine

and the advent of HIV/AIDS in the early 1980s, were frequent, and wherever they occurred, the incidence of new cases soared (Amaral *et al.*, 2010). In New York City during the early 1990s, it became clear that new cases of pulmonary tuberculosis had quadrupled, that more than half of these cases were resistant to the two most effective anti-tuberculosis drugs, INH and RIF (Moss *et al.*, 1997), and that the vast majority of these new cases of multidrug-resistant *M. tuberculosis* (MDR-TB) were found in the migrant population (Tornieporth *et al.*, 1997). Rapid measures were taken and within 5 years the incidence of new cases was decreased to levels below that of the 1950s (Driver *et al.*, 2007). These measures involved vast improvements in the manner by which the laboratory identified *M. tuberculosis* in the sputum of infected patients, the rapid culture of the products of sputum in liquid media and antibiotic susceptibility to at least four antibiotics commonly employed for the therapy of MDR-TB, using such systems as the BACTEC 460TB System (Salfinger and Pfyffer, 1994). The establishment of a fast-track programme that placed the sputum specimen at the highest level of priority for subsequent laboratory examinations and the creation of directly observable therapy (DOT) that ensured the patient would indeed take the medication were the landmark programmes that yielded success (Salfinger and Pfyffer, 1994). But this was not to last, for within a few years, clinical isolates that were resistant to INH and RIF, to any fluoroquinolone and to at least one of the injectable anti-*M. tuberculosis* drugs (capreomycin, kanamycin and amikacin) began to appear with increasing frequency (Migliori *et al.*, 2009). These extensively drug-resistant strains were termed XDR-TB, and the therapy of the XDR-TB patient is far more problematic than that posed by infections produced by MDR-TB (London, 2009). In areas of the USA where the frequency of HIV/AIDS is high, co-infection with XDR-TB strains and HIV result in mortality within a year of diagnosis, regardless of the therapy employed (Chan and Iseman, 2008). At the time of writing, there is no effective anti-XDR-TB standardized treatment, unless we consider alternative therapies such as thioridazine (TZ), an inexpensive drug used for over 40 years for the therapy of psychosis and as safe as any other more current neuroleptic (Thanacoody, 2007). It is the intent of this chapter to provide the rationale and experimental basis for its consideration as a new effective anti-XDR-TB drug.

18.2 Development of Antibiotic Resistance in *Mycobacterium tuberculosis*

The development of resistance to antibiotics used for the therapy of tuberculosis may take place via a variety of ways. Because of the extraordinary length of the therapy period, involving a minimum of 2–3 months for patients whose tuberculin or purified protein derivative (PPD) skin test converted from negative to positive, the spontaneous mutation occurred in a gene for a given

antibiotic target may take place. However, it is well known that in *M. tuberculosis*, chromosomal mutations can be responsible for the resistance seen in several strains and that the MDR phenotype is due to the accumulation of random mutations in the genes involved in the resistance to the most effective anti-tuberculous drugs (INH and RIF). Resistance to RIF is attributed to point mutations in the *rpoB* gene and is almost always associated with resistance to INH (Viveiros *et al.*, 2005; Migliori *et al.*, 2010). The main mechanism of resistance to INH is due to mutations in the *KatG* gene (Migliori *et al.*, 2009, 2010). The rates of mutation in these genes contribute to approximately 75% of the cases of resistance to INH obtained in the clinical setting (Guo *et al.*, 2006).

Therapy consisting of the antibiotic to which the strain is now resistant promotes selection of that strain if the effectiveness of other antibiotics is reduced due to non-compliance (Lipsitch and Levin, 1998), poor management of the patient (Victor *et al.*, 2002) or establishment of mutations that contribute to the drug-resistance mechanisms in the strains.

The selected strain may undergo further mutation that renders the strain resistant to another antibiotic within the same infected patient (Victor *et al.*, 2002), or within another patient who was infected by the first mutated strain (Iademarco and Castro, 2003). Because the two most effective anti-*M. tuberculosis* antibiotics are INH and RIF, resistance to these two antibiotics (MDR-TB) from serial mutations constitutes the major threat for successful therapy. Further serial mutations result in further resistance to other antibiotics, such that today, XDR-TB strains are emerging globally (Migliori *et al.*, 2010). The dissemination of these highly drug-resistant strains is of obvious concern. The need for effective anti-MDR- and XDR-TB agents is urgent.

However, resistance to one antibiotic may not involve a mutation. As early as 2001, experimentally induced resistance of INH susceptible *M. tuberculosis* to INH could be brought about by prolonged exposure of the strain to increasing concentrations of INH (Viveiros *et al.*, 2002). Because this induced resistance could be eliminated by transfer to drug-free medium or by the addition of known efflux pump inhibitors, the putative presence of an overexpressed efflux pump that extruded the INH prodrug, or its prodrug product, prior to reaching its intended target seemed plausible. Since that demonstration, others have shown that the overexpression of given efflux pumps in mycobacteria render resistance to given antibiotics such as INH, clarithromycin, RIF and clofazimine (Ramón-García *et al.*, 2009; Rodrigues *et al.*, 2009).

The role of efflux pumps in MDR-TB and XDR-TB is of obvious interest and, at the time of writing, is pursued vigorously. Agents that can inhibit the efflux pumps responsible for antibiotic resistance are needed for possible adjuvant use.

Dormant *M. tuberculosis* strains commonly reside in macrophages of the lung and are considered to be in a non-replicating stage (Ehlers, 2009). Dormant *M. tuberculosis* can be induced readily from the incubation of antibiotic-susceptible *M. tuberculosis in vitro*, by the addition of oxygen-coupling agents into the medium and incubation of the culture in the absence of oxygen (Sohaskey, 2008). Because dormant *M. tuberculosis* are resistant to most antibiotics (Sohaskey, 2008) and because they may be the prominent strains that infect the human but do not produce an active infection until many decades later (reactivated tuberculosis) (Wayne and Sohaskey, 2001), therapy with INH and RIF of a patient who has sero-converted to a positive PPD test may not provide a cure and, therefore, the possibility of reactivated tuberculosis in later life is a possibility. Agents that have activity against dormant *M. tuberculosis* are therefore of great interest for use whenever PPD sero-conversion has taken place.

18.3 Criteria for an Effective Anti-MDR/XDR-TB, Anti-latent *M. tuberculosis* Agent

Pulmonary tuberculosis is essentially an intracellular infection of the pulmonary macrophage of the alveolar sac caused by a strain of *M. tuberculosis* with the capacity to dis-seminate to other sites of the body once it escapes its macrophage prison (Mogga *et al.*, 2002; El-Masry *et al.*, 2007; Yoshida *et al.*, 2009). Prior to escape, the organism lays dormant for many years, if not decades. Diagnosis may be made with a simple skin test (PPD) in countries that do not immunize routinely and boost the young with the Bacillus Calmette–Guérin (BCG). This test, also known as the Mantoux test, is now standardized by the WHO and continues to be used as the standard method for detecting latent infection with *M. tuberculosis*. It is widely used to support clinical and radiological findings in the evaluation of patients with suspected tuberculosis. A positive result can help in the decision to start treatment while bacteriological confirmation is awaited or lacking. The test uses PPD, a combination of mycobacterial antigens obtained from *M. tuberculosis* culture and which share a large number of antigens, both with BCG and with environmental mycobacteria. It consists of an intradermal injection of 0.1 ml of tuberculin (100 units/ml). This combination elicits delayed-type hypersensitivity response or type IV hypersensitivity reaction that is mediated by specific T lymphocytes. Such effector cells function in essentially the same way as during a response to an infectious agent. When small amounts of PPD are injected, a T cell-mediated local inflammatory reaction evolves in individuals who have previously responded to *M. tuberculosis*. This indicates the presence of antibodies or lymphocytes that are specific for PPD. This cell-mediated immunity can then be detected as a local response when the individual's skin is injected with a small amount of PPD. The response typically appears a day or two after the injection and consists of a raised, red and hard (or indurated) area. This induration can be measured 2–7 days afterwards and disappears as the PPD is degraded.

Vaccination with BCG can result in a positive PPD test and even though many claim that the size of indurations is related to a recent infection by *M. tuberculosis* of a BCG-immunized subject, this claim is not faithfully realized. The poor sensitivity of the Mantoux test in young children and immunosuppressed people makes it impossible to interpret negative results in these groups. Moreover, up to 25% of immunocompetent adults with active tuberculosis may have a negative or ambiguous result (Gooding *et al.*, 2007).

Regardless, until the organism breaks free of its macrophage prison, the infected patient is not infectious and therapy is desirable only to obviate the progression of latent infection to active disease – the infectious phase of tuberculosis. This stage is accompanied by the presence of acid-fast stained bacteria present in the sputum of the subject who is presenting with some or all of the symptoms of active disease. Confirmation that the sputum does indeed contain *M. tuberculosis* is made from culture and identification, or by direct identification with the use of specific molecular probes or PCR-type tests (Parsons *et al.*, 2004; Viveiros *et al.*, 2005).

If the laboratory and radiological tests support the diagnosis of a pulmonary tuberculosis infection and the responsible strain is susceptible to INH and RIF, the patient is treated with these antibiotics. This therapy may apparently cure the patient of overt symptoms related to the destruction of pulmonary tissue, such as the immune responses that result in inflammation and physical symptoms such as night sweats, loss of appetite, loss of weight, morbidity, respiratory stress, due to killing of intracellular bacteria that have begun their replicative phase and, hence, are susceptible to INH and RIF. However, those that are still in the dormant phase are not affected and, therefore, when therapy is deemed 'complete', and ended, the recurrence of symptoms may take place due to the progression of the intracellular strain from the quiescent to the replicative state, and destruction of pulmonary tissue and the extracellular phase begins anew. If the infection is caused by MDR or XDR *M. tuberculosis*, therapy is problematic, and even for those few successful cases, a real cure is not probable due to the presence of dormant mycobacteria.

The criterion that an agent must satisfy to be a truly successful anti-tuberculosis drug that provides a cure for antibiotic-susceptible MDR, XDR and latent *M. tuberculosis* is to have activity against these forms of *M. tuberculosis* when the organism is intracellular.

To do this, the agent must first be shown to have *in vitro* activity against all forms of *M. tuberculosis*, it must traverse the plasma membrane of the macrophage, reach the phagosome (vacuole formed by the fusion of the cell membrane around the phagocytosed bacteria) or phagolysosome (cellular compartment that results from the fusion of the phagosome with lysosomes during their maturation process) where the organism resides and retain its proven *in vitro* activity against the organism *in situ*. Is there such a compound? Is there such a compound that exists and which has been used relatively safely for the past 40 years for the therapy of a non-infectious pathology? Is this agent ready for clinical trials at sites of the globe where tuberculosis, MDR, XDR and their latent forms produce a high prevalence of pulmonary tuberculosis infections? The answer is yes.

18.4 Phenothiazines and Their Anti-tuberculosis Activity

Phenothiazines have a long history of antimicrobial activity that began with studies conducted by Paul Ehrlich in the late 19th century (Kristiansen and Amaral, 1997; Amaral and Kristiansen, 2000). However, because the first phenothiazine studied was methylene blue, and this turned patients blue, it was only after its colourless derivative, chlorpromazine (CPZ), was introduced in 1957 for the therapy of psychosis that its anti-mycobacteriological properties were noted (Pleasure, 1956; Alcozer and Lingiardi, 1957; Hyvert *et al.*, 1957; Marchand and Reuter, 1957; Shubin *et al.*, 1957; Zamfir and Ionesco, 1958; Santopadre and Silanos, 1959; Filippov, 1960; Hollister *et al.*, 1960; Amaral *et al.*, 2001a). However, because therapy of tuberculosis was very successful with IHN and RIF, and CPZ produced a series of nasty side effects (Amaral *et al.*, 2001b), interest in CPZ as an anti-tuberculosis agent was limited to intellectual curiosity (Molnár *et al.*, 1977; Kristiansen and Vergmann, 1986). However, with the global resurgence of tuberculosis during the 1980s and the emergence of MDR-TB, especially at the beginning of the

1990s, and its problematic therapy, attention was now being paid to the possibility that CPZ could have a special role for therapy of MDR-TB. That the anti-mycobacterial activity of CPZ took place at concentrations that were extremely high (minimum inhibitory concentrations (MICs) in excess of 20–30 mg/l) and clinically irrelevant (maximum plasma concentration that can be achieved safely is c.0.4–0.5 mg/l), meant the use of CPZ for therapy was out of the question. However, resurgence in the interest of CPZ took place momentarily with the demonstration that CPZ could promote the killing of intracellular M. tuberculosis when its concentration in the macrophage was lower than that present in the plasma of a CPZ chronically treated patient (Amaral et al., 2001b). Nevertheless, the problems posed by the serious side effects produced by CPZ presented an insurmountable barrier for its use. The demonstration that a derivative of this compound, TZ, the equal to CPZ for therapy of psychosis but far less problematic with respect to serious side effects, could inhibit the in vitro replication of XDR-TB strains (Amaral et al., 1996) led to the consideration of a phenothiazine for use, albeit limited only by the fact that its in vitro activity took place with concentrations that were well beyond those achievable in the patient. This latter limitation was eliminated with the demonstration that CPZ and TZ could enhance the killing of intracellular antibiotic-susceptible and antibiotic-resistant strains (MDR- and XDR-TB) at concentrations that were well below those present in the plasma of patients treated initially with TZ (Crowle et al., 1992; Ordway et al., 2003; Amaral et al., 2007; Martins et al., 2007a). Demonstration of the ability of TZ to cure mice infected with M. tuberculosis soon followed (Martins et al., 2007b; van Ingen et al., 2009). The ability of TZ to effect complete cures of 10 out of 12 XDR-TB patients when used as an adjuvant to therapy with three antibiotics, as previously recommended (Bettencourt et al., 2000), was demonstrated in 2007 by Eduardo Abbate and his group (Abbate et al., 2007). Since that time, a global call for clinical trials for therapy of XDR-TB with TZ has been made (Amaral et al., 2010) and has resulted in a number of Phase IV studies in India. These trials are also known as post-marketing surveillance trials and involve the safety surveillance, namely pharmacovigilance, and ongoing technical support of a drug after it receives permission to be sold. Phase IV clinical trials may be required by regulatory authorities, or alternatively may be undertaken by the sponsoring companies (for example, in the case that the drug has not been tested for interactions with other drugs). In this case, safety surveillance is designed to detect any rare or long-term adverse effects over a much larger patient population and longer period than was possible during the Phase I–III clinical trials. Harmful effects identified during Phase IV trials may result in a drug no longer being sold, or restricted to certain uses.

18.4.1 Targeting the macrophage: a unique concept for the therapy of MDR- and XDR-TB infections

The mechanism by which TZ enhances the killing of intracellular mycobacteria appears to be one related to the inhibition of the Ca^{2+}/K^+ transport of the macrophage (Martins et al., 2008a). The sequence of events by which this mechanism is believed to take place is as follows:

1. The mycobacterium binds to the plasma membrane of the macrophage, thereby activating the phagocytosis process (García et al., 2005; Plaza et al., 2007; Chapeton-Montes et al., 2008; Link et al., 2010). This process results in the invagination of the plasma membrane, resulting in a vacuole that contains the mycobacterium; the phagosome. It is important to note that the plasma membrane contains Ca^{2+}/K^+ transporters that bind Ca^{2+}/K^+ and pump it into the cytoplasm of the cell against a gradient. The invaginated plasma membrane therefore contains Ca^{2+}/K^+ transporters. However, after the internalization of the bacteria, they now pump Ca^{2+}/K^+ from the phagosome to the cytoplasm of the cell.

2. The phagosome and the lysosome will fuse eventually, but because Ca^{2+}/K^+ is pumped out from the phagolysosome, the acidification of the phagolysosome needed for the activation of hydrolases does not take

place (Reeves *et al.*, 2002; Ahluwalia *et al.*, 2004; Segal, 2005). This could be one of the reasons why the pulmonary macrophage does not kill phagocytosed mycobacteria.

3. TZ (Eilam, 1983; Kongsamut *et al.*, 2002), as well as other phenothiazines (Moriyama *et al.*, 1993; Chattopadhyay *et al.*, 1998; Sampaio-Maia *et al.*, 2001; Choi *et al.*, 2005), is known to inhibit the Ca^{2+}/K^+ transporters (Traykov *et al.*, 1997).

4. TZ, as well as other neuroleptic phenothiazines, is concentrated by macrophages that are rich in vesicles (Wójcikowski and Daniel, 2002; Daniel, 2003). This process takes place via pinocytosis and results in a TZ-containing vesicle formed from the invagination of the plasma membrane.

5. The phenothiazine is concentrated by the macrophage vesicles (Daniel and Wójcikowski, 1999; Daniel *et al.*, 2001).

6. The fusion of the phagosome and the TZ-containing vesicle takes place.

7. TZ inhibits the Ca^{2+}/K^+ flux of the phagolysosome and therefore the energy needed by the Ca^{2+}/K^+ transporter for pumping out Ca^{2+}/K^+ from the phagolysosome is obviated.

8. The build-up of Ca^{2+}/K^+ takes place, with cytosolic homeostasis mechanisms activated, leading to an increased activity of V-ATPases that will acidify the phagolysosome, and subsequently the activation of the hydrolases takes place and the mycobacterium is finally degraded and killed.

The mechanism by which a phenothiazine enhances the killing of intracellular mycobacteria invokes a totally new concept for the therapy of a pulmonary tuberculosis infection, as well as for other bacterial infections of the non-killing pulmonary macrophage. This concept targets the macrophage rather than the intracellular bacterium (Amaral *et al.*, 2008; Martins *et al.*, 2008b, 2009; Amaral and Molnar, 2010) and so bypasses any mutational response directed by the organism against TZ. One would therefore expect that the use of TZ for the therapy of MDR- and XDR-TB infections would not suffer the expected consequences of resistance that result from exposure of the mycobacterium to the agent.

18.4.2 *In vitro* activity of TZ against induced latent *M. tuberculosis*

TZ has been shown to kill *in vitro* non-replicating *M. tuberculosis* as well as induced dormant *M. tuberculosis* (Sohaskey, 2008). This suggests that if the agent is equally effective against these forms of *M. tuberculosis* when the organism is intracellular, then the use of TZ for therapy of an infection that had been demonstrated decades earlier, and which is probably latent, has the potential to reduce, if not obviate, reactivated tuberculosis.

18.4.3 TZ as an inhibitor of efflux pumps in antibiotic resistance in *M. tuberculosis*

INH-susceptible *M. tuberculosis* can be induced readily to high-level resistance to this antibiotic (Viveiros *et al.*, 2002). The induced resistance is due to the overexpression of efflux pumps of the organism that extrudes INH prior to either its conversion to the active drug by peroxidases or prior to the active drug reaching its intended target (Viveiros *et al.*, 2003). A number of efflux pumps of *M. tuberculosis* have been characterized (Aínsa *et al.*, 1998; Choudhuri *et al.*, 1999; De Rossi *et al.*, 2002). Moreover, these efflux pumps appear to bestow antibiotic resistance to the organism (De Rossi *et al.*, 2002, 2006; De La Iglesia *et al.*, 2006; Gupta *et al.*, 2006, 2010; Escribano *et al.*, 2007; Gumbo *et al.*, 2007; Jiang *et al.*, 2008; Ramón-García *et al.*, 2008a). TZ has been shown to inhibit efflux pumps of mycobacteria (Viveiros *et al.*, 2002; Amaral *et al.*, 2008; Rodrigues *et al.*, 2009) and so therapy of MDR infections caused by *M. tuberculosis* that overexpress efflux pumps is promising.

18.4.4 Compassionate therapy of the XDR-TB patient with TZ

Therapy of antibiotic-susceptible infections with TZ is not recommended at this time. Rather, therapy should be restricted to selected cases of MDR- and XDR-TB that have not responded to therapy and whose prognosis is poor (Amaral *et al.*, 2010). At the time of writing, 10 XDR-TB patients in Mumbai, India, who were deemed terminal, were selected for monotherapy with TZ. Prior to therapy, the patients were monitored for cardiac functions for at least 4 consecutive days, for the first 2 weeks of therapy and periodically thereafter. Monitoring of cardiac functions is mandatory since TZ may, on rare occasions, produce a prolongation of the QT interval, which, if significant, can cause death. The therapeutic protocol consisted of a daily dose of 25 mg/day for 1 week, followed by weekly increments of 25 mg/day until a daily dose of 75 mg/day was reached. Within 1 week, symptoms such as night sweats, loss of appetite, depression and anxiety were obviated and patients began to gain weight. The number of acid-fast positive organisms in sputa was decreased.

However, at the time of writing, 6 weeks of therapy had not yet resulted in negative cultures. It is still too early to tell if a cure is under way. However, the quality of life of the patients could be improved significantly.

18.5 Conclusion

The emergence of MDR- and XDR-TB represents a major threat to public health worldwide, as many of these strains are untreatable with the current arsenal of drugs. Treatment of these infections with existing antibiotics is only marginally effective. Nevertheless, they remain the only available therapeutic option in the clinical setting. To design and implement new approaches that can reduce the concentration of these drugs at the site of infection while maintaining efficacy is a substantial challenge. It is now widely accepted that the intrinsic drug resistance (i.e. low-level resistance) exhibited by many eukaryotic and prokaryotic cells is due to the maintenance of active efflux pumps, and the magnitude of this resistance can be reduced by the use of effective efflux pump inhibitors. Enhanced killing by the human macrophage using compounds that can act as efflux pump inhibitors proceeds via a mechanism that promotes the acidification of the phago-lysosome wherein the eukaryotic Ca^{2+} and K^+

pumps are inactivated. CPZ and TZ have been shown to be effective efflux pump inhibitors with clinically relevant activity against mycobacteria. These compounds are ideal candidates that can be tested in combination with conventional antibiotics. Combined therapies will decrease the critical concentration of antibiotics *in vitro* and in infected human macrophages, thereby reducing toxicity, one of the main problems associated with clinically significant levels of these drugs. Since they can transform the non-killing macrophage into an effective killer, they provide an exciting new approach for the therapy of these MDR-TB infections and may contribute to limiting the emergence of XDR-TB.

Acknowledgements

This work was supported by grants SDH. IC.I.01.17-TB Task Force for Greater Lisbon (2001), TB-Fast-Track Programme (2004) and XDRTB Early Detection in Greater Lisbon (2009) from the Calouste Gulbenkian Foundation. The work was also supported by the EU-FSE/FEDER-POCI/SAU-MMO/59370/2004 and the EU-FSE/FEDER-PTDC/BIA-MIC/71280/2006 grants provided by the Fundação para a Ciência e a Tecnologia (FCT) of Portugal. M. Martins was a recipient of grant SFRH/BD/14319/2003 provided by FCT (Portugal).

References

Abbate, E., Vescovo, M., Natiello, M., Cufré, M., Garcia, A., Ambroggi, M., *et al.* (2007) Tuberculosis extensamente resistente (XDR-TB) en Argentina: aspectos destacables epidemiológicos, bacteriológicos, terapéuticos y evolutivos. *Revista Argentina de Medicina Respiratoria* 1, 19–25.

Ahluwalia, J., Tinker, A., Clapp, L.H., Duchen, M.R., Abramov, A.Y., Pope, S., *et al.* (2004) The large-conductance Ca2+-activated K+ channel is essential for innate immunity. *Nature* 427, 853–858.

Aínsa, J.A., Blokpoel, M.C., Otal, I., Young, D.B., De Smet, K.A. and Martín, C. (1998) Molecular cloning and characterization of Tap, a putative multidrug efflux pump present in *Mycobacterium fortuitum* and *Mycobacterium tuberculosis*. *The Journal of Bacteriology* 180, 5836–5843.

Alcozer, G. and Lingiardi, G. (1957) Chlorpromazine in therapy of pulmonary tuberculosis. *Archivio 'E. Maragliano' di Patologia e Clinica* 13, 1247–1264.

Amaral, L. and Kristiansen, J.E. (2000) Phenothiazines: an alternative to conventional therapy for the initial management of suspected multidrug resistant tuberculosis. A call for studies. *International Journal of Antimicrobial Agents* 14, 173–176.

Amaral, L. and Molnar, J. (2010) Therapy of XDRTB with thioridazine a drug beyond patent protection but eligible for patent 'As New Use'. *Recent Patents on Anti-infective Drug Discovery* 5, 109–114.

Amaral, L., Kristiansen, J.E., Abebe, L.S. and Millett, W. (1996) Inhibition of the respiration of multi-drug resistant clinical isolates of *Mycobacterium tuberculosis* by thioridazine: potential use for initial therapy of freshly diagnosed tuberculosis. *Journal of Antimicrobial Chemotherapy* 38, 1049–1053.

Amaral, L., Kristiansen, J.E., Viveiros, M. and Atouguia, J. (2001a) Activity of phenothiazines against antibiotic-resistant *Mycobacterium tuberculosis*: a review supporting further studies that may elucidate the potential use of thioridazine as anti-tuberculosis therapy. *Journal of Antimicrobial Chemotherapy* 47, 505–511.

Amaral, L., Viveiros, M. and Kristiansen, J.E. (2001b) Phenothiazines: potential alternatives for the management of antibiotic resistant infections of tuberculosis and malaria in developing countries. *Tropical Medicine and International Health* 6, 1016–1022.

Amaral, L., Martins, M. and Viveiros, M. (2007) Phenothiazines as anti-multi-drug resistant tubercular agents. *Infectious Disorders – Drug Targets* 7, 257–265.

Amaral, L., Martins, M., Viveiros, M., Molnar, J. and Kristiansen, J.E. (2008) Promising therapy of XDR-TB/MDR-TB with thioridazine an inhibitor of bacterial efflux pumps. *Current Drug Targets* 9, 816–819.

Amaral, L., Boeree, M.J., Gillespie, S.H., Udwadia, Z.F. and van Soolingen, D. (2010) Thioridazine cures extensively drug-resistant tuberculosis (XDR-TB) and the need for global trials is now! *International Journal of Antimicrobial Agents* 35, 524–526.

Bettencourt, M.V., Bosne-David, S. and Amaral, L. (2000) Comparative *in vitro* activity of phenothiazines against multidrug-resistant *Mycobacterium tuberculosis*. *International Journal of Antimicrobial Agents* 16, 69–71.

Chan, E.D. and Iseman, M.D. (2008) Multidrug-resistant and extensively drug-resistant tuberculosis: a review. *Current Opinion in Infectious Diseases* 21, 587–595.

Chapeton-Montes, J.A., Plaza, D.F., Curtidor, H., Forero, M., Vanegas, M., Patarroyo, M.E., *et al.* (2008) Characterizing the *Mycobacterium tuberculosis* Rv2707 protein and determining its sequences which specifically bind to two human cell lines. *Protein Science* 17, 342–351.

Chattopadhyay, D., Mukherjee, T., Pal, P., Saha, B. and Bhadra, R. (1998) Altered membrane permeability as the basis of bactericidal action of methdilazine. *Journal of Antimicrobial Chemotherapy* 42, 83–86.

Choi, S.Y., Koh, Y.S. and Jo, S.H. (2005) Inhibition of human ether-a-go-go-related gene K+ channel and IKr of guinea pig cardiomyocytes by antipsychotic drug trifluoperazine. *Journal of Pharmacology and Experimental Therapeutics* 313, 888–895.

Choudhuri, B.S., Sen, S. and Chakrabarti, P. (1999) Isoniazid accumulation in *Mycobacterium smegmatis* is modulated by proton motive force-driven and ATP-dependent extrusion systems. *Biochemical and Biophysical Research Communications* 256, 682–684.

Crowle, A.J., Douvas, G.S. and May, M.H. (1992) Chlorpromazine: a drug potentially useful for treating mycobacterial infections. *Chemotherapy* 38, 410–419.

Daniel, W.A. (2003) Mechanisms of cellular distribution of psychotropic drugs. Significance for drug action and interactions. *Progress in Neuro-Psychopharmacology and Biological Psychiatry* 27, 65–73.

Daniel, W.A. and Wójcikowski, J. (1999) The role of lysosomes in the cellular distribution of thioridazine and potential drug interactions. *Toxicology and Applied Pharmacology* 158, 115–124.

Daniel, W.A., Wójcikowski, J. and Pałucha, A. (2001) Intracellular distribution of psychotropic drugs in the grey and white matter of the brain: the role of lysosomal trapping. *British Journal of Pharmacology* 134, 807–814.

Danilchanka, O., Mailaender, C. and Niederweis, M. (2008a) Identification of a novel multidrug efflux pump of *Mycobacterium tuberculosis*. *Antimicrobial Agents and Chemotherapy* 52, 2503–2511.

Danilchanka, O., Pavlenok, M. and Niederweis, M. (2008b) Role of porins for uptake of antibiotics by *Mycobacterium smegmatis*. *Antimicrobial Agents and Chemotherapy* 52, 3127–3134.

De La Iglesia, A.I. and Morbidoni, H.R. (2006) Mechanisms of action of and resistance to rifampicin and isoniazid in *Mycobacterium tuberculosis*: new information on old friends. *Revista Argentina de Microbiología* 38, 97–109.

De Rossi, E., Arrigo, P., Bellinzoni, M., Silva, P.A., Martín, C., Aínsa, J.A., *et al.* (2002) The multidrug transporters belonging to major facilitator superfamily in *Mycobacterium tuberculosis*. *Molecular Medicine* 8, 714–724.

De Rossi, E., Aínsa, J.A. and Riccardi, G. (2006) Role of mycobacterial efflux transporters in drug resistance: an unresolved question. *FEMS Microbiology Reviews* 30, 36–52.

Driver, C.R., Kreiswirth, B., Macaraig, M., Clark, C., Munsiff, S.S., Driscoll, J., *et al.* (2007) Molecular epidemiology of tuberculosis after declining incidence, New York City, 2001-2003. *Epidemiology and Infection* 135, 634–643.

Ehlers, S. (2009) Lazy, dynamic or minimally recrudescent? On the elusive nature and location of the mycobacterium responsible for latent tuberculosis. *Infection* 37, 87–95.

Eilam, Y. (1983) Membrane effects of phenothiazines in yeasts. I. Stimulation of calcium and potassium fluxes. *Biochimica et Biophysica Acta* 733, 242–248.

El-Masry, S., Lotfy, M., Nasif, W.A., El-Kady, I.M. and Al-Badrawy, M. (2007) Elevated serum level of interleukin (IL)-18, interferon (IFN)-gamma and soluble Fas in patients with pulmonary complications in tuberculosis. *Acta Microbiologica et Immunologica Hungarica* 54, 65–77.

Escribano, I., Rodríguez, J.C., Llorca, B., García-Pachon, E., Ruiz, M. and Royo, G. (2007) Importance of the efflux pump systems in the resistance of *Mycobacterium tuberculosis* to fluoroquinolones and linezolid. *Chemotherapy* 53, 397–401.

Filippov, Mi. (1960) Aminazin therapy of active forms of tuberculosis in mental patients. (Preliminary communication). *Zhurnal nevropatologii i psikhiatrii imeni S.S. Korsakova* 60, 1024–1026.

García, J., Puentes, A., Rodríguez, L., Ocampo, M., Curtidor, H., Vera, R., *et al.* (2005) *Mycobacterium tuberculosis* Rv2536 protein implicated in specific binding to human cell lines. *Protein Science* 14, 2236–2245.

Gooding, S., Chowdhury, O., Hinks, T., Richeldi, L., Losi, M., Ewer, K., *et al.* (2007) Impact of a T cell-based blood test for tuberculosis infection on clinical decision-making in routine practice. *Journal of Infection* 54, e169–174.

Gumbo, T., Louie, A., Liu, W., Ambrose, P.G., Bhavnani, S.M., Brown, D., *et al.* (2007) Isoniazid's bactericidal activity ceases because of the emergence of resistance, not depletion of *Mycobacterium tuberculosis* in the log phase of growth. *The Journal of Infectious Diseases* 195, 194–201.

Guo, H., Seet, Q., Denkin, S., Parsons, L. and Zhang, Y. (2006) Molecular characterization of isoniazid-resistant clinical isolates of *Mycobacterium tuberculosis* from the USA. *Journal of Medical Microbiology* 55, 1527–1531.

Gupta, A.K., Chauhan, D.S., Srivastava, K., Das, R., Batra, S., Mittal, M., *et al.* (2006) Estimation of efflux mediated multi-drug resistance and its correlation with expression levels of two major efflux pumps in mycobacteria. *The Journal of Communicable Diseases* 38, 246–254.

Gupta, A.K., Katoch, V.M., Chauhan, D.S., Sharma, R., Singh, M., Venkatesan, K., *et al.* (2010) Microarray analysis of efflux pump genes in multidrug-resistant *Mycobacterium tuberculosis* during stress induced by common anti-tuberculous drugs. *Microbial Drug Resistance* 16, 21–28.

Hollister, Le., Eikenberry, Dt., and Raffel, S. (1960) Chlorpromazine in nonpsychotic patients with pulmonary tuberculosis. *American Review of Respiratory Disease* 81, 562–566.

Hyvert, M., Le Cloarec, J. and Carrer, J. (1957) Chlorpromazine and atypical tuberculosis in 578 chronic mental patients; need for combined therapy. *Annales Médico-Psychologiques (Paris)* 115, 296–300.

Iademarco, M.F. and Castro, K.G. (2003) Epidemiology of tuberculosis. *Seminars in Respiratory Infections* 18, 225–240.

James, C.E., Mahendran, K.R., Molitor, A., Bolla, J.M., Bessonov, A.N., Winterhalter, M., *et al.* (2009) How beta-lactam antibiotics enter bacteria: a dialogue with the porins. *PLoS One* 4, e5453.

Jiang, X., Zhang, W., Zhang, Y., Gao, F., Lu, C., Zhang, X., *et al.* (2008) Assessment of efflux pump gene expression in a clinical isolate *Mycobacterium tuberculosis* by real-time reverse transcription PCR. *Microbial Drug Resistance* 14, 7–11.

Kongsamut, S., Kang, J., Chen, X.L., Roehr, J. and Rampe, D. (2002) A comparison of the receptor binding and HERG channel affinities for a series of antipsychotic drugs. *European Journal of Pharmacology* 450, 37–41.

Kristiansen, J.E. and Amaral, L. (1997) The potential management of resistant infections with non-antibiotics. *Journal of Antimicrobial Chemotherapy* 40, 319–327.

Kristiansen, J.E. and Vergmann, B. (1986) The antibacterial effect of selected phenothiazines and thioxanthenes on slow-growing mycobacteria. *Acta Pathologica et Microbiologica Scandinavica – Section B* 94, 393–398.

Link, T.M., Park, U., Vonakis, B.M., Raben, D.M., Soloski, M.J. and Caterina, M.J. (2010) TRPV2 has apivotal role in macrophage particle binding and phagocytosis. *Nature Immunology* 11, 232–239.

Lipsitch, M. and Levin, B.R. (1998) Population dynamics of tuberculosis treatment: mathematical models of the roles of non-compliance and bacterial heterogeneity in the evolution of drug resistance. *International Journal of Tubercle and Lung Diseases* 2, 187–199.

London, L. (2009) Confinement for extensively drug-resistant tuberculosis: balancing protection of health systems, individual rights and the public's health. *International Journal of Tubercle and Lung Diseases* 13, 1200–1209.

Marchand, H. and Reuter, C. (1957) Phenothiazine derivatives in treatment of pulmonary tuberculosis. *Tuberkulosearzt* 11, 19–27.

Martins, M., Schelz, Z., Martins, A., Molnar, J., Hajös, G., Riedl, Z., *et al.* (2007a) *In vitro* and *ex vivo* activity of thioridazine derivatives against *Mycobacterium tuberculosis. International Journal of Antimicrobial Agents* 29, 338–340.

Martins, M., Viveiros, M., Kristiansen, J.E., Molnar, J. and Amaral, L. (2007b) The curative activity of thioridazine on mice infected with *Mycobacterium tuberculosis. In Vivo* 21, 771–775.

Martins, M., Viveiros, M. and Amaral, L. (2008a) Inhibitors of Ca^{2+} and K^+ transport enhance intracellular killing of *M. tuberculosis* by nonkilling macrophages. *In Vivo* 22, 69–75.

Martins, M., Viveiros, M. and Amaral, L. (2008b) The TB laboratory of the future: macrophage-based selection of XDR-TB therapeutics. *Future Microbiology* 3, 135–144.

Martins, M., Viveiros, M., Couto, I. and Amaral, L. (2009) Targeting human macrophages for enhanced killing of intracellular XDR-TB and MDR-TB. *The International Journal of Tuberculosis and Lung Disease* 13, 569–573.

Migliori, G.B., D'Arcy Richardson, M., Sotgiu, G. and Lange, C. (2009) Multidrug-resistant and extensively drug-resistant tuberculosis in the West. Europe and United States: epidemiology, surveillance, and control. *Clinics In Chest Medicine* 30, 637–665.

Migliori, G.B., Centis, R., Lange, C., Richardson, M.D. and Sotgiu, G. (2010) Emerging epidemic of drug-resistant tuberculosis in Europe, Russia, China, South America and Asia: current status and global perspectives. *Current Opinion in Pulmonary Medicine* 16, 171–179.

Mogga, S.J., Mustafa, T., Sviland, L. and Nilsen, R. (2002) Increased Bcl-2 and reduced Bax expression in infected macrophages in slowly progressive primary murine *Mycobacterium tuberculosis* infection. *Scandinavian Journal of Immunology* 56, 383–391.

Molnár, J., Béládi, I. and Földes, I. (1977) Studies on antituberculotic action of some phenothiazine derivatives *in vitro. Zentralblatt für Bakteriologie, Parasitenkunde, Infektionskrankheiten und Hygiene. Erste Abteilung Originale. Reihe A: Medizinische Mikrobiologie und Parasitologie* 239, 521–526.

Moriyama, Y., Tsai, H.L. and Futai, M. (1993) Energy-dependent accumulation of neuron blockers causes selective inhibition of neurotransmitter uptake by brain synaptic vesicles. *Archives of Biochemistry and Biophysics* 305, 278–281.

Moss, A.R., Alland, D., Telzak, E., Hewlett, D. Jr, Sharp, V., Chiliade, P., *et al.* (1997) A city-wide outbreak of a multiple-drug-resistant strain of *Mycobacterium tuberculosis* in New York. *International Journal of Tubercle and Lung Diseases* 1, 115–121.

Ordway, D., Viveiros, M., Leandro, C., Bettencourt, R., Almeida, J., Martins, M., *et al.* (2003) Clinical concentrations of thioridazine kill intracellular multidrug-resistant *Mycobacterium tuberculosis. Antimicrobial Agents and Chemotherapy* 47, 917–922.

Parsons, L.M., Somoskövi, A., Urbanczik, R. and Salfinger, M. (2004) Laboratory diagnostic aspects of drug resistant tuberculosis. *Frontiers in Bioscience* 9, 2086–2105.

Plaza, D.F., Curtidor, H., Patarroyo, M.A., Chapeton-Montes, J.A., Reyes, C., Barreto, J., *et al.* (2007) The *Mycobacterium tuberculosis* membrane protein Rv2560 – biochemical and functional studies. *FEBS Journal* 274, 6352–6364.

Pleasure, H. (1956) Chlorpromazine (thorazine) for mental illness in the presence of pulmonary tuberculosis. *The Psychiatric Quarterly* 30, 23–30.

Purdy, G.E., Niederweis, M. and Russell, D.G. (2009) Decreased outer membrane permeability protects mycobacteria from killing by ubiquitin-derived peptides. *Molecular Microbiology* 73, 844–857.

Ramón-García, S., Martín, C., Thompson, C.J. and Aínsa, J.A. (2009) Role of the *Mycobacterium tuberculosis* P55 efflux pump in intrinsic drug resistance, oxidative stress responses, and growth. *Antimicrobial Agents and Chemotherapy* 53, 3675–3682.

Reeves, E.P., Lu, H., Jacobs, H.L., Messina, C.G., Bolsover, S., Gabella, G., *et al.* (2002) Killing activity of neutrophils is mediated through activation of proteases by K⁺ flux. *Nature* 416, 291–297.

Rodrigues, L., Sampaio, D., Couto, I., Machado, D., Kern, W.V., Amaral, L., *et al.* (2009) The role of efflux pumps in macrolide resistance in *Mycobacterium avium* complex. *International Journal of Antimicrobial Agents* 34, 529–533.

Salfinger, M. and Pfyffer, G.E. (1994) The new diagnostic mycobacteriology laboratory. *European Journal of Clinical Microbiology and Infectious Diseases* 13, 961–979.

Sampaio-Maia, B. and Soares-Da-Silva, P. (2001) Inhibition of calcium-independent luminal uptake of L-dopa by calmodulin antagonists in immortalized rat capillary cerebral endothelial cells. *Cell Biology International* 25, 245–252.

Santopadre, I. and Silanos, G. (1959) Neuroplegics as a therapeutic aid in treatment of tuberculous meningitis. *La Clinica Pediatrica (Bologna)* 41, 925–936.

Segal, A.W. (2005) How neutrophils kill microbes. *Annual Review of Immunology* 23, 197–223.

Shubin, H., Heiken, Ca., Glaskin, A., Pennes, E. and Arsenian, J. (1957) Chlorpromazine as an adjunct in managing tuberculous patients. *International Record of Medicine and General Practice Clinics* 170, 369–373.

Siroy, A., Mailaender, C., Harder, D., Koerber, S., Wolschendorf, F., Danilchanka, O., *et al.* (2008) Rv1698 of *Mycobacterium tuberculosis* represents a new class of channel-forming outer membrane proteins. *The Journal of Biological Chemistry* 283, 17827–17837.

Sohaskey, C.D. (2008) Nitrate enhances the survival of *Mycobacterium tuberculosis* during inhibition of respiration. *The Journal of Bacteriology* 190, 2981–2986.

Svetlíková, Z., Skovierová, H., Niederweis, M., Gaillard, J.L., McDonnell, G. and Jackson, M. (2009) Role of porins in the susceptibility of *Mycobacterium smegmatis* and *Mycobacterium chelonae* to aldehyde-based disinfectants and drugs. *Antimicrobial Agents and Chemotherapy* 53, 4015–4018.

Thanacoody, H.K. (2007) Thioridazine: resurrection as an antimicrobial agent? *British Journal of Clinical Pharmacology* 64, 566–574.

Tornieporth, N.G., Ptachewich, Y., Poltoratskaia, N., Ravi, B.S., Katapadi, M., Berger, J.J., *et al.* (1997) Tuberculosis among foreign-born persons in New York City, 1992–1994: implications for tuberculosis control. *International Journal of Tubercle and Lung Diseases* 1, 528–535.

Traykov, T., Hadjimitova, V., Goliysky, P. and Ribarov, S. (1997) Effect of phenothiazines on activated macrophage-induced luminol-dependent chemiluminescence. *General Physiology and Biophysics* 16, 3–14.

van Ingen, J., van der Laan, T., Amaral, L., Dekhuijzen, R., Boeree, M.J. and van Soolingen, D. (2009) *In vitro* activity of thioridazine against mycobacteria. *International Journal of Antimicrobial Agents* 34, 190–191.

Victor, T.C., Lee, H., Cho, S.N., Jordaan, A.M., van der Spuy, G., van Helden, P.D., *et al.* (2002) Molecular detection of early appearance of drug resistance during *Mycobacterium tuberculosis* infection. *Clinical Chemistry and Laboratory Medicine* 40, 876–881.

Viveiros, M., Portugal, I., Bettencourt, R., Victor, T.C., Jordaan, A.M., Leandro, C., *et al.* (2002) Isoniazid-induced transient high-level resistance in *Mycobacterium tuberculosis*. *Antimicrobial Agents and Chemotherapy* 46, 2804–2810.

Viveiros, M., Leandro, C. and Amaral, L. (2003) Mycobacterial efflux pumps and chemotherapeutic implications. *International Journal of Antimicrobial Agents* 22, 274–278.

Viveiros, M., Leandro, C., Rodrigues, L., Almeida, J., Bettencourt, R., Couto, I., *et al.* (2005) Direct application of the INNO-LiPA Rif.TB line-probe assay for rapid identification of *Mycobacterium tuberculosis* complex strains and detection of rifampin resistance in 360 smear-positive respiratory specimens from an area of high incidence of multidrug-resistant tuberculosis. *Journal of Clinical Microbiology* 43, 4880–4884.

Viveiros, M., Dupont, M., Rodrigues, L., Couto, I., Davin-Regli, A., Martins, M., *et al.* (2007) Antibiotic stress, genetic response and altered permeability of *E. coli*. *PLoS One* 2, e365.

Wayne, L.G. and Sohaskey, C.D. (2001) Non-replicating persistence of *Mycobacterium tuberculosis*. *Annual Review of Microbiology* 55, 139–163.

Wójcikowski, J. and Daniel, W.A. (2002) Thioridazine-fluoxetine interaction at the level of the distribution process *in vivo*. *Polish Journal of Pharmacology* 54, 647–654.

Yoshida, A., Inagawa, H., Kohchi, C., Nishizawa, T. and Soma, G. (2009) The role of toll-like receptor 2 in survival strategies of *Mycobacterium tuberculosis* in macrophage phagosomes. *Anticancer Research* 29, 907–910.

Zamfir, D. and Ionesco, G. (1958) Healing of tuberculous caverns of the lung, with persistence of the cavitary image, after treatment by antibiotics associated with chlorpromazine and phenylsemicarbazide. *Le Poumon et le Coeur* 14, 1093–1097.

19 Vaccines for Tuberculosis

Helen McShane

The Jenner Institute, University of Oxford, Oxford, UK

19.1 Existing Vaccines

The only licensed vaccine against tuberculosis is an attenuated strain of *Mycobacterium bovis*, named Bacille Calmette–Guérin (BCG) after the French scientists who were responsible for developing it. BCG was first used *per os* in 1921 and has been routinely administered intradermally or subcutaneously in many countries throughout the world for many decades. It forms an integral part of the Expanded Programme on Immunization (EPI) infant vaccination schedule and is administered at birth throughout the developing world. BCG has never been routinely used in the USA for the prevention of tuberculosis, but is widely used in a variety of vaccination schedules throughout Europe. Since BCG was first developed, many efficacy trials have been conducted with the aim of evaluating protective efficacy in different populations. It is clear that BCG immunization in infancy confers significant protection against disseminated disease (Rodrigues *et al.*, 1993; Trunz *et al.*, 2006). However, the level of efficacy demonstrated against pulmonary disease varies widely across the many trials conducted in tuberculosis-endemic countries throughout the world (Colditz *et al.*, 1994). In temperate climates, trials such as the British MRC study, conducted in the 1950s, show a clear and significant degree of protective efficacy (Hart and Sutherland, 1977). As a result of this trial, routine BCG administration to adolescent schoolchildren was introduced throughout the UK, a practice which has only recently been revised (Fine, 2005). In contrast, many large-scale efficacy trials conducted in the USA and in various countries in the developing world failed to demonstrate any protective efficacy at all (Comstock and Palmer, 1966; Baily, 1980).

Understanding the scientific basis for this variability in protective efficacy poses one of the biggest challenges in tuberculosis vaccine development. An understanding of why BCG appears to work well in some populations but not in others is important for the design of new tuberculosis vaccines. Any new vaccine ideally would work across all populations throughout the world.

Many potential hypotheses have been proposed to explain why BCG is less effective in tropical climates than in temperate ones. Some of these key hypotheses are listed in Box 19.1.

There are many different substrains of BCG in use throughout the world that have evolved through distribution and repeated subculture (Ritz and Curtis, 2009). With modern genetic sequencing tools, it is possible to identify genetic differences in these BCG subtypes (Behr *et al.*, 1999). Levels of gene expression also differ, particularly between BCG strains derived early on in the development and strains which were derived

Box 19.1.

Potential explanations for variability in BCG across geographical areas
Genetic sequence differences between BCG strains in clinical use
Microbiological differences in BCG formulation
Nutritional status of population
Pre-existing exposure to non-tuberculous mycobacteria

later (Brosch *et al.*, 2007). It is not a simple task to relate these genetic differences to the variability in protective efficacy, as the efficacy trials have been conducted in genetically diverse populations with differing exposure to mycobacteria and different trial designs. As well as evaluating different substrains of BCG, these trials used different formulations of BCG, with different routes of delivery. Some of the early studies used a mid-log phase of growth formulation, where the mycobacteria were most likely to be replicating, whereas some of the later studies used a lyophilized formulation. These different formulations may have different proportions of live and dead bacilli, which may impact on immunogenicity and protective efficacy (Behr, 2002). Data from preclinical animal models where direct comparisons can be performed more easily demonstrate that the different BCG substrains result in different levels of immunogenicity and protective efficacy in some, but not all, studies (Freudenstein *et al.*, 1979; Smith *et al.*, 1979; Lagranderie *et al.*, 1996; Horwitz *et al.*, 2009). Data from clinical studies where the immunogenicity of different BCG strains has been directly compared also reveal some studies which demonstrate differences and some which do not (Brindle *et al.*, 1972; Davids *et al.*, 2006; Gorak-Stolinska *et al.*, 2006). Nevertheless, strain differences cannot explain all the variability in protective efficacy, as Danish BCG gave significant protection in the UK but not in Southern India (Hart and Sutherland, 1977; Baily, 1980).

Nutritional factors may also be relevant in contributing to an explanation regarding the variability in BCG efficacy. However, while it is likely that no vaccine would work well in a profoundly malnourished population, many of the populations in which BCG does not work well are not severely malnourished and there is no evidence that BCG protects less well in malnourished individuals (Fine and Rodrigues, 1990).

Another potential explanation for the variability in efficacy across temperate and tropical climates is that exposure to non-tuberculous mycobacteria (NTM) may offer some degree of protective immunity. Such exposure varies according to geographical latitude, being greater in more tropical climates. This NTM exposure may also interfere directly with the protective efficacy conferred by subsequent BCG vaccination. The first demonstration that NTM exposure can protect against a subsequent *M. tuberculosis* challenge was in guinea pigs (Palmer and Long, 1966). In clinical studies, work by Dockrell *et al.* has demonstrated a high degree of pre-existing exposure to NTM in BCG-naïve adolescents in Malawi, where BCG is known not to work well, and very little pre-existing exposure in a population of BCG-naïve adolescents in the UK, where BCG has previously been shown to be highly effective (Black *et al.*, 2002). In this study, BCG vaccination in each of these populations had a very different effect on anti-mycobacterial immune responses. In the UK, where there was little pre-existing exposure, vaccination with BCG induced a potent Th-1 cellular immune response. In contrast, in the Malawian adolescents who had a high pre-existing level of anti-mycobacterial immune responses, vaccination with BCG did not alter this level of immunity significantly (Black *et al.*, 2002). This phenomenon is referred to as 'masking', whereby the anti-mycobacterial immunity induced by NTM exposure 'masks' the immunity induced by BCG. The implication from these data is also that vaccination with BCG cannot boost this NTM-induced immunity. Subsequent work has demonstrated a dramatic difference in the pro- and anti-inflammatory profile induced by BCG in the UK and Malawian adolescents studied (Weir *et al.*, 2004). A related hypothesis is that NTM-induced immunity inhibits BCG replication, and hence interferes with or 'blocks' the induction of a BCG-induced protective immune response. There are some data from preclinical studies which support this explanation, and it is known that inhibiting BCG replication with isoniazid inhibits the induction of a protective immune response (Dworski, 1973; Brandt *et al.*, 2002).

More recently, a further limitation of routine BCG vaccination in infancy has been identified. A rare but well-recognized side effect of BCG vaccination is disseminated BCG disease. Over the past few years, it has become clear that the incidence of disseminated BCG disease is higher than initially thought in populations with a high prevalence of HIV infection (Hesseling *et al.*, 2007). Such data have led the World Health Organization (WHO) to amend the BCG vaccination guidelines, and these guidelines now recommend withholding BCG vaccination in infancy in areas where HIV is prevalent, until the HIV status of the infant is known (WHO, 2007). Such a strategy is far from ideal, as many areas where HIV is prevalent do not have optimal testing facilities and any strategy which requires determining HIV status before vaccination will result in a reduced vaccine uptake rate. There is, therefore, an urgent need for a safe vaccination regimen for all infants, including those who are HIV infected.

19.2 Nature of the Protective Immune Response

In order to design an effective vaccine against *M. tuberculosis*, it is necessary to understand the nature of protective immunity to mycobacteria. Only one in ten immunocompetent people infected with *M. tuberculosis* develop disease. Ideally, a new vaccine would mimic this naturally occurring protective immunity.

An effective early innate immune response at the site of infection is responsible for the clearance of pathogen in most people who are exposed to *M. tuberculosis*. Natural killer cells and neutrophils have both been implicated in this early protective effect (Feng *et al.*, 2006; Korbel *et al.*, 2008). Gamma-delta T cells, a subpopulation of T cells thought to have a role in the non-adaptive, early host immune response to foreign pathogens, also appear to have a protective role against mycobacteria (Shen *et al.*, 2002; Spencer *et al.*, 2008). Once infected, *M. tuberculosis* is an intracellular pathogen, residing primarily inside macrophages. Such an intracellular organism is resistant to antibody-mediated immune defence mechanisms, and the primary protective immune response against mycobacteria is a T cell-mediated immune response. Herein lies the first challenge. With the exception of BCG, there are no vaccines licensed and in routine use which induce the cellular arm of the immune response. All of the vaccines used today work via, or were licensed on the basis of, the induction of a humoral immune response. Developing the next generation of vaccines which induce strong cellular immunity represents one of the significant hurdles in the field.

Within the cellular immune response, there are many subsets of T cells and cytokines which are implicated in this protective immune response. We know of the importance of Class II-restricted CD4+ T cells from preclinical studies in gene-deleted animals and from adoptive transfer experiments (Orme, 1987; Caruso *et al.*, 1999). However, the best evidence for an essential role for CD4+ T cells comes from HIV-infected populations: as the absolute CD4+ count declines, the risk of developing tuberculosis disease increases (Jones *et al.*, 1993). HIV-uninfected people have a 10% lifetime risk of reactivating latent infection. In contrast, HIV-infected people have a 10% annual risk of reactivation (Corbett and De Cock, 1996).

There is also evidence for the importance of Class I-restricted CD8+ T cells in protective immunity against *M. tuberculosis*. Evidence for a role for CD8+ T cells comes from preclinical studies in gene-depleted mice and adoptive transfer experiments (Sousa *et al.*, 2000). In addition, there is some evidence from studies in non-human primates for an essential role for CD8+ T cells in BCG-induced protection against *M. tuberculosis* challenge

(Chen *et al.*, 2009). While there is accumulating evidence for a role for CD8+ T cells, the exact mechanism by which they confer protection remains unclear. There is some evidence that they may be more important in controlling latent infection than in containing the acute phase of infection (van Pinxteren *et al.*, 2000). The primary action of CD8+ T cells may be via the secretion of cytokines (Tascon *et al.*, 1998; Brookes *et al.*, 2003). However, human cytotoxic T lymphocytes can kill *M. tuberculosis*, and this is dependent on the presence of granulysin in cytotoxic vesicles (Stenger *et al.*, 1998).

A newly defined subset of T cells, called Th-17 cells, may also be involved in protective immunity. There is some evidence from preclinical and clinical studies to support a role for these cells, which secrete the cytokine IL-17, in protection against *M. tuberculosis*. Levels of IL-17 pre-challenge correlate with protection in cattle; in mice, IL-17 was necessary for the accumulation of interferon gamma (IFN-γ)-secreting CD4+ T cells in the lungs; and in humans, tuberculin skin test (TST)-positive subjects had lower levels of IL-17 than TST-negative subjects (Khader *et al.*, 2007; Vordermeier *et al.*, 2009; Babu *et al.*, 2010).

There are many cytokines which are required for protective immunity against mycobacteria. The essential nature of IFN-γ has been demonstrated by studies in both preclinical animal models and in human subjects deficient in this pathway (Flynn *et al.*, 1993; Newport *et al.*, 1996). However, it is increasingly clear that IFN-γ alone is not sufficient for protection and, moreover, absolute levels of this cytokine, as measured by a variety of immunological assays, do not appear to correlate with protection (Langermans *et al.*, 2001; Mittrucker *et al.*, 2007; Wedlock *et al.*, 2007). There is evidence from preclinical studies for the importance of tumour necrosis factor alpha (TNF-α) in protective immunity against *M. tuberculosis*. Mice deficient in TNF-α are more susceptible to *M. tuberculosis* challenge than their wild-type counterparts (Flynn *et al.*, 1995). Furthermore, monoclonal antibodies against TNF-α, used as therapy for rheumatoid arthritis, increase reactivation of latent *M.*

tuberculosis (Keane *et al.*, 2001). Other cytokines such as interleukin-2 (IL-2) are known to be important for the generation and maintenance of central memory T-cell responses, which are necessary for durable protection against *M. tuberculosis* (Sallusto *et al.*, 2004; Harari *et al.*, 2005).

More recently, there has been increasing interest in so-called multifunctional T cells, which express the Th-1 cytokines IFN-γ, TNF-α and IL-2 on intracellular cytokine staining. Such multifunctional T cells appear to be important in protection in preclinical models of leishmania and tuberculosis (Darrah *et al.*, 2007; Forbes *et al.*, 2008). However, recent evidence from a randomized controlled clinical trial of BCG vaccination in South African infants found that the level of BCG-induced multifunctional T cells did not differ in protected and unprotected infants (Kagina *et al.*, 2010). Additional work in both clinical and preclinical studies is required to define further the role of these T cells in protective immunity.

19.3 Target Populations for a New Tuberculosis Vaccine

There are several different points on the tuberculosis clinical disease spectrum at which one might intervene with an effective vaccine, and hence a number of different target populations for such a vaccine. Vaccines administered at or soon after birth would be administered predominantly to *M. tuberculosis*-uninfected infants and therefore could potentially prevent infection and/or primary disease. Infants in the developing world are an important target population, as disease rates in this group are high (Moyo *et al.*, 2010). A vaccine administered during adolescence/early adulthood would be administered to a mixture of *M. tuberculosis* infected and *M. tuberculosis* uninfected adolescents, depending on the prevalence of infection in any particular population. Adolescents and young adults form a second important target population, as disease incidence throughout most of the world is highest in this age group. Finally, HIV-infected people form an important population for deployment of an effective tuberculosis vaccine, given the high rate of disease in HIV co-infected subjects. The HIV-infected population would also consist of a mixture of *M. tuberculosis*-infected and -uninfected individuals.

One further potential use for an effective tuberculosis vaccine is as a therapeutic vaccine for administration as an adjunct to chemotherapy in patients with tuberculosis disease. There are safety concerns about administering vaccines which induce a potent anti-mycobacterial immune response in patients with a heavy bacillary burden, as there is some preclinical data which demonstrate the induction of immunopathology (so-called Koch phenomenon) in animals with a heavy bacillary burden (Taylor *et al.*, 2003). It is likely that any potential therapeutic vaccine would be evaluated in conjunction with conventional chemotherapy.

19.4 Vaccine Evaluation

In general, most candidate tuberculosis vaccines follow a well-established development programme through preclinical animal testing in different species to early-stage clinical testing in Phase I/IIa safety and immunogenicity studies and finally through to Phase IIb/III efficacy testing in the target populations. Any new vaccine is first evaluated in a series of preclinical animal models, and some level of efficacy within more than one species is usually required before clinical evaluation begins. All the animal models used in tuberculosis vaccine development have utility but also limitations, and until we have an effective human vaccine, we will not know how representative any of these models are of human disease.

In general, preclinical evaluation begins in the murine model and then moves in sequence through into guinea pigs and non-human primates. Cattle are also a relevant animal model for a new tuberculosis vaccine and, importantly, are a target species for a new tuberculosis vaccine in their own right. As well as evaluating the protective efficacy of a new vaccine, these animal models can be used to identify potential immunological

correlates of protection, which can be further evaluated in clinical efficacy trials to (i) validate the relevance of the preclinical animal model for human disease and (ii) validate the correlate of protection. Most of these animal models are used to evaluate the effects of prophylactic immunization in naïve animals, and this represents vaccination best in *M. tuberculosis*-uninfected subjects, most obviously in infancy. However, with increased interest in developing vaccines which specifically target the latent phase of *M. tuberculosis* infection, there are animal models of latency in development (Scanga *et al.*, 1999; Botha and Ryffel, 2002; Capuano *et al.*, 2003).

Once sufficient preclinical efficacy data have been obtained, preclinical safety and toxicology studies conducted under Good Laboratory Practice conditions are also required before any new vaccine can be evaluated in early-stage clinical trials. The clinical trials typically begin in small numbers of subjects and primarily evaluate safety and immunogenicity in different target populations. Once sufficient data have been obtained, these trials then progress through to Phase IIb/Phase III efficacy testing in large numbers of subjects within a particular target population.

19.5 Potential Approaches to the Development of a New Tuberculosis Vaccine

The established protective efficacy of BCG against disseminated tuberculosis, when administered in infancy, has resulted in most global effort focusing on the development of vaccination strategies to improve BCG rather than replace it completely. Efforts to improve BCG have been either by adding a second subunit vaccine, designed to enhance the immune response and protective efficacy of BCG, or by improving BCG itself in some way. A further approach is to replace BCG with an attenuated strain of *M. tuberculosis* in order to improve the efficacy. The leading new vaccination approaches currently being explored in preclinical and clinical studies are outlined in Table 19.1.

Table 19.1. Summary of tuberculosis vaccine candidates undergoing clinical evaluation.

Type of vaccine		Vaccine name	Stage of development	References
BCG replacements	Recombinant BCG	rBCG30	Phase I	Hoft et al., 2008
		rBCGΔureChly	Phase I	Grode et al., 2005
Subunit vaccines	Recombinant viral vectors	MVA85A	Phase IIb	Brookes et al., 2003; McShane et al., 2004; Ibanga et al., 2006; Pathan et al., 2007; Hawkridge et al., 2008; Sander et al., 2009; Scriba et al., 2010
		Aeras-402	Phase IIb	Abel et al., 2010
	Protein and adjuvant	M72	Phase IIa	Von Eschen et al., 2009
		Hybrid I	Phase IIa	van Dissel et al., 2010
		HyVAC IV	Phase I	Dietrich et al., 2005
Other		M. vaccae	Phase III	von Reyn et al., 2010
		RUTI	Phase I	Vilaplana et al., 2010

The general strategies and leading vaccine candidates are discussed in detail below, with a focus on those candidates currently being evaluated, or close to commencing evaluation, in clinical trials.

19.5.1 BCG replacements

There have been two WHO working group meetings on so-called 'live vaccines' which encompassed the BCG replacement vaccines in development, in 2004 and 2009, in order to facilitate development and help define a regulatory pathway forward (Kamath et al., 2005; Walker et al., 2010). An important goal of the live vaccine approach is to demonstrate improved safety over BCG, particularly given the concerns with using BCG in HIV-infected infants (Hesseling et al., 2007). Preclinical models such as severe combined immunodeficiency (SCID) mice can be used to demonstrate improved safety when compared to wild-type BCG strains. In addition, levels of efficacy equivalent or superior to the wild-type strain should also be demonstrated in preclinical models. The scale of clinical trial needed to demonstrate non-inferiority over wild-type strains means that such a trial may not be feasible. One of the challenges for the field is, therefore, to devise an alternative clinical pathway for product registration which is sufficiently robust.

Recombinant BCG strains

Broadly, there are two general approaches being investigated. The first is whether the construction of recombinant strains of BCG which overexpress certain immunodominant antigens will lead to an enhancement in protective efficacy. One such vaccine, which demonstrates improved efficacy over the wild-type parent strain in guinea pigs, is rBCG30 (Horwitz et al., 2000). A Phase I clinical trial with this vaccine in the USA demonstrated comparable safety profile and enhanced immunogenicity when compared to the parentral strain of BCG (Tice) used alone (Hoft et al., 2008). A second potential candidate, BCG::RD1-2F9, replaces the region of deletion 1 (RD-1) which is missing from BCG (Pym et al., 2003). Although this recombinant BCG confers greater protection against aerosol M. tuberculosis challenge in mice and guinea pigs, there are safety concerns regarding the virulence of such a strain of BCG and, in addition, this vaccine could be likely to confound the new interferon gamma release assays (IGRAs), Quantiferon Gold and T-Spot TB, which are based on a T-cell response to two antigens in the RD-1 gene, ESAT-6 and CFP-10 and are now in routine clinical use as diagnostic tests (see Chapter 4) (Pym *et al.*, 2002; Pai *et al.*, 2004). The second approach being pursued is to generate recombinant strains of BCG which express molecules such as listeriolysin or perfringolysin (Grode *et al.*, 2005; Sun *et al.*, 2009). The scientific rationale behind these candidates is to enhance cross-priming and hence improve the induction of a CD8+ T-cell response. One of these vaccines has been evaluated in a Phase I clinical trial in Europe (clinicaltrials.gov trial identifier NCT00749034) and is currently in a Phase I trial in South African adults (clinicaltrials. gov trial identifier NCT01113281). It is possible to combine these two approaches, and recombinant strains of BCG which express perfringolysin and immunodominant antigens are currently in development (Sun *et al.*, 2009).

Attenuated M. tuberculosis strains

An alternative approach to modifying BCG is to develop a rationally attenuated strain of *M. tuberculosis*. The potential advantage in using *M. tuberculosis* as the starting organism rather than BCG is that some of the genes which are present in *M. tuberculosis* but deleted in BCG may be relevant for protection (Hernandez Pando *et al.*, 2006). There are two distinct approaches currently being developed. One candidate is an attenuated strain of *M. tuberculosis* with a disrupted Pho-P gene, which has demonstrated superior efficacy when compared to BCG in the guinea pig and non-human primate models (Williams *et al.*, 2005b; Verreck *et al.*, 2009). The safety and efficacy of two other attenuated *M. tuberculosis* vaccine strains, mc^26020 and mc^26030, in non-human primates has also been demonstrated (Larsen *et al.*, 2009).

There are significant safety concerns regarding the clinical evaluation of attenuated strains of *M. tuberculosis*. However, the WHO working group has defined a pathway forward for early-stage clinical evaluation of such vaccines and these vaccine candidates represent an important proof-of-concept in tuberculosis vaccine development.

19.5.2 BCG booster vaccines

These vaccine candidates are designed to be given after BCG immunization, in order to enhance the protective efficacy of BCG. They are more advanced than the potential BCG replacements described above and there are currently five vaccine candidates undergoing evaluation in clinical trials. These candidates involve the delivery of an immunodominant antigen or antigens, either as a recombinant protein with adjuvant or as a recombinant viral vector. Both antigen(s) and the antigen delivery system need to be identified. Regarding antigen selection, there has been a focus on the well-characterized and immuno-dominant antigens such as the antigen 85 complex, and RD-1 genes such as ESAT-6 and TB10.4. The antigen 85 complex (A, B and C) constitutes a major portion of the secreted proteins from *M. tuberculosis*, BCG and all other mycobacteria sequenced to date (Andersen *et al.*, 1992). The antigen 85 complex is protective against *M. tuberculosis* challenge in small animals, either as a DNA vaccine or as protein (Horwitz *et al.*, 1995; Huygen *et al.*, 1996). Inclusion of genes from the RD-1, either in a subunit vaccine or in a recombinant BCG strain, may potentially confound the new IGRA diagnostic tests and this may limit the development of candidates containing these antigens, as these IGRAs rely on detecting a T-cell response to the RD-1 antigens, ESAT-6 and CFP-10 (Pym *et al.*, 2002; Pai *et al.*, 2004).

There is increasing interest in the inclusion of so-called 'dormancy' or hypoxia-induced antigens, which may be preferentially upregulated and expressed during latent infection. Inclusion of such antigens into a subunit vaccine may be necessary for optimal efficacy of a post-exposure vaccine administered to latently infected subjects (Roupie *et al.*, 2007). In addition, while the most advanced candidates have focused on protein antigens, there is now an increasing interest in non-protein, glycolipid antigens as well (Guiard *et al.*, 2009).

In terms of antigen delivery systems, there are two main approaches being pursued and the leading candidates using each approach are discussed below.

Recombinant viral vectors

This approach to antigen delivery requires the selection of antigen. This approach clones the antigen(s) of choice into a viral vector and uses the virus itself as an endogenous adjuvant. Many viruses have been used as vectors for antigen delivery, such as pox viruses, adenoviruses, flaviviruses and lentiviruses (Prevec et al., 1989; Paoletti, 1996; Bonaldo et al., 2010; Draper and Heeney, 2010; Negri et al., 2010). Safety concerns with the use of replicating vectors means that the challenge is to develop an attenuated viral vector which induces a persistent immune response. One significant limitation of virally vectored vaccines is the presence of immunity to the vector (virus), which limits the ability of the recombinant virus to induce or boost the immune response. This is relevant for naturally occurring antivector immunity (as with human adenoviral strains, particularly AdHu5) (Tatsis and Ertl, 2004) but also for repeated use of a single vector, both for boosting an immune response to a single pathogen and for multiple usage of the same vector as a vaccine for different pathogens. Heterologous prime-boost immunization regimens, where two different viral vectors encoding the same antigen are delivered sequentially, are an effective way to induce high levels of cellular immunity for both CD4+ and CD8+ T cells and circumvent the problems of antivector immunity (Schneider et al., 1998; Hanke et al., 1999; McShane et al., 2001). For the development of a tuberculosis vaccine, BCG becomes the priming immunization in such a strategy and many groups, including our own, have focused on developing an effective 'boost' for BCG. Such a strategy retains the protective efficacy of BCG conferred against disseminated disease and aims to improve protection against pulmonary disease. There are two leading approaches using viral vectors currently being developed.

MVA85A (OXFORD UNIVERSITY; OXFORD EMERGENT TUBERCULOSIS CONSORTIUM) This approach uses the modified vaccinia virus Ankara (MVA), an attenuated strain of vaccinia, to induce a potent cell-mediated immune response. Recombinant MVAs are known to be effective at boosting pre-existing T-cell responses (Schneider et al., 1998; Hanke et al., 1999; Amara et al., 2001; McConkey et al., 2003). In MVA85A, the antigen expressed by the MVA vector is antigen 85A. Preclinical studies with MVA85A have demonstrated that MVA85A can improve BCG-induced protection in animal models (McShane et al., 2002; Williams et al., 2005a; Verreck et al., 2009; Vordermeier et al., 2009). The last of these references demonstrates that both MVA85A and an adenovirus expressing antigen 85A can both improve BCG-induced protection against M. bovis challenge in cattle (Vordermeier et al., 2009). This cattle study identified two potential correlates of protection: both levels of antigen 85A-specific IL-17 and cultured ELISPOT responses to antigen 85A on the day of challenge correlated with subsequent protection in this experiment. These correlates are now being evaluated in the ongoing clinical studies.

MVA85A was the first new tuberculosis subunit vaccine to enter into clinical trials in September 2002 and is currently the most clinically advanced new tuberculosis vaccine. Since 2002, a series of Phase I/IIa clinical trials in the UK, The Gambia and South Africa have been conducted with this vaccine candidate in populations including BCG naïve adults, BCG vaccinated adults, adolescents, children and infants, M. tuberculosis-infected adults and, most recently, HIV-infected adults (Brookes et al., 2003; McShane et al., 2004; Ibanga et al., 2006; Pathan et al., 2007; Hawkridge et al., 2008; Sander et al., 2009; Scriba et al., 2010; Minassian et al., unpublished data). These trials have all demonstrated this vaccine candidate to be safe and immunogenic, and to be particularly potent at stimulating an antigen-specific CD4+ T-cell response. More detailed characterization of the vaccine-induced immune response demonstrates a high level of polyfunctional CD4+ T cells, which are positive on intracellular cytokine staining performed on either peripheral blood mononuclear cells (PBMCs) or whole blood samples for interferon gamma, TNF-α, IL-2, IL-17 and MiP1b (Beveridge et al., 2007). These antigen-specific T cells proliferate and have a non-terminally differentiated phenotype (Beveridge *et al.*, 2007). It is also possible to detect a modest antigen-specific CD8+ T-cell response after vaccination with this candidate (Whelan *et al.*, 2009). Furthermore, it is clear that a regulatory T-cell response is also induced after vaccination (Fletcher *et al.*, 2008). This last study demonstrates the importance of characterizing the regulatory T-cell response as well as the effector T-cell response in early-stage vaccine trials, as any effective immune response will be the result of a balance between these different aspects of the cellular immune response. A Phase IIb proof-of-concept efficacy trial with MVA85A commenced in South African BCG-vaccinated infants in 2009 (clinicaltrials.gov trial identifier NCT00953927; http://clinicaltrials.gov/ct2/show/NCT00953927?term=NCT00953927&rank=1).

AERAS-402 (AERAS; CRUCELL) This vaccine candidate is a recombinant, replication-deficient adenovirus, serotype 35, expressing a fusion protein created from the sequences of the antigens Ag85A, B and TB10.4 from *M. tuberculosis*. One of the limitations of using adenoviruses as viral vectors for vaccines in general is the level of pre-existing, naturally occurring antivector immunity. Immunity to the commonest serotype, AdHu5, exists at levels of up to 90% in some populations (Xiang *et al.*, 2006). Pre-existing immunity to AdHu35, a rarer serotype, is known to be considerably lower (Kostense *et al.*, 2004). Aeras-402 is a recombinant strain of AdHu35 expressing antigens 85A, B and TB10.4 (Abel *et al.*, 2010). Preclinical studies in mice have demonstrated this vaccine confers levels of protection comparable with BCG when administered by either the systemic or the mucosal route (Radosevic *et al.*, 2007). This vaccine is also immunogenic in non-human primates following either BCG or recombinant BCG prime (Magalhaes *et al.*, 2008). A clinical trial with this vaccine in BCG-vaccinated South African adults has demonstrated a good safety profile, together with high levels of antigen-specific CD8+ T cells and more modest levels of CD4+ T cells (Abel *et al.*, 2010). In this trial, a second booster vaccination administered 2 months

after the primary immunization did not result in higher levels of antigen-specific T cells, likely because of antivector immunity to the AdHu35 induced by the first dose (Abel *et al.*, 2010). This vaccine is now being evaluated in a Phase II safety, immunogenicity and efficacy study in HIV-infected adults in South Africa (clinicaltrials.gov trial identifier NCT01017536; http://clinicaltrials.gov/ct2/show/NCT01017536?term=NCT01017536&rank=1).

Protein/adjuvant combinations

Using recombinant protein is one other method of developing a subunit vaccine based on one or a few immunodominant antigens. Recombinant protein delivered alone is a poor inducer of a cellular immune response. However, recombinant protein which is co-administered with an adjuvant can be an effective way to induce a cellular immune response. The challenge is in developing adjuvants which are good at stimulating the Th-1 pathway. The most widely used adjuvant, aluminium salts, induces primarily antibody responses and a Th-2 biased cellular immune response (HogenEsch, 2002). There are new adjuvants being developed which induce a Th-1 biased cellular immune response and some of these are being evaluated with mycobacterial proteins for use as a tuberculosis vaccine. These protein/adjuvant combinations are also being developed as booster vaccines to enhance the protective efficacy conferred by BCG. To date, there are three such protein/adjuvant candidate tuberculosis vaccines which have entered into clinical testing:

HYBRID I (STATUM SERUM INSTITUTE, SSI) This vaccine consists of a fusion protein of antigen 85B and ESAT-6. Preclinical studies with this protein, administered intranasally with the mucosal adjuvant LTK63, a non-toxic mutant of the *Escherichia coli* heat labile enterotoxin, demonstrated an improvement on BCG-induced protection in mice (Dietrich *et al.*, 2006). However, no improvement on BCG-induced protection was demonstrated in the guinea pig (Williams *et al.*, 2005b). A clinical trial of this vaccine candidate in BCG naïve subjects has now been completed (van Dissel *et al.*, 2010). When administered alone, this protein was only very weakly immunogenic. When co-administered with a high dose of a novel adjuvant, IC31, a synthetic formulation which combines an antimicrobial peptide, KLK, and an immunostimulatory oligodeoxynocleotide, ODN1a, significantly higher immunogenicity was demonstrated using a short-term cultured ELISPOT assay (van Dissel *et al.*, 2010). Further studies are now being conducted in purified protein derivative (PPD)-positive subjects (clinical trials.gov trial identifier NCT00929396; http://clinicaltrials.gov/ct2/show/NCT00929396?term=NCT00929396&rank=1); and with another novel adjuvant, CAF01 (clinicaltrials.gov trial identifier NCT00922363; http://clinicaltrials.gov/ct2/show/NCT00922363?term=NCT00922363&rank=1). One potential limitation with this protein/adjuvant vaccine candidate is the potential for the T-cell response to ESAT-6 to interfere with the new IGRAs, as discussed above. To date, the available clinical data demonstrate a low level of Quantiferon positivity (one of the new IGRA tests) after vaccination with Hybrid I; however, this construct has not yet been evaluated in tuberculosis-endemic countries (van Dissel *et al.*, 2010). A Phase I study evaluating the safety of this candidate administered intranasally was terminated for safety reasons (clinicaltrials.gov trial identifier NCT00440544; http://clinicaltrials.gov/ct2/show/NCT00440544?term=NCT00440544&rank=1).

HYVAC IV (SSI) In this second-generation fusion protein from SSI, the ESAT-6 antigen has been replaced with another immunodominant antigen from *M. tuberculosis*, TB10.4, in order to avoid the problems of confounding the diagnostic IGRA assays (Dietrich *et al.*, 2005). Preclinical data with this construct show levels of protection comparable to BCG in mice and guinea pigs (Dietrich *et al.*, 2005; Skeiky *et al.*, 2010).

M72 (GSK) This vaccine candidate consists of a fusion protein of two antigens from *M. tuberculosis*, the 32 kDa and the 39 kDa antigens (Alderson *et al.*, 2000). In preclinical models, this fusion protein, when admini-

stered with the adjuvant AS02A, a proprietary oil in water emulsion with the immunostimulants, monophosphoryl lipid A and *Quillaja saponaria* fraction 21, has demonstrated comparable efficacy to BCG in mice and guinea pigs (Skeiky *et al.*, 2004) and to improve BCG-induced protection in guinea pigs but not mice (Brandt *et al.*, 2004). A Phase I clinical trial with M72, administered with AS02A, demonstrated this candidate to be modestly reactogenic, with a significant induction of an antigen-specific CD4+ T-cell response but no detectable CD8+ T-cell responses (Von Eschen *et al.*, 2009). Further studies are under way in tuberculosis-endemic regions (clinicaltrials.gov trial identifier NCT00600782; http://clinicaltrials.gov/ct2/show/NCT00600782?term=NCT00600782&rank=1).

Other tuberculosis vaccines in development

MYCOBACTERIUM VACCAE *M. vaccae* is a whole cell lysate of a culture of *M. vaccae*, which has been evaluated in many clinical trials as a therapeutic vaccine over the past 10 years. The results from most of these trials have been variable (Stanford *et al.*, 1990; Durban Immunotherapy Trial Group, 1999; Johnson *et al.*, 2000). More recently, a Phase III study in HIV-infected adults in Tanzania evaluating repeated immunizations with *M. vaccae* demonstrated a modest degree of efficacy against culture-positive tuberculosis (von Reyn *et al.*, 2010). The primary end point in this study was disseminated disease, and too few cases were accrued for this end point to be met. Further studies are required to demonstrate the reproducibility of this result, where culture-positive disease is the primary end point. If these results are reproducible, this study represents an important proof-of-concept that vaccine-induced protection against tuberculosis, even in immunosuppressed subjects, is achievable.

RUTI RUTI is a potential therapeutic vaccine for tuberculosis which consists of detoxified and liposomal cellular fragments of *M. tuberculosis* (Vilaplana *et al.*, 2010). A Phase I clinical trial in healthy subjects has recently demonstrated that this vaccine is safe and modestly immunogenic for the induction of antigen-specific IFN-γ (Vilaplana *et al.*, 2010).

19.6 Major Challenges to Tuberculosis Vaccine Development

As vaccine candidates are advanced through preclinical studies to clinical evaluation, the major challenges in the field become more apparent. These are discussed below.

19.6.1 Lack of immunological correlates of protection

The identification of an immunological correlate of protection would greatly facilitate vaccine development. Although we understand broadly the nature of a protective immune response to *M. tuberculosis*, we do not yet have a simple, validated measure of immunogenicity that will predict vaccine success in human clinical trials. The only way to evaluate whether a vaccine is effective is in large-scale, expensive and time-consuming efficacy trials. The early-stage clinical trials are essential for the demonstration of safety, and also immunogenicity, in order to be sure that the vaccine candidate in question is inducing what is thought to be a protective immune response. However, in the absence of predefined correlates, such data do not necessarily predict efficacy. It is only possible to validate an immunological correlate once we have an effective vaccine. It would be too resource- and time-inefficient to perform detailed immunology on all subjects in efficacy trials. However, if peripheral blood mononuclear cells and serum samples from all subjects are stored in such trials, at the end of the trial samples from diseased (i.e. not protected) subjects and matched healthy exposed controls can be analysed in order to identify potential immunological correlates. Any potential correlates can then be validated subsequently in a Phase III trial. However, protective immunity to mycobacteria is complex, and it is perhaps unlikely that a single, simple immunological correlate will be identified in such trials. It may also be that

any immune correlate is vaccine specific. Results from a recent randomized controlled trial of BCG vaccination in South African infants demonstrated that neither frequency nor function of antigen-specific T cells, measured 10 weeks after BCG vaccination, correlated with protection (Kagina *et al.*, 2010). The challenge with these studies, particularly in infants where blood volumes are limited, is to identify the optimal time point for evaluation. BCG is a complex whole organism vaccine, known to induce a robust innate immune response. Further work is required to evaluate correlates of protection in the ongoing efficacy trials with the new candidates.

19.6.2 Lack of validated animal models

Although there are many preclinical animal models of tuberculosis vaccine evaluation, we do not yet know which, if any, of these models predicts vaccine success in humans. It is only once we have a vaccine which protects against human disease that we can go back to the animal models and evaluate which one(s) predicts success best in humans. It is only by moving forward in an iterative way, evaluating several candidates in proof-of-concept efficacy trials, that we can reach a clearer understanding as to the nature of protective immunity and the most useful animal models with which to evaluate subsequent vaccine candidates. Such models can be utilized for the identification of potential immunological correlates, which can then be evaluated in clinical efficacy trials.

19.6.3 Lack of high-incidence field sites

Although the global prevalence of tuberculosis disease is high, the incidence in any particular population is relatively low. Any efficacy trial needs to be conducted in a population with as high an incidence as possible, in order for the trial to be conducted as quickly as possible. In addition, the epidemiological data which underpin the incidence data need to be robust and recent, in order that the efficacy trials can be powered with confidence. Such epidemiological studies in themselves take considerable time and resources. A more pragmatic way forward may be to use less robust incidence data in an adaptive trial design, and to plan for a Data and Safety Monitoring Board review of the real-time case accrual rate in the control arm of any vaccine study, and for the sample size and/or follow-up time to be adjusted accordingly (Luce *et al.*, 2009).

There are very few sites throughout the world which are currently capable of conducting an efficacy trial with a new tuberculosis vaccine. The limitations are due to lack of sites both with a sufficiently high (and well-defined) incidence and with a sufficient clinical trial infrastructure for the conduct of a regulatory standard, International Conference on Harmonization Good Clinical Practice (ICH-GCP)-compliant clinical trial. It is important that, in parallel with vaccine development, a commitment is made to the funding and development of clinical trial sites capable of evaluating these vaccine candidates. Such sites will necessarily be in high-burden countries; however, it is important that such sites are not limited to sub-Saharan Africa. The BCG efficacy data demonstrate a striking variability in efficacy across different geographical latitudes and it is important that efficacy testing of the new vaccine candidates is conducted in different continents.

19.6.4 End point definitions in efficacy trials

The end points in a clinical trial are critical. Such end points must be clearly defined and acceptable to the regulatory agencies. For efficacy trials, the end points must relate to tuberculosis disease and the gold standard is a positive culture for *M. tuberculosis*. For clinical trials in infants, this poses a problem as, in infants, most of the tuberculosis disease diagnosed in routine clinical practice is not culture positive (Moyo *et al.*, 2010). Efficacy trials in infants therefore require end points which are defined by a complex algorithm of clinical, radiological, microbiological and immunological factors, which together con-

stitute a case definition of tuberculosis. Some link to the causative organism is important from a regulatory viewpoint. In the absence of a positive *M. tuberculosis* culture, factors such as TST positivity, IGRA positivity (or conversion) or Ziehl–Neelsen (ZN)-positive sputum smears, need to be considered. Newer molecular diagnostic tests such as PCR-based tests offer real promise in providing specificity without a loss of sensitivity. One of the important aspects to explore in Phase IIb proof-of-concept trials is which end points work best and which are most acceptable to regulatory agencies. The challenge of defining appropriate and meaningful end points is not just in infant trials. With other indications, for example HIV-infected adults, the end points can also be challenging, as HIV-associated tuberculosis is also less likely to be sputum smear positive than in HIV-negative people, and HIV-infected adults are more likely to have extra-pulmonary disease (Sterling *et al.*, 2010).

19.7 Conclusions

The last decade has been an exciting time in tuberculosis vaccine development. After decades of inadequate funding, there are now several vaccine candidates being evaluated in clinical trials and the most advanced of these are being evaluated in efficacy trials. These proof-of-concept efficacy trials are essential for vaccine development, and ultimately for the registration of a new tuberculosis vaccine. However, there is much more than individual vaccine efficacy that we can learn from such trials. These trials allow the opportunity to feedback iteratively into immunological analysis and preclinical animal models, to allow us to establish models which are more predictive of human disease and also to identify potential correlates within which subsequent vaccines can be evaluated.

References

Abel, B., Tameris, M., Mansoor, N., Gelderbloem, S., Hughes, J., Abrahams, D., *et al.* (2010) The novel tuberculosis vaccine, AERAS-402, induces robust and polyfunctional CD4+ and CD8+ T cells in adults. *American Journal of Respiratory and Critical Care Medicine* 181, 1407–1417.

Alderson, M.R., Bement, T., Day, C.H., Zhu, L., Molesh, D., Skeiky, Y.A., *et al.* (2000) Expression cloning of an immunodominant family of *Mycobacterium tuberculosis* antigens using human CD4(+) T cells. *Journal of Experimental Medicine* 191, 551–560.

Amara, R.R., Villinger, F., Altman, J.D., Lydy, S.L., O'Neil, S.P., Staprans, S.I., *et al.* (2001) Control of a mucosal challenge and prevention of AIDS by a multiprotein DNA/MVA vaccine. *Science* 292, 69–74.

Andersen, P., Askgaard, D., Gottschau, A., Bennedsen, J., Nagai, S. and Heron, I. (1992) Identification of immunodominant antigens during infection with *Mycobacterium tuberculosis*. *Scandinavian Journal of Immunology* 36, 823–831.

Babu, S., Bhat, S.Q., Kumar, N.P., Kumaraswami, V. and Nutman, T.B. (2010) Regulatory T cells modulate Th17 responses in patients with positive tuberculin skin test results. *Journal of Infectious Diseases* 201, 20–31.

Baily, G.V. (1980) Tuberculosis prevention trial, Madras. *Indian Journal of Medical Research* 72(Suppl), 1–74.

Behr, M.A. (2002) BCG – different strains, different vaccines? *The Lancet Infectious Diseases* 2, 86–92.

Behr, M.A., Wilson, M.A., Gill, W.P., Salamon, H., Schoolnik, G.K., Rane, S., *et al.* (1999) Comparative genomics of BCG vaccines by whole-genome DNA microarray. *Science* 284, 1520–1523.

Beveridge, N.E., Price, D.A., Casazza, J.P., Pathan, A.A., Sander, C.R., Asher, T.E., *et al.* (2007) Immunisation with BCG and recombinant MVA85A induces long-lasting, polyfunctional *Mycobacterium tuberculosis*-specific CD4+ memory T lymphocyte populations. *European Journal of Immunology* 37, 3089–3100.

Black, G.F., Weir, R.E., Floyd, S., Bliss, L., Warndorff, D.K., Crampin, A.C., *et al.* (2002) BCG-induced increase in interferon-gamma response to mycobacterial antigens and efficacy of BCG vaccination in Malawi and the UK: two randomised controlled studies. *The Lancet* 359, 1393–1401.

Bonaldo, M.C., Martins, M.A., Rudersdorf, R., Mudd, P.A., Sacha, J.B., Piaskowski, S.M., *et al.* (2010) Recombinant yellow fever vaccine virus 17D expressing simian immunodeficiency virus SIVmac239 gag induces SIV-specific CD8+ T-cell responses in rhesus macaques. *Journal of Virology,* 84, 3699–3706.

Botha, T. and Ryffel, B. (2002) Reactivation of latent tuberculosis by an inhibitor of inducible nitric oxide synthase in an aerosol murine model. *Immunology* 107, 350–357.

Brandt, L., Feino Cunha, J., Weinreich Olsen, A., Chilima, B., Hirsch, P., Appelberg, R., *et al.* (2002) Failure of the *Mycobacterium bovis* BCG vaccine: some species of environmental mycobacteria block multiplication of BCG and induction of protective immunity to tuberculosis. *Infection and Immunity* 70, 672–678.

Brandt, L., Skeiky, Y.A., Alderson, M.R., Lobet, Y., Dalemans, W., Turner, O.C., *et al.* (2004) The protective effect of the *Mycobacterium bovis* BCG vaccine is increased by coadministration with the *Mycobacterium tuberculosis* 72-kilodalton fusion polyprotein Mtb72F in *M. tuberculosis*-infected guinea pigs. *Infection and Immunity* 72, 6622–6632.

Brindle, T.W., Griffiths, M.I., Holme, T., Stalker, R., Burland, W.L., Coates, G.A., *et al.* (1972) A trial to compare United Kingdom strength BCG vaccine with vaccine of double the moist weight content. *Tubercle* 53, 106–110.

Brookes, R.H., Pathan, A.A., McShane, H., Hensmann, M., Price, D.A. and Hill, A.V. (2003) CD8+ T cell-mediated suppression of intracellular *Mycobacterium tuberculosis* growth in activated human macrophages. *European Journal of Immunology* 33, 3293–3302.

Brosch, R., Gordon, S.V., Garnier, T., Eiglmeier, K., Frigui, W., Valenti, P., *et al.* (2007) Genome plasticity of BCG and impact on vaccine efficacy. *Proceedings of the National Academy of Sciences* 104, 5596–5601.

Capuano, S.V. 3rd, Croix, D.A., Pawar, S., Zinovik, A., Myers, A., Lin, P.L., *et al.* (2003) Experimental *Mycobacterium tuberculosis* infection of cynomolgus macaques closely resembles the various manifestations of human *M. tuberculosis* infection. *Infection and Immunity* 71, 5831–5844.

Caruso, A.M., Serbina, N., Klein, E., Triebold, K., Bloom, B.R. and Flynn, J.L. (1999) Mice deficient in CD4 T cells have only transiently diminished levels of IFN-gamma, yet succumb to tuberculosis. *Journal of Immunology* 162, 5407–5416.

Chen, C.Y., Huang, D., Wang, R.C., Shen, L., Zeng, G., Yao, S., *et al.* (2009) A critical role for CD8 T cells in a nonhuman primate model of tuberculosis. *PLoS Pathogens* 5, e1000392.

Colditz, G.A., Brewer, T.F., Berkey, C.S., Wilson, M.E., Burdick, E., Fineberg, H.V., *et al.* (1994) Efficacy of BCG vaccine in the prevention of tuberculosis. Meta-analysis of the published literature. *Journal of the American Medical Association* 271, 698–702.

Comstock, G.W. and Palmer, C.E. (1966) Long-term results of BCG vaccination in the southern United States. *American Review of Respiratory Disease* 93, 171–183.

Corbett, E.L. and De Cock, K.M. (1996) Tuberculosis in the HIV-positive patient. *British Journal of Hospital Medicine* 56, 200–204.

Darrah, P.A., Patel, D.T., De Luca, P.M., Lindsay, R.W., Davey, D.F., Flynn, B.J., *et al.* (2007) Multifunctional TH1 cells define a correlate of vaccine-mediated protection against *Leishmania major*. *Nature Medicine* 13, 843–850.

Davids, V., Hanekom, W.A., Mansoor, N., Gamieldien, H., Gelderbloem, S.J., Hawkridge, A., *et al.* (2006) The effect of bacille Calmette–Guerin vaccine strain and route of administration on induced immune responses in vaccinated infants. *Journal of Infectious Diseases* 193, 531–536.

Dietrich, J., Aagaard, C., Leah, R., Olsen, A.W., Stryhn, A., Doherty, T.M., *et al.* (2005) Exchanging ESAT6 with TB10.4 in an Ag85B fusion molecule-based tuberculosis subunit vaccine: efficient protection and ESAT6-based sensitive monitoring of vaccine efficacy. *Journal of Immunology* 174, 6332–6339.

Dietrich, J., Andersen, C., Rappuoli, R., Doherty, T.M., Jensen, C.G. and Andersen, P. (2006) Mucosal administration of Ag85B-ESAT-6 protects against infection with *Mycobacterium tuberculosis* and boosts prior bacillus Calmette–Guerin immunity. *Journal of Immunology* 177, 6353–6360.

Draper, S.J. and Heeney, J.L. (2010) Viruses as vaccine vectors for infectious diseases and cancer. *Nature Reviews Microbiology* 8, 62–73.

Durban Immunotherapy Trial Group (1999) Immuno-therapy with *Mycobacterium vaccae* in patients with newly diagnosed pulmonary tuberculosis: a randomised controlled trial. *The Lancet* 354, 116–119.

Dworski, M. (1973) Efficacy of bacillus Calmette–Guerin and isoniazid-resistant bacillus Calmette–Guerin with and without isoniazid chemoprophylaxis from day of vaccination. I. Experimental findings in guinea pigs. *American Review of Respiratory Disease* 108, 294–300.

Feng, C.G., Kaviratne, M., Rothfuchs, A.G., Cheever, A., Hieny, S., Young, H.A., *et al.* (2006) NK cell-derived IFN-gamma differentially regulates innate resistance and neutrophil response in T cell-deficient hosts infected with *Mycobacterium tuberculosis*. *Journal of Immunology* 177, 7086–7093.

Fine, P. (2005) Stopping routine vaccination for tuberculosis in schools. *British Medical Journal* 331, 647–648.

Fine, P.E. and Rodrigues, L.C. (1990) Modern vaccines. Mycobacterial diseases. *The Lancet* 335, 1016–1020.

Fletcher, H.A., Pathan, A.A., Berthoud, T.K., Dunachie, S.J., Whelan, K.T., Alder, N.C., *et al.* (2008) Boosting BCG vaccination with MVA85A down-regulates the immunoregulatory cytokine TGF-beta1. *Vaccine* 26, 5269–5275.

Flynn, J.L., Chan, J., Triebold, K.J., Dalton, D.K., Stewart, T.A. and Bloom, B.R. (1993) An essential role for interferon gamma in resistance to *Mycobacterium tuberculosis* infection. *Journal of Experimental Medicine* 178, 2249–2254.

Flynn, J.L., Goldstein, M.M., Chan, J., Triebold, K.J., Pfeffer, K., Lowenstein, C.J., *et al.* (1995) Tumor necrosis factor-alpha is required in the protective immune response against *Mycobacterium tuberculosis* in mice. *Immunity* 2, 561–572.

Forbes, E.K., Sander, C., Ronan, E.O., McShane, H., Hill, A.V., Beverley, P.C., *et al.* (2008) Multifunctional, high-level cytokine-producing Th1 cells in the lung, but not spleen, correlate with protection against *Mycobacterium tuberculosis* aerosol challenge in mice. *Journal of Immunology* 181, 4955–4964.

Freudenstein, H., Pranter, W. and Schweinsberg, H. (1979) Assessment of several BCG vaccines in different animal test systems (additional studies to an IABS collaborative assay). *Journal of Biological Standardisation* 7, 203–212.

Gorak-Stolinska, P., Weir, R.E., Floyd, S., Lalor, M.K., Stenson, S., Branson, K., *et al.* (2006) Immunogenicity of Danish-SSI 1331 BCG vaccine in the UK: comparison with Glaxo-Evans 1077 BCG vaccine. *Vaccine* 24, 5726–5733.

Grode, L., Seiler, P., Baumann, S., Hess, J., Brinkmann, V., Nasser Eddine, A., *et al.* (2005) Increased vaccine efficacy against tuberculosis of recombinant *Mycobacterium bovis* bacille Calmette–Guerin mutants that secrete listeriolysin. *Journal of Clinical Investigation* 115, 2472–2479.

Guiard, J., Collmann, A., Garcia-Alles, L.F., Mourey, L., Brando, T., Mori, L., *et al.* (2009) Fatty acyl structures of mycobacterium tuberculosis sulfo-glycolipid govern T cell response. *Journal of Immunology* 182, 7030–7037.

Hanke, T., Samuel, R.V., Blanchard, T.J., Neumann, V.C., Allen, T.M., Boyson, J.E., *et al.* (1999) Effective induction of simian immunodeficiency virus-specific cytotoxic T lymphocytes in macaques by using a multiepitope gene and DNA prime-modified vaccinia virus Ankara boost vaccination regimen. *Journal of Virology* 73, 7524–7532.

Harari, A., Vallelian, F., Meylan, P.R. and Pantaleo, G. (2005) Functional heterogeneity of memory

CD4 T cell responses in different conditions of antigen exposure and persistence. *Journal of Immunology* 174, 1037–1045.

Hart, P.D. and Sutherland, I. (1977) BCG and vole bacillus vaccines in the prevention of tuberculosis in adolescence and early adult life. *British Medical Journal* 2, 293–295.

Hawkridge, T., Scriba, T.J., Gelderbloem, S., Smit, E., Tameris, M., Moyo, S., *et al.* (2008) Safety and immunogenicity of a new tuberculosis vaccine, MVA85A, in healthy adults in South Africa. *Journal of Infectious Diseases* 198, 544–552.

Hernandez Pando, R., Aguilar, L.D., Infante, E., Cataldi, A., Bigi, F., Martin, C., *et al.* (2006) The use of mutant mycobacteria as new vaccines to prevent tuberculosis. *Tuberculosis (Edinburgh)* 86, 203–210.

Hesseling, A.C., Marais, B.J., Gie, R.P., Schaaf, H.S., Fine, P.E., Godfrey-Faussett, P., *et al.* (2007) The risk of disseminated Bacille Calmette–Guerin (BCG) disease in HIV-infected children. *Vaccine* 25, 14–18.

Hoft, D.F., Blazevic, A., Abate, G., Hanekom, W.A., Kaplan, G., Soler, J.H., *et al.* (2008) A new recombinant bacille Calmette–Guerin vaccine safely induces significantly enhanced tuberculosis-specific immunity in human volunteers. *Journal of Infectious Diseases* 198, 1491–1501.

HogenEsch, H. (2002) Mechanisms of stimulation of the immune response by aluminum adjuvants. *Vaccine* 20(Suppl 3), S34–39.

Horwitz, M.A., Lee, B.W., Dillon, B.J. and Harth, G. (1995) Protective immunity against tuberculosis induced by vaccination with major extracellular proteins of *Mycobacterium tuberculosis*. *Proceedings of the National Academy of Sciences* 92, 1530–1534.

Horwitz, M.A., Harth, G., Dillon, B.J. and Maslesa-Galic, S. (2000) Recombinant bacillus Calmette–Guerin (BCG) vaccines expressing the *Mycobacterium tuberculosis* 30-kDa major secretory protein induce greater protective immunity against tuberculosis than conventional BCG vaccines in a highly susceptible animal model. *Proceedings of the National Academy of Sciences* 97, 13853–13858.

Horwitz, M.A., Harth, G., Dillon, B.J. and Maslesa-Galic, S. (2009) Commonly administered BCG strains including an evolutionarily early strain and evolutionarily late strains of disparate genealogy induce comparable protective immunity against tuberculosis. *Vaccine* 27, 441–445.

Huygen, K., Content, J., Denis, O., Montgomery, D.L., Yawman, A.M., Deck, R.R., *et al.* (1996) Immunogenicity and protective efficacy of a tuberculosis DNA vaccine. *Nature Medicine* 2, 893–898.

Ibanga, H.B., Brookes, R.H., Hill, P.C., Owiafe, P.K., Fletcher, H.A., Lienhardt, C., *et al.* (2006) Early clinical trials with a new tuberculosis vaccine, MVA85A, in tuberculosis-endemic countries: issues in study design. *The Lancet Infectious Diseases* 6, 522–528.

Johnson, J.L., Kamya, R.M., Okwera, A., Loughlin, A.M., Nyole, S., Hom, D.L., *et al.* (2000) Randomized controlled trial of *Mycobacterium vaccae* immunotherapy in non-human immunodeficiency virus-infected Ugandan adults with newly diagnosed pulmonary tuberculosis. The Uganda-Case Western Reserve University Research Collaboration. *Journal of Infectious Diseases* 181, 1304–1312.

Jones, B.E., Young, S.M., Antoniskis, D., Davidson, P.T., Kramer, F. and Barnes, P.F. (1993) Relationship of the manifestations of tuberculosis to CD4 cell counts in patients with human immunodeficiency virus infection. *American Review of Respiratory Disease* 148, 1292–1297.

Kagina, B.M., Abel, B., Scriba, T.J., Hughes, E.J., Keyser, A., Soares, A., *et al.* (2010) Specific T cell frequency and cytokine expression profile do not correlate with protection against tuberculosis, following BCG vaccination of newborns. *American Journal of Respiratory and Critical Care Medicine* 182(8), 1073–1079.

Kamath, A.T., Fruth, U., Brennan, M.J., Dobbelaer, R., Hubrechts, P., Ho, M.M., *et al.* (2005) New live mycobacterial vaccines: the Geneva consensus on essential steps towards clinical development. *Vaccine* 23, 3753–3761.

Keane, J., Gershon, S., Wise, R.P., Mirabile-Levens, E., Kasznica, J., Schwieterman, W.D., *et al.* (2001) Tuberculosis associated with infliximab, a tumor necrosis factor alpha-neutralizing agent. *New England Journal of Medicine* 345, 1098–1104.

Khader, S.A., Bell, G.K., Pearl, J.E., Fountain, J.J., Rangel-Moreno, J., Cilley, G.E., *et al.* (2007) IL-23 and IL-17 in the establishment of protective pulmonary CD4+ T cell responses after vaccination and during *Mycobacterium tuberculosis* challenge. *Nature Immunology* 8, 369–377.

Korbel, D.S., Schneider, B.E. and Schaible, U.E. (2008) Innate immunity in tuberculosis: myths and truth. *Microbes and Infection* 10, 995–1004.

Kostense, S., Koudstaal, W., Sprangers, M., Weverling, G.J., Penders, G., Helmus, N., *et al.* (2004) Adenovirus types 5 and 35 seroprevalence in AIDS risk groups supports type 35 as a vaccine vector. *AIDS* 18, 1213–1216.

Lagranderie, M.R., Balazuc, A.M., Deriaud, E., Leclerc, C.D. and Gheorghiu, M. (1996) Comparison of immune responses of mice immunized with five different *Mycobacterium bovis* BCG vaccine strains. *Infection and Immunity* 64, 1–9.

Langermans, J.A., Andersen, P., Van Soolingen, D., Vervenne, R.A., Frost, P.A., Van der Laan, T., *et al.* (2001) Divergent effect of bacillus Calmette–Guerin (BCG) vaccination on *Mycobacterium tuberculosis* infection in highly related macaque species: implications for primate models in tuberculosis vaccine research. *Proceedings of the National Academy of Sciences* 98, 11497–11502.

Larsen, M.H., Biermann, K., Chen, B., Hsu, T., Sambandamurthy, V.K., Lackner, A.A., *et al.* (2009) Efficacy and safety of live attenuated persistent and rapidly cleared *Mycobacterium tuberculosis* vaccine candidates in non-human primates. *Vaccine* 27, 4709–4717.

Luce, B.R., Kramer, J.M., Goodman, S.N., Connor, J.T., Tunis, S., Whicher, D., *et al.* (2009) Rethinking randomized clinical trials for comparative effectiveness research: the need for transformational change. *Annals of Internal Medicine* 151, 206–209.

McConkey, S.J., Reece, W.H., Moorthy, V.S., Webster, D., Dunachie, S., Butcher, G., *et al.* (2003) Enhanced T-cell immunogenicity of plasmid DNA vaccines boosted by recombinant modified vaccinia virus Ankara in humans. *Nature Medicine* 9, 729–735.

McShane, H., Brookes, R., Gilbert, S.C. and Hill, A.V. (2001) Enhanced immunogenicity of CD4(+) t-cell responses and protective efficacy of a DNA-modified vaccinia virus Ankara prime-boost vaccination regimen for murine tuberculosis. *Infection and Immunity* 69, 681–686.

McShane, H., Behboudi, S., Goonetilleke, N., Brookes, R. and Hill, A.V. (2002) Protective immunity against *Mycobacterium tuberculosis* induced by dendritic cells pulsed with both CD8(+)- and CD4(+)-T-cell epitopes from antigen 85A. *Infection and Immunity* 70, 1623–1626.

McShane, H., Pathan, A.A., Sander, C.R., Keating, S.M., Gilbert, S.C., Huygen, K., *et al.* (2004) Recombinant modified vaccinia virus Ankara expressing antigen 85A boosts BCG-primed and naturally acquired antimycobacterial immunity in humans. *Nature Medicine* 10, 1240–1244.

Magalhaes, I., Sizemore, D.R., Ahmed, R.K., Mueller, S., Wehlin, L., Scanga, C., *et al.* (2008) rBCG induces strong antigen-specific T cell responses in rhesus macaques in a prime-boost setting with an adenovirus 35 tuberculosis vaccine vector. *PLoS One* 3, e3790.

Mittrucker, H.W., Steinhoff, U., Kohler, A., Krause, M., Lazar, D., Mex, P., *et al.* (2007) Poor correlation between BCG vaccination-induced T cell responses and protection against tuberculosis. *Proceedings of the National Academy of Sciences* 104, 12434–12439.

Moyo, S., Verver, S., Mahomed, H., Hawkridge, A., Kibel, M., Hatherill, M., *et al.* (2010) Age-related tuberculosis incidence and severity in children under 5 years of age in Cape Town, South Africa. *International Journal of Tuberculosis and Lung Disease* 14, 149–154.

Negri, D.R., Michelini, Z., Baroncelli, S., Spada, M., Vendetti, S., Bona, R., *et al.* (2010) Non-integrating lentiviral vector-based vaccine efficiently induces functional and persistent CD8+ T cell responses in mice. *Journal of Biomedicine and Biotechnology* 2010, Article 534501.

Newport, M.J., Huxley, C.M., Huston, S., Hawrylowicz, C.M., Oostra, B.A., Williamson, R., *et al.* (1996) A mutation in the interferon-gamma-receptor gene and susceptibility to mycobacterial infection. *New England Journal of Medicine* 335, 1941–1949.

Orme, I.M. (1987) The kinetics of emergence and loss of mediator T lymphocytes acquired in response to infection with *Mycobacterium tuberculosis*. *Journal of Immunology* 138, 293–298.

Pai, M., Riley, L.W. and Colford, J.M. Jr (2004) Interferon-gamma assays in the immuno-diagnosis of tuberculosis: a systematic review. *The Lancet Infectious Diseases* 4, 761–776.

Palmer, C.E. and Long, M.W. (1966) Effects of infection with atypical mycobacteria on BCG vaccination and tuberculosis. *American Review of Respiratory Disease* 94, 553–568.

Paoletti, E. (1996) Applications of pox virus vectors to vaccination: an update. *Proceedings of the National Academy of Sciences* 93, 11349–11353.

Pathan, A.A., Sander, C.R., Fletcher, H.A., Poulton, I., Alder, N.C., Beveridge, N.E., *et al.* (2007) Boosting BCG with recombinant modified vaccinia Ankara expressing antigen 85A: different boosting intervals and implications for efficacy trials. *PLoS ONE* 2, e1052.

Prevec, L., Schneider, M., Rosenthal, K.L., Belbeck, L.W., Derbyshire, J.B. and Graham, F.L. (1989) Use of human adenovirus-based vectors for antigen expression in animals. *Journal of General Virology* 70(Pt 2), 429–434.

Pym, A.S., Brodin, P., Brosch, R., Huerre, M. and Cole, S.T. (2002) Loss of RD1 contributed to the attenuation of the live tuberculosis vaccines *Mycobacterium bovis* BCG and *Mycobacterium microti*. *Molecular Microbiology* 46, 709–717.

Pym, A.S., Brodin, P., Majlessi, L., Brosch, R., Demangel, C., Williams, A., *et al.* (2003) Recombinant BCG exporting ESAT-6 confers enhanced protection against tuberculosis. *Nature Medicine* 9, 533–539.

Radosevic, K., Wieland, C.W., Rodriguez, A., Weverling, G.J., Mintardjo, R., Gillissen, G., *et al.* (2007) Protective immune responses to a recombinant adenovirus type 35 tuberculosis vaccine in two mouse strains: CD4 and CD8 T-cell epitope mapping and role of gamma interferon. *Infection and Immunity* 75, 4105–4115.

Ritz, N. and Curtis, N. (2009) Mapping the global use of different BCG vaccine strains. *Tuberculosis (Edinburgh)* 89, 248–251.

Rodrigues, L.C., Diwan, V.K. and Wheeler, J.G. (1993) Protective effect of BCG against tuberculous meningitis and miliary tuberculosis: a meta-analysis. *International Journal of Epidemiology* 22, 1154–1158.

Roupie, V., Romano, M., Zhang, L., Korf, H., Lin, M.Y., Franken, K.L., *et al.* (2007) Immunogenicity of eight dormancy regulon-encoded proteins of *Mycobacterium tuberculosis* in DNA-vaccinated and tuberculosis-infected mice. *Infection and Immunity* 75, 941–949.

Sallusto, F., Geginat, J. and Lanzavecchia, A. (2004) Central memory and effector memory T cell subsets: function, generation, and maintenance. *Annual Reviews of Immunology* 22, 745–763.

Sander, C.R., Pathan, A.A., Beveridge, N.E., Poulton, I., Minassian, A., Alder, N., *et al.* (2009) Safety and immunogenicity of a new tuberculosis vaccine, MVA85A, in *Mycobacterium tuberculosis*-infected individuals. *American Journal of Respiratory and Critical Care Medicine* 179, 724–733.

Scanga, C.A., Mohan, V.P., Joseph, H., Yu, K., Chan, J. and Flynn, J.L. (1999) Reactivation of latent tuberculosis: variations on the Cornell murine model. *Infection and Immunity* 67, 4531–4538.

Schneider, J., Gilbert, S.C., Blanchard, T.J., Hanke, T., Robson, K.J., Hannan, C.M., *et al.* (1998) Enhanced immunogenicity for CD8+ T cell induction and complete protective efficacy of malaria DNA vaccination by boosting with modified vaccinia virus Ankara. *Nature Medicine* 4, 397–402.

Scriba, T.J., Tameris, M., Mansoor, N., Smit, E., Van der Merwe, L., Isaacs, F., *et al.* (2010) Modified vaccinia Ankara-expressing Ag85A, a novel tuberculosis vaccine, is safe in adolescents and children, and induces polyfunctional CD4+ T cells. *European Journal of Immunology* 40, 279–290.

Shen, Y., Zhou, D., Qiu, L., Lai, X., Simon, M., Shen, L., *et al.* (2002) Adaptive immune response of Vgamma2Vdelta2+ T cells during mycobacterial infections. *Science* 295, 2255–2258.

Skeiky, Y.A., Alderson, M.R., Ovendale, P.J., Guderian, J.A., Brandt, L., Dillon, D.C., *et al.* (2004) Differential immune responses and protective efficacy induced by components of a tuberculosis polyprotein vaccine, Mtb72F, delivered as naked DNA or recombinant protein. *Journal of Immunology* 172, 7618–7628.

Skeiky, Y.A., Dietrich, J., Lasco, T.M., Stagliano, K., Dheenadhayalan, V., Goetz, M.A., *et al.* (2010) Non-clinical efficacy and safety of HyVac4:IC31 vaccine administered in a BCG prime-boost regimen. *Vaccine* 28, 1084–1093.

Smith, D., Harding, G., Chan, J., Edwards, M., Hank, J., Muller, D., *et al.* (1979) Potency of 10 BCG vaccines as evaluated by their influence on the bacillemic phase of experimental airborne tuberculosis in guinea-pigs. *Journal of Biological Standardisation* 7, 179–197.

Sousa, A.O., Mazzaccaro, R.J., Russell, R.G., Lee, F.K., Turner, O.C., Hong, S., *et al.* (2000) Relative contributions of distinct MHC class I-dependent cell populations in protection to tuberculosis infection in mice. *Proceedings of the National Academy of Sciences* 97, 4204–4208.

Spencer, C.T., Abate, G., Blazevic, A. and Hoft, D.F. (2008) Only a subset of phosphoantigen-responsive gamma9delta2 T cells mediate protective tuberculosis immunity. *Journal of Immunology* 181, 4471–4484.

Stanford, J.L., Bahr, G.M., Rook, G.A., Shaaban, M.A., Chugh, T.D., Gabriel, M., *et al.* (1990) Immunotherapy with *Mycobacterium vaccae* as an adjunct to chemotherapy in the treatment of pulmonary tuberculosis. *Tubercle* 71, 87–93.

Stenger, S., Hanson, D.A., Teitelbaum, R., Dewan, P., Niazi, K.R., Froelich, C.J., *et al.* (1998) An antimicrobial activity of cytolytic T cells mediated by granulysin. *Science* 282, 121–125.

Sterling, T.R., Pham, P.A. and Chaisson, R.E. (2010) HIV infection-related tuberculosis: clinical manifestations and treatment. *Clinical Infectious Disease* 50(Suppl 3), S223–230.

Sun, R., Skeiky, Y.A., Izzo, A., Dheenadhayalan, V., Imam, Z., Penn, E., *et al.* (2009) Novel recombinant BCG expressing perfringolysin O and the over-expression of key immunodominant antigens; pre-clinical characterization, safety and protection against challenge with *Mycobacterium tuberculosis*. *Vaccine* 27, 4412–4423.

Tascon, R.E., Stavropoulos, E., Lukacs, K.V. and Colston, M.J. (1998) Protection against *Mycobacterium tuberculosis* infection by CD8+ T cells requires the production of gamma interferon. *Infection and Immunity* 66, 830–834.

Tatsis, N. and Ertl, H.C. (2004) Adenoviruses as vaccine vectors. *Molecular Therapy* 10, 616–629.

Taylor, J.L., Turner, O.C., Basaraba, R.J., Belisle, J.T., Huygen, K. and Orme, I.M. (2003) Pulmonary necrosis resulting from DNA vaccination against tuberculosis. *Infection and Immunity* 71, 2192–2198.

Trunz, B.B., Fine, P. and Dye, C. (2006) Effect of BCG vaccination on childhood tuberculous meningitis and miliary tuberculosis worldwide: a meta-analysis and assessment of cost-effectiveness. *The Lancet* 367, 1173–1180.

Van Dissel, J.T., Arend, S.M., Prins, C., Bang, P., Tingskov, P.N., Lingnau, K., *et al.* (2010) Ag85B-ESAT-6 adjuvanted with IC31 promotes strong and long-lived *Mycobacterium tuberculosis* specific T cell responses in naive human volunteers. *Vaccine* 28, 3571–3581.

Van Pinxteren, L.A., Cassidy, J.P., Smedegaard, B.H., Agger, E.M. and Andersen, P. (2000) Control of latent *Mycobacterium tuberculosis* infection is dependent on CD8 T cells. *European Journal of Immunology* 30, 3689–3698.

Verreck, F.A., Vervenne, R.A., Kondova, I., Van Kralingen, K.W., Remarque, E.J., Braskamp, G., *et al.* (2009) MVA.85A boosting of BCG and an attenuated, phoP deficient *M. tuberculosis* vaccine both show protective efficacy against tuberculosis in rhesus macaques. *PLoS One* 4, e5264.

Vilaplana, C., Montane, E., Pinto, S., Barriocanal, A.M., Domenech, G., Torres, F., *et al.* (2010) Double-blind, randomized, placebo-controlled Phase I Clinical Trial of the therapeutical antituberculous vaccine RUTI. *Vaccine* 28, 1106–1116.

Von Eschen, K., Morrison, R., Braun, M., Ofori-Anyinam, O., De Kock, E., Pavithran, P., *et al.* (2009) The candidate tuberculosis vaccine Mtb72F/AS02A: tolerability and immunogenicity in humans. *Human Vaccines* 5, 475–482.

Von Reyn, C.F., Mtei, L., Arbeit, R.D., Waddell, R., Cole, B., Mackenzie, T., *et al.* (2010) Prevention of tuberculosis in Bacille Calmette–Guerin-primed, HIV-infected adults boosted with an inactivated whole-cell mycobacterial vaccine. *AIDS* 24, 675–685.

Vordermeier, H.M., Villarreal-Ramos, B., Cockle, P.J., McAulay, M., Rhodes, S.G., Thacker, T., *et al.* (2009) Viral booster vaccines improve *Mycobacterium bovis* BCG-induced protection against bovine tuberculosis. *Infection and Immunity*, 77, 3364–3373.

Walker, K.B., Brennan, M.J., Ho, M.M., Eskola, J., Thiry, G., Sadoff, J., *et al.* (2010) The second Geneva Consensus: recommendations for novel live TB vaccines. *Vaccine* 28, 2259–2270.

Wedlock, D.N., Denis, M., Vordermeier, H.M., Hewinson, R.G. and Buddle, B.M. (2007) Vaccination of cattle with Danish and Pasteur strains of *Mycobacterium bovis* BCG induce different levels of IFNgamma post-vaccination, but induce similar levels of protection against bovine tuberculosis. *Veterinary Immunology and Immunopathology* 118, 50–58.

Weir, R.E., Black, G.F., Dockrell, H.M., Floyd, S., Fine, P.E., Chaguluka, S.D., *et al.* (2004) Mycobacterial purified protein derivatives stimulate innate immunity: Malawians show enhanced tumor necrosis factor alpha, interleukin-1beta (IL-1beta), and IL-10 responses compared to those of adolescents in the United Kingdom. *Infection and Immunity* 72, 1807–1811.

Whelan, K.T., Pathan, A.A., Sander, C.R., Fletcher, H.A., Poulton, I., Alder, N.C., *et al.* (2009) Safety and immunogenicity of boosting BCG vaccinated subjects with BCG: comparison with boosting with a new TB vaccine, MVA85A. *PLoS One* 4, e5934.

WHO (2007) *Weekly Epidemiological Record* 3, 17–24.

Williams, A., Goonetilleke, N.P., McShane, H., Clark, S.O., Hatch, G., Gilbert, S.C., *et al.* (2005a) Boosting with poxviruses enhances *Mycobacterium bovis* BCG efficacy against tuberculosis in guinea pigs. *Infection and Immunity* 73, 3814–3816.

Williams, A., Hatch, G.J., Clark, S.O., Gooch, K.E., Hatch, K.A., Hall, G.A., *et al.* (2005b) Evaluation of vaccines in the EU TB Vaccine Cluster using a guinea pig aerosol infection model of tuberculosis. *Tuberculosis (Edinburgh)* 85, 29–38.

Xiang, Z., Li, Y., Cun, A., Yang, W., Ellenberg, S., Switzer, W.M., *et al.* (2006) Chimpanzee adenovirus antibodies in humans, sub-Saharan Africa. *Emerging Infectious Diseases* 12, 1596–1599.

Index